FUNCTIONAL ULTRASTRUCTURE
OF THE KIDNEY

edited by

ARVID B. MAUNSBACH   T. STEEN OLSEN
ERIK ILSØ CHRISTENSEN

University of Aarhus
Aarhus, Denmark

1980

ACADEMIC PRESS

A Subsidiary of Harcourt Brace Jovanovich, Publishers

London New York Toronto Sydney San Francisco

ACADEMIC PRESS INC. (LONDON) LTD
24/28 Oval Road,
London NW1

United States Edition published by
ACADEMIC PRESS INC.
111 Fifth Avenue,
New York, New York 10003

British Library Cataloguing in Publication Data

Functional ultrastructure of the kidney.
1. Kidneys
I. Maunsbach, A N   II. Olsen, T S
III. Christensen, E
599'.08'72   QP249   80–41247
ISBN 0–12–481250–3

Filmset by Northumberland Press Ltd, Gateshead, Tyne and Wear
Printed in England by Fletcher and Son Ltd, Norwich

List of Contributors

Numbers in parentheses indicate the pages on which the authors' contributions begin.

JAMES L. ATKINS *Department of Physiology, University of Maryland School of Medicine, Baltimore, Maryland 21201, USA* (411)

RICHARD BAUER *Department of Physiology, University of Munich, 8000 Munich, German Federal Republic* (177)

JEAN BARIÉTY *Department of Medicine, Hôpital Broussais, 75674 Paris, Cedex 14, France* (53, 303)

KARL BAUMANN *Department of Cell Physiology, Institute of Physiology, University of Hamburg, 2000 Hamburg, German Federal Republic* (291)

FRANZ BECK *Department of Physiology, University of Munich, 8000 Munich, German Federal Republic* (177)

MARIE-FRANCE BELAIR *Department of Medicine, Hôpital Broussais, 75674 Paris, Cedex 14, France* (53, 303)

DONALD R. BELL *Department of Physiology, University of Maryland School of Medicine, Baltimore, Maryland 21201, USA* (411)

FOLKERT BODE *Department of Cell Physiology, Institute of Physiology, University of Hamburg, 2000 Hamburg, German Federal Republic* (291, 385)

SVEN-OLOF BOHMAN *Karolinska Institutet, Department of Pathology at Huddinge Hospital, 14186 Huddinge, Sweden* (457)

EMILE BOULPAEP *Department of Physiology, School of Medicine, Yale University, New Haven, Connecticut 06510, USA* (207)

LEONARDO CAGNOLI *Department of Nephrology and Dialysis, Ospedale M. Malpighi, Bologna, Italy* (151)

FRANK A. CARONE *Northwestern Memorial Hospital, Department of Pathology, Chicago, Illinois 60611, USA* (327)

SILVIA CASANOVA *Department of Nephrology and Dialysis, Ospedale M. Malpighi, Bologna, Italy* (151)

ERIK ILSØ CHRISTENSEN *Department of Cell Biology, Institute of Anatomy, University of Aarhus, 8000 Aarhus C, Denmark* (341)

THOMAS G. COTTER *Department of Biochemistry, South Parks Road, Oxford OX1 3QV, United Kingdom* (75)

CHARLES A. DECHENNE *Departments of Medicine and Pathology, State University of Liège, 4020 Liège, Belgium* (133)

PHILIPPE DRUET *Department of Medicine, Hôpital Broussais, 75674 Paris, Cedex 14, France* (53, 303)

ADOLF DÖRGE *Department of Physiology, University of Munich, 8000 Munich, German Federal Republic* (177)

MARILYN G. FARQUHAR *Section of Cell Biology, Yale University School of Medicine, New Haven, Connecticut 06510, USA* (31)

GERT-JAN FLEUREN *Centre for Medical Electron Microscopy, 9713 EZ Groningen, The Netherlands* (105)

JACQUELINE B. FOIDART *Department of Medicine, State University of Liège, 4020 Liège, Belgium* (133)

REINHARD GEIGER *Department of Clinical Chemistry and Biochemistry, University of Munich, 8000 Munich, German Federal Republic* (375)

HANS JØRGEN G. GUNDERSEN *2nd University Clinic of Internal Medicine, Kommunehospitalet, 8000 Aarhus C, Denmark* (143)

HANS-G. HEIDRICH *Max-Planck-Institut für Biochemie, 8033 Martiensried b. München, German Federal Republic* (375)

KARIN HERMANSSON *Departments of Physiology and Medical Biophysics, University of Uppsala, 75123 Uppsala, Sweden* (65)

PHILIP J. HOEDEMAEKER *Centre for Medical Electron Microscopy, 9713 EZ Groningen, The Netherlands* (105)

BRIGITTE KAISSLING *Institute of Anatomy I and Institute of Physiology I, University of Heidelberg, 6900 Heidelberg, German Federal Republic* (239)

MORRIS J. KARNOVSKY *Department of Pathology, Harvard Medical School, Boston, Massachusetts 02115, USA* (119)

JEFFREY I. KREISBERG *Department of Pathology, Harvard Medical School, Boston, Massachusetts 02115, USA* (119)

WILHELM KRIZ *Institute of Anatomy I, University of Heidelberg, 6900 Heidelberg, German Federal Republic* (239)

JENS PETER KROUSTRUP *Department of Connective Tissue Research, Institute of Anatomy, University of Aarhus, 8000 Aarhus C, Denmark* (143)

FRANÇOIS LALIBERTÉ *Department of Medicine, Hôpital Broussais, 75674 Paris, Cedex 14, France* (303)

KARL HEINZ LANGER *Institute of Pathology, Johannes Gutenberg University, 6500 Mainz, German Federal Republic* (431)

MIKAEL LARSON *Department of Physiology and Medical Biophysics, University of Uppsala, 751 23 Uppsala, Sweden* (65)

LARS LARSSON *Department of Paediatrics, Karolinska Institute, St Görans Children's Hospital, 104 01 Stockholm, Sweden* (223)

HARRISON LATTA *Department of Pathology, University of California School of Medicine, Los Angeles, 90024 California, USA* (3)

KIRSTEN M. MADSEN *Division of Nephrology, University of Florida, Gainesville, Florida 32610, USA* (291, 385)

PHILIPPE R. MAHIEU *Department of Medicine, State University of Liège, 4020 Liège, Belgium* (133)

KLAUS MANN *Department of Clinical Chemistry and Biochemistry, University of Munich, 8000 Munich, German Federal Republic* (375)

SEPPO O. MARKKANEN *Department of Anatomy, University of Kuopio, 70101 Kuopio 10, Finland* (361)

JUNE MASON *Department of Physiology, University of Munich, 8000 Munich, German Federal Republic* (177)

ARVID B. MAUNSBACH *Department of Cell Biology, Institute of Anatomy, University of Aarhus, 8000 Aarhus C, Denmark* (207, 291, 341, 385, 443)

CARL ERIK MOGENSEN *Medical Department I, Aarhus Amtssygehus, 8000 Aarhus C, Denmark* (143, 269)

IZAÄK MOLENAAR *Centre for Medical Electron Microscopy, 9713 EZ Groningen, The Netherlands* (105)

KJELD MØLLGÅRD *Anatomy Department A, University of Copenhagen, 2100 Copenhagen Ø, Denmark* (251)

CATHERINE SAPIN *Department of Medicine, Hôpital Broussais, 75674 Paris, Cedex 14, France* (53, 303)

MAURO SASDELLI *Department of Nephrology and Dialysis and Laboratory of Electron Microscopy, Department of Pathology, Ospedale M. Malpighi, Bologna, Italy* (151)

AUGUST SCHILLER *Institute of Physiology I, University of Heidelberg, 6900 Heidelberg, German Federal Republic* (239, 315)

JACOB W. SCHURER *Centre for Medical Electron Microscopy, 9713 EZ Groningen, The Netherlands* (105)

KJARTAN SEYER-HANSEN *2nd University Clinic of Internal Medicine, Kommunehospitalet, 8000 Aarhus C, Denmark* (143)

MATS SJÖQUIST *Department of Physiology and Medical Biophysics, University of Uppsala, 751 23 Uppsala, Sweden* (65)

JENS CHR. SKOU *Institute of Biophysics, University of Aarhus, 8000 Aarhus C, Denmark* (165)

JOHN E. STORK *Department of Physiology, School of Medicine, University of Maryland at Baltimore, Baltimore, Maryland 21201, USA* (411, 423)

ROLAND TAUGNER *Institute of Physiology I, University of Heidelberg, 6900 Heidelberg, German Federal Republic* (239, 315)

KLAUS THURAU *Department of Physiology, University of Munich, 8000 Munich, German Federal Republic* (177)

C. CRAIG TISHER *Division of Nephrology, University of Florida, Gainesville, Florida 32610, USA* (191)

N. GUNNAR WESTBERG *Department of Medicine V, Sahlgren's Hospital, University of Gothenburg, 413 45 Gothenburg, Sweden* (91)

P. DAVID WILSON *Department of Preventive Medicine, School of Medicine, University of Maryland at Baltimore, Baltimore, Maryland 21201, USA* (411, 423)

MATS WOLGAST *Department of Physiology and Medical Biophysics, University of Uppsala, 75123 Uppsala, Sweden* (65)

PIETRO ZUCCHELLI *Department of Nephrology and Dialysis, Ospedale M. Malpighi, Bologna, Italy* (151)

RUTH ØSTERBY *Institute of Experimental Clinical Research and Department of Cell Biology, Institute of Anatomy, University of Aarhus, 8000 Aarhus C, Denmark*   (143)

Preface

The ultrastructure of the kidney has been extensively studied over the last several years and much effort is directed at present towards elucidating the correlations between renal ultrastructure and function. The contributions to this book discuss and review areas where such correlations have been found fruitful and of particular importance. The book is based in part on the presentations at an international symposium, "Correlation of Renal Ultrastructure and Function", which was arranged in Aarhus, Denmark, on 21–23 August 1978 in connection with the 50th anniversary of the University of Aarhus. We gratefully acknowledge the financial support for the symposium from the Faculty of Medicine at the University of Aarhus, the Research Fund of the University of Aarhus and the Danish Medical Research Council.

We would like to thank Miss Anne-Marie Lassen and Dr Kirsten Madsen for generous assistance during the organization of the symposium and Miss Kirsten Svendsen and Dr Elisabeth Skriver for valuable help in the editing of this book.

Aarhus, January 1980

Arvid B. Maunsbach
T. Steen Olsen
Erik Ilsø Christensen

Contents

Part II: Tubules: Ion and Fluid Pathways

Part III: Tubule: Handling of Macromolecules

Part IV: Interstitium

Part V: Concluding Remarks

Part I

Glomerulus

1
Filtration Barriers in the Glomerular Capillary Wall

Harrison Latta

Introduction

A major function of this international symposium is to establish areas of agreement and to pinpoint important problems remaining to be clarified in the field of glomerular permeability. Investigators in this area come from the far corners of the world, and many of them have worked in two or three countries, often widely separated. This is truly an international field.

It is also a multidisciplinary field. It is a timely and critical area of molecular biology because of the many recent advances and the fact that investigators are working at the limits of their techniques. The techniques involve such different disciplines that it is difficult for one investigator to understand the problems, errors, and limits of the conclusions of an investigator in a different discipline. Yet integration of much diverse information will be required to understand glomerular permeability in terms of the characteristics and behavior of various macromolecules and the different structures in the glomerular capillary wall.

Studies of glomerular permeability encompass a wide range. Physiologic techniques were used initially to establish the fact of glomerular filtration. They have been refined to the quantitation of various hemodynamic factors on which filtration depends and determination of fractional clearances of various test molecules (Brenner *et al.*, 1978). Much study of the molecular characteristics of endogenous and exogenous macromolecules has demonstrated the importance of molecular size, shape, flexibility or rigidity, and surface charge at pH 7·4. From these it was inferred that the glomerular filter had sieving characteristics with some type of pore structure restricting serum albumin and larger molecules. Light and electron microscopic studies have identified cellular and extracellular layers in the capillary wall. Biochemical and histochemical studies have revealed the glycoprotein nature and negative charge of the extracellular layers. Electron microscopic studies have shown various tracers to be restricted at three different levels in the capillary wall under different conditions. Changes in experimental or disease conditions associated with proteinuria show focal changes in the glomerular capillary walls.

A few words of caution may be advisable before we start a more detailed consideration of the evidence. Technical limitations need to be considered, but it is not safe to disregard any evidence that does not fit our conceptual framework. In this particular field we have had to change our ideas several times in the past. Even artifacts have a message for us if we can find out why they occur. There are advantages to reviewing earlier work in the light of our present knowledge. Finally it has become increasingly apparent that we cannot regard the glomerular capillary wall as a fixed structure with fixed permeability characteristics. It is a dynamic structure quite sensitive in a living animal to conditions varying from daily activity and mild stress to overt disease. This means that the barriers are not absolute, but variable.

This review is limited by space and time. Other reviews will serve for more detailed information and guides to the literature (Karnovsky and Ainsworth, 1972; Latta, 1973; Schneeberger, 1974; Farquhar, 1975; Rennke and Venkatachalam, 1977b; Brenner et al., 1978; Karnovsky, 1979). This review will consider some of the macromolecules which have been used to study glomerular filtration. It will examine the nature of restrictive barriers found at three different levels in the capillary wall. It will note some points that have been little discussed by others, and it will put more emphasis on recent work.

Physiologic Considerations of Permeability

Glomerular filtration results in a filtrate which is similar to blood plasma except for the plasma proteins, which are normally largely retained in the circulation. Up to a third of the plasma that enters the kidney is driven into the glomerular filtrate by the blood pressure (Brenner and Humes, 1977). Glomerular ultrafiltration is determined by the initial plasma flow rate, the mean transcapillary hydraulic pressure difference (largely dependent on blood pressure), the ultrafiltration coefficient (water permeability of the capillary wall times the surface area available for filtration), and the afferent plasma protein concentration.

Physiologists usually compare the excretion of test substances to inulin

(Brenner *et al.*, 1978). Inulin is considered the ideal reference substance because it appears in the glomerular filtrate in the same concentration as in the glomerular plasma water and is neither reabsorbed nor secreted by the tubules. The ratio of clearance of a test substance compared to inulin clearance is the fractional clearance of that substance. Neutral dextrans do not show restriction to filtration (or a fractional clearance less than 1) until their effective hydrodynamic radii are greater than 20 Å. Fractional clearances of neutral dextrans decrease as their radii increase and approach zero at radii greater than 42 Å. The great importance of charge is shown by comparing fractional clearances of dextrans of similar effective radii, but with a different molecular charge. Negatively charged or anionic dextran is restricted much more than neutral dextran, and the latter is restricted more than positively charged or cationic dextran.

Physiologists have long regarded serum albumin as a protein molecule usually retained in the circulation. In general, larger protein molecules are retained and smaller ones are excreted. The appearance of albuminuria with exercise, heart failure, and in some people on just standing up (orthostatic proteinuria) indicates the ease with which the retention mechanisms are broken down. Pollack and Pesce (1972) have presented evidence that some serum albumin passes into the glomerular filtrate in apparently normal animals and human beings and is reabsorbed into lysosomes by proximal tubule cells. The reabsorption mechanism seems to have a low capacity which accounts for a trace of albumin normally appearing in the urine and the rapidity with which frank albuminuria appears after mild stress.

Because serum albumin has long been regarded as a critical molecule in glomerular permeability, physiologists have used its effective hydrodynamic (Einstein–Stokes) radius ($a_e = 36$ Å) to estimate the size of the openings or "pores" in the glomerular filter. On this basis Renkin and Gilmore (1973) have proposed three theoretical models for the filter: long slits 72 Å wide, circular pores 72 Å in diameter, and randomly oriented fibers with a mean interspace of 52 Å. Evidence given below will suggest that the barrier to albumin is more like a three-dimensional network. Moreover, a molecule of serum albumin is really quite asymmetric or cigar-shaped. Hydrated bovine serum albumin monomer has been represented as a prolate ellipsoid of revolution with a major axis of 140 Å and minor axes of 40 Å (Squire *et al.*, 1968). It is also considered to be stiff or rigid. When data from diffusion of linear polymers in hyaluronate solutions was considered (Laurent *et al.*, 1975) it was found that linear molecules were less retarded than globular particles of equal hydrodynamic radii. They seem to pentrate a network preferentially by end on movements which would offer fewer obstacles in their path. This would suggest that the effective openings in the glomerular network have a radius smaller than 36 Å but larger than 20 Å, the radius of the minor axis

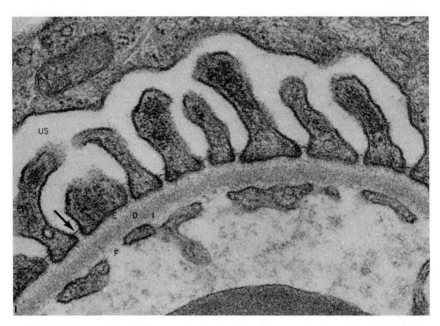

FIG. 1. *Glomerular capillary wall of a rat. The filtration path includes the fenestrations (F) of the endothelium, three layers of the basement membrane (lamina rara interna (I), lamina densa (D), and lamina rara externa (E)), the slit diaphragm (arrow) and the filtration slits between the sides of the foot processes which open into the urinary space (US). Glycoproteins do not stain with osmium tetroxide. (From Latta (1970).) × 64 000.*

of albumin. In addition, the labile mechanisms suggested by Ryan and Karnovsky (1976) with cessation of blood flow have to be considered. The site and magnitude of hydraulic resistance also need to be determined before a more accurate model for the albumin barrier consistent with all the evidence can be proposed. Finally, when conditions are such that the albumin barrier breaks down, other barriers then become important.

The Glomerular Capillary Wall

It is generally agreed as a result of the earlier work with tracers that the path of glomerular filtrate is through endothelial fenestrations and basement membrane layers and then between epithelial foot processes into the urinary space (Figs 1 and 2) (Farquhar and Palade, 1961; Graham and Karnovsky, 1966). The subsequent discussion will follow this sequence. There is also evidence that glomerular filtration takes place through the mesangial region.

The capillary wall does not appear to present a barrier to several tracers

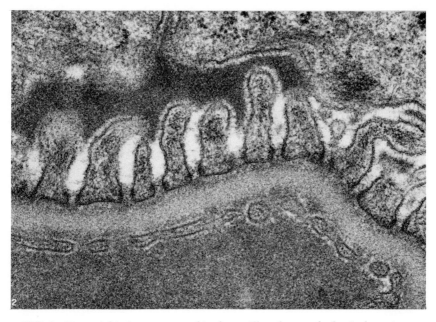

FIG. 2. *Hemoglobin is concentrated in the capillary lumen, the lamina rara interna, the lamina rara externa and the urinary space. This demonstrates that the laminae rara interna and externa have looser structures than the lamina densa. The hemoglobin in the urinary space outlines the free surface coat of the foot processes. The surface coat is so compact that very little hemoglobin can accumulate in it. The absence of hemoglobin in the filtration slits between foot processes indicates that their surface coats were in contact* in vivo. (*From Latta (1973)*.) × 64 000.

studied with electron microscopy. We will consider three of the larger tracers that penetrate easily without apparent restriction in electron microscopic studies (Table I). Horseradish peroxidase passes from the capillary lumen to the urinary space rapidly in high concentration without demonstrating a concentration gradient (Graham and Karnovsky, 1966). Its effective radius is 30 Å but its shape is not known. Neutral graded dextrans of 32 000 daltons also appear in the urinary space in high concentrations soon after intravenous injection (Caulfield and Farquhar, 1974). Their radius ($a_e = 38$ Å) cannot be used to determine a pore size, because it is thought that they unfold and become linear as they pass through the wall. We should note that fractional clearances show some restriction to filtration of dextrans with effective radii greater than 20 Å (Brenner *et al.*, 1978).

Hemoglobin is a better molecule to measure pore size because it can be visualized when concentrated in the basement membrane (Fig. 2) (Latta, 1970) and it is a globular anionic protein molecule with an effective radius

TABLE I
No apparent filtration barrier

Tracer	Molecular weight (daltons)	Effective radius, a_e (Å)	Shape or dimensions (Å)	pI	Charge[a]	References[b]
Horseradish peroxidase	40 000	30		7·2–7·4	N	Graham and Karnovsky (1966)
Hemoglobin	64 500	32	50 × 55 × 64	6·8	–	Latta (1970)
Dextran	32 000	38	Flexible		N	Caulfield and Farquhar (1974)

[a] N = neutral, − = negatively charged, and + = positively charged at pH 7·4.
[b] Most of the figures are taken from the references given, but some are modified by Rennke and Venkatachalam (1977) and Karnovsky (1979).

TABLE II
The lamina rara interna as an apparent filtration barrier

Tracer	Molecular weight (daltons)	Effective radius, a_e (Å)	Shape or dimensions (Å)	pI	Charge[a]	References[a]
Serum albumin (good blood flow)	66 700	36	40 × 40 × 140	4·9	–	Ryan and Karnovsky (1975), Squire et al. (1968)
Thorotrast		> 70	Globular		N	Latta et al. (1960)
Thorotrast (partial barrier)		45–70	Globular		N	Latta et al. (1960)
Ferritin (partial barrier)	480 000	61	Globular	4·1–4·7	–	Farquhar et al. (1961)
Dextran (partial barrier)	125 000	78	Flexible		N	Caulfield and Farquhar (1974)
Dextran	250 000	100	Flexible		N	Caulfield and Farquhar (1974)

[a] See footnotes for Table I.

of 32 Å and dimensions of 50 Å × 55 Å × 64 Å. The rather extreme conditions in which it dissociates into subunits do not occur in the body (Leltman and Huntsman, 1974). From the effective radius we might infer pores over 64 Å wide, but perhaps it would be more accurate to say the pores should be over 50 Å × 55 Å. Such pores would be expected to allow albumin to penetrate end on. Perhaps the higher negative charge on albumin restricts it more, or the barrier network may have enough cross-linking to render it less permeable than hyaluronate solutions to a rigid linear molecule.

Lamina rara interna and glomerular endothelial fenestrations
The inner less dense layer of the basement membrane (lamina rara interna) appears to be either an effective barrier or a partial barrier in electron microscopic studies to the tracers listed in Table II.

A very significant study locating a filtration barrier in the glomerulus with electron microscopy is that of Ryan and Karnovsky (1976) who fixed superficial glomeruli in Munich-Wistar rats *in vivo* and localized rat serum albumin with an immunoperoxidase technique. They found that rats with normal blood flow had serum albumin confined to the glomerular capillary lumen and endothelial fenestrations. Interrupting the blood flow or fixing by immersion allowed albumin to penetrate the basement membrane and pass into the urinary space. If the blood flow was restored for 10 min. the basement membrane became impermeable again.

Similar experiments have been performed by Laliberté *et al.* (1978) and the results after *in vivo* fixation were similar to those observed after immersion fixation by them and by Ryan and Karnovsky (1976). Technical problems abound and it remains to be seen which group is more nearly correct for animals with good blood flow. If a barrier for serum albumin does not normally occur at the level of the fenestrations, as Ryan and Karnovsky (1976) indicate, then no other barrier has been demonstrated in the glomerular capillary wall, because electron micrographs of both groups show albumin to have passed into the urinary space without apparent restriction.

If serum albumin stops at the endothelial fenestrations under normal hemodynamic conditions, this suggests that the inner layer of the basement membrane (lamina rara interna) contributes to the barrier function (Latta and Johnston, 1976). What is the nature of the lamina rara interna? Early studies using immersion fixation showed that particles in the circulating blood such as thorotrast (Latta *et al.*, 1960) and ferritin (Farquhar *et al.*, 1961) could pass through endothelial fenestrations and spread out along the subendothelial surface of the dense layer of the basement membrane (lamina densa) in smaller concentrations than in the lumen. This indicated that the lamina rara interna was not a shrinkage artifact but a functionally signifi-

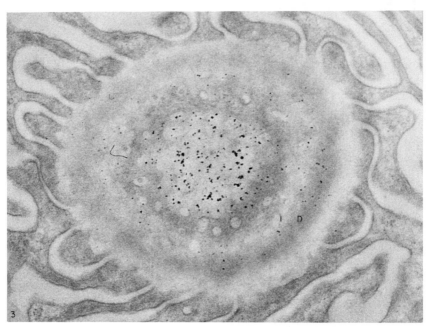

FIG. 3. *Thorotrast particles of various sizes demonstrate sieving by the two inner layers of the basement membrane. Although particles up to several hundred Ångstroms in diameter are in the circulation, only particles 140 Å or less in diameter pass into the lamina rara interna (I). Particles 90–100 Å in diameter are stopped by the lamina densa (D). This tangential section of a rat capillary wall shows blood plasma in the center, then fenestrated endothelium, the three layers of the basement membrane, and the foot processes. (From Latta et al. (1960).) × 29 000.*

cant structure with properties different from the lamina densa. The lamina rara interna seemed to have a sieving property because thorotrast particles up to several hundred Ångstroms in diameter were seen in the capillary lumen but only particles up to about 70 Å radius were found in this inner layer (Fig. 3). Particles from about 45 to 70 Å radius were seen here in smaller concentrations than in the lumen. The ferritin particles have since been considered to have an effective hydrodynamic radius of 61 Å and a diameter of 122 Å. The two protein molecules, hemoglobin (Fig. 2) and horseradish peroxidase, accumulate in the lamina rara interna, showing that it is loose enough for this to occur.

Similar observations have been made subsequently with dextrans of 125 000 daltons molecular weight ($a_e = 78$ Å) (Caulfield and Farquhar, 1974); that is, they are seen in the lamina rara interna in smaller amounts than in the lumen. Smaller dextran molecules concentrate more readily in the lamina rara interna. One problem with the technique of visualizing the dextrans is that they are seen best in the capillary lumen or urinary space, where they are thought to aggregate, but they are demonstrated less well in the basement membrane layers, where they are probably unfolded and aggregation is prevented. Small dextrans of 32 000 daltons are clearly demonstrated in the lamina rara interna and the urinary space but not in the lamina densa or lamina rara externa. This suggests that the two outer layers are too dense for aggregation to occur.

The effects of molecular charge, shape, and deformability will be discussed further below.

Diaphragms across endothelial fenestrations have not been found in most mice or rats and have not been seen in rabbits, monkeys, or human beings (Latta, 1973; Latta et al., 1975). A block to most of the tracers mentioned above is not seen after immersion fixation. For these reasons diaphragms are not considered to play a significant role in glomerular filtration.

A layer in the position of the lamina rara interna has been found with stains for polyanionic polysaccharides or glycoproteins (Latta et al., 1975). With ruthenium red this layer stained with moderate intensity, like the surface coat of the endothelium (Figs 4 and 5), but unlike the latter most of it seemed to wash away with perfusion fixation (Fig. 6). It stained faintly with colloidal iron (Jones, 1969). It was shown that it passed under the fenestrations and could be relatively homogeneous (Latta and Johnston, 1976). The layer is composed of crossing (and possibly branching) fibrils 12–25 Å wide, which are similar to and may be derived from the surface coat of the endothelial cells. The amount of cross-linking is unknown, but it is likely that there is cohesion between oligosaccharide side chains (Latta et al., 1975). This polyanionic gel seemed to be in the right place and to have the right charge to contribute to a permeability barrier to serum albumin and other anionic macromolecules (Latta and Johnston, 1976; Rennke and Venkatachalam, 1977b). Ryan and Karnovsky (1976) have proposed three hypotheses to explain the pentration of albumin when the blood stops flowing: (1) as the hydrostatic pressure falls, pores may dilate; (2) the high flux of filtrate through pores may inhibit the passage of albumin (molecular sieving); and (3) the pores through which albumin passes may normally be blocked by larger molecules concentrated from the blood plasma on one side of the barrier (concentration polarization). When filtration stops, these large molecules could diffuse away. (Such molecules might also come from the endothelial cells.)

In summary, the lamina rara interna seems to be a polyanionic gel with a moderate negative charge and a labile and potentially loose structure, and to possess an impermeability to albumin that is lost when the blood stops flowing.

The evidence considered above makes such a consistent story that the

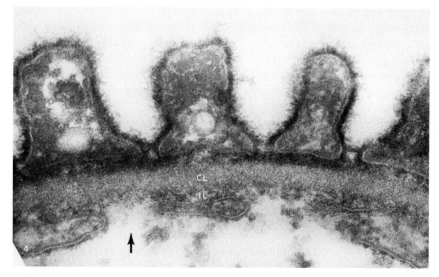

FIG. 4. *Glycoproteins in a rat glomerular capillary wall stained with ruthenium red and osmium tetroxide. The inner layer (IL) of the basement membrane (lamina rara interna) forms a continuous layer inside the central layer (CL) (lamina densa). The inner layer is more homogeneous beneath the left fenestration (arrow) which approximates what would be expected for a finer filtration barrier. The poor staining of the central layer indicates that it has a low negative charge, while the heavier staining of the outer layer (lamina rara externa) and the free surface coat indicates that they have a greater negative charge. Counterstained with uranyl acetate and lead citrate. (From Latta and Johnston (1976).) × 114 000.*

recent observations of Ryan *et al.* (1978) are quite surprising. They examined the location of anionic groups under different hemodynamic conditions using a colloidal iron technique, and they found good staining of structures in the capillary wall after immersion fixation similar to earlier observations (Latta and Johnston, 1976). However, after fixation during good blood flow, little labeling was seen in the lamina rara interna, although the surface coat of endothelial cells still showed moderate staining and the free surface coat of foot processes was heavily stained. They explained the appearance of a negative charge in the lamina rara interna after immersion fixation as probably an artifact due to clumping of albumin and other plasma polyanions after diffusion into the capillary wall when the blood flow stops. They postulated that under normal conditions of good blood flow the negative charge in the lamina rara externa and the surface coats of the foot processes has a field effect which is exerted across the lamina densa and lamina rara interna.

This explanation seems unlikely to the present author, but it is difficult

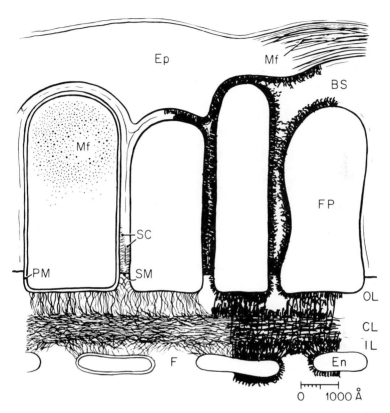

FIG. 5. *Diagram of glomerular capillary wall. The left side represents the appearance after metal staining probably of protein portions of the basement membrane. The right side shows the appearance of polyanionic glycoproteins in the capillary wall stained with ruthenium red and osmium tetroxide. The inner layer of the basement membrane (IL) (lamina rara interna) seems to consist largely of glycoproteins continuous with the cell coat of endothelial cells (En). It lies beneath endothelial fenestrations (F). Some glycoprotein fibrils lie in the central layer (CL) (lamina densa) probably bound to small collagenous fibrils. The outer layer (OL) (lamina rara externa) has a portion of the foot processes (FP) embedded in it. The surface coat of the latter seems to contribute glycoprotein to the rest of this layer. The slit membrane (SM) (slit diaphragm) marks the outer boundary of the basement membrane. It is covered by a dense surface coat (SC) which continues over the plasma membrane (PM) of adjacent foot processes. The surface coats partially or completely fill the filtration slits in the living animal. The epithelial cell cytoplasm (Ep) and the foot processes contain myofilaments (Mf) which probably function during retraction and loss of the foot processes. The urinary space is also known as Bowman's space (BS). (From Latta and Johnston (1976).)*

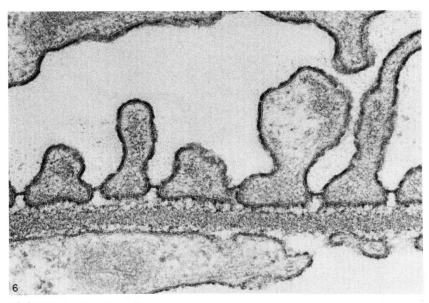

FIG. 6. *After perfusion fixation much of the glycoproteins in the capillary wall seems to have been lost. This is particularly true of the lamina rara interna and the free surface coat over the foot processes. A dense surface coat layer still covers the slit diaphragm. Compare this figure with the denser and thicker layers seen in Figs 4, 7, and 8. (From Latta* et al. *(1975).*) × 79 000.

to propose a better one. The colloidal iron technique does not reveal as fine detail as ruthenium red but it is regarded as a good stain for acidic polysaccharides (Luft, 1976). Neuraminidase eliminates staining of the epithelial coat but not the faint staining of the basement membrane, which was eliminated by hyaluronidase (Jones, 1969). Luft (1976) commented on our studies (Latta *et al.*, 1975) and emphasized the lability of surface coats and the possibility that they may contain material absorbed from the blood plasma or produced locally by cells. Certainly the possible addition, loss, or movement of molecules in the capillary wall needs to be examined in more detail, as well as the evidence that charge is operating at the same level as the effective pores for molecules of critical size (Renkin and Gilmore, 1973).

Lamina densa

The central layer of the basement membrane (lamina densa) acts as a fairly effective barrier or a partial barrier to the tracers listed in Table III. It blocks most thorotrast particles with a radius of 45–50 Å (Fig. 3) (Latta *et al.*, 1960). The thorotrast particles were suspended in dextran, so that their

TABLE III

The lamina densa as an apparent filtration barrier

Tracer	Molecular weight (daltons)	Effective radius, a_e (Å)	Shape or dimensions (Å)	pI	Charge[a]	References[a]
Thorotrast		45–50	Globular		N	Latta *et al.* (1960)
Catalase (partial barrier)	240 000	52	$70 \times 80 \times 95$	5·7	–	Venkatachalam *et al.* (1970)
Dextran (partial barrier)	62 000	55	Flexible		N	Caulfield and Farquhar (1974)
Ferritin	480 000	61	Globular	4·1–4·7	–	Farquhar *et al.* (1961)

[a] See footnotes to Table I.

surface charge was probably neutral. The lamina densa is also a good but imperfect barrier to native anionic ferritin ($a_e = 61$ Å) (Farquhar *et al.*, 1961). Catalase ($a_e = 52$ Å) shows a concentration gradient across the dense layer, indicating that it is a partial barrier for this protein (Venkatachalam *et al.*, 1970). The dense layer was named for its appearance after metal staining (Fig. 1) but it also seems to be structurally dense, because hemoglobin cannot concentrate in it at a time when the two adjacent layers are filled with hemoglobin (Fig. 2) (Latta, 1970). Neutral dextran of 62 000 daltons ($a_e = 55$ Å) appears to penetrate the lamina densa with difficulty and relatively little appears in the urinary space (Caulfield and Farquhar, 1974). Dextran of 125 000 daltons ($a_e = 78$ Å) seems to be largely held up by the lamina densa.

The lamina densa seems to constitute most of the portion analyzed by biochemists (Kefalides, 1973; Misra and Berman, 1966; Sato and Spiro, 1976; Carlson *et al.*, 1978). One component contains non-collagenous glycoproteins with a low sialic acid content. Sialic acid together with an excess of acidic amino acids (Carlson *et al.*, 1978) could account for a slight negative charge and would explain the minimal staining with ruthenium red (Figs 4 and 7) (Latta *et al.*, 1975). Most of the fibrils in this layer are 12–25 Å wide and generally run in the plane of the membrane. There is some crossing of fibrils, and branching is possible but difficult to determine by electron microscopy. Considerable cross-linking of polypeptide chains by disulfide bonds holds the basement membrane together as an insoluble structure (Sato and Spiro, 1976). Thus, the lamina densa should be regarded more like a three-dimensional network than a group of parallel or randomly oriented fibers. Occasional fibrils up to 50 Å wide have been seen (Latta *et al.*, 1975). Most spacings between fibrils are less than 50 Å, but occasional larger spacings have been found. This is consistent with the ability to block the passage of ferritin and thorotrast and allow the slow passage of smaller molecules like native catalase (Latta *et al.*, 1975).

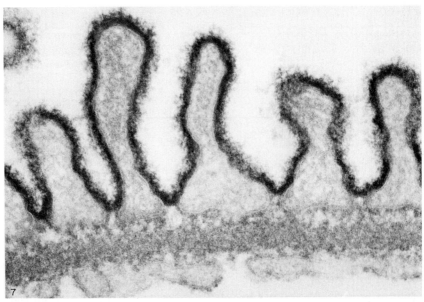

FIG. 7. *The glycoprotein in the free surface coat has a greater negative charge and stains more heavily than the glycoproteins in the basement membrane and on the endothelium. The fuzzy free surface coat extends over the slit diaphragms. Fixed by immersion in contrast to Fig. 6. (From Latta* et al. *(1975).) × 69 000.*

Lamina rara externa

The outer layer of the basement membrane (lamina rara externa) seems to have the structure of a moderately loose gel because it permits hemoglobin (Fig. 2) and peroxidases to accumulate in it as well as in the lamina rara interna (Latta, 1970, 1973). However, the lamina rara externa seems somewhat denser than the lamina rara interna, because dextrans of smaller size do not aggregate and become stained in it as they do in the lamina rara interna. The lamina rara externa stains like polysaccharides or glycoproteins with a moderate negative charge, and is similar to (and may be derived from) the surface coat on the foot processes embedded in it. This surface coat also binds cationic (basic) proteins like myeloperoxidase (Graham and

Karnovsky, 1966) and lysozyme (Farquhar, 1975). Fibrils run across this layer and appear to anchor the foot processes to the lamina densa more firmly than the endothelium is anchored (Latta, 1970).

Slit diaphragm
The slit diaphragm (previously called the slit membrane or the outer limiting membrane) runs between the outer leaflets of the plasma membrane of adjacent foot processes and is about 40–60 Å thick with metal stains (Fig. 1) (Latta, 1973). A remarkable zipper-like structure has been found in it with tannic acid fixation in rat, mouse (Rodewald and Karnovsky, 1974), and human (Schneeberger *et al.*, 1975) glomeruli. It is about 70 Å thick and contains a series of rectangular pores about 40 Å × 140 Å. The dimensions may be in part artifactual, but the complex shapes assumed by the slit diaphragm when the foot processes are lost indicate a stable underlying structure (Ryan *et al.*, 1975). The pore width would need to be wider than 50 Å to allow passage of hydrated hemoglobin molecules whose smallest dimension is 50 Å. Perfusion with tannic acid gave a slit diaphragm width of 394 Å (Rodewald and Karnovsky, 1974). This is over 100 Å more than the widths found with immersion fixation, which in cross-sections averaged 283 Å and in tangential sections 258 Å (Latta *et al.*, 1975). With the latter figures the pore length would be between 101 and 92 Å. Part of the increased width of the diaphragm may be due to increased contraction of foot processes with tannic acid and part may be due to perfusion fixation. Perfusion with glutaraldehyde gave a width of 327 Å (Latta *et al.*, 1975). If this more nearly approximates the state in the living animal, the pore length may be estimated as about 116 Å. Thus, the pores here are probably between 92 and 116 Å long and over 50 Å wide.

Surface coat of foot processes
The free surface coat (glycocalyx) of glomerular visceral epithelium (podocytes) has long been known to be especially prominent and to stain differently from other substances in the glomerulus (Latta and Cook, 1962). It stains particularly well with ruthenium red and osmium tetroxide because of its sialic acid content (Figs 4, 7, and 8) (Latta *et al.*, 1975). The high negative charge of sialic acid accounts for its staining with colloidal iron (Groniowsky *et al.*, 1969; Jones, 1969; Luft, 1976). The surface coat is now considered a polyanionic sialoglycoprotein anchored in the plasma membrane (Latta *et al.*, 1975). It is expansible and compressable. In the living animal it usually fills the filtration slits between the foot processes. It contains filaments 12–25 Å wide that are so densely packed that anionic hemoglobin ($a_e = 32$ Å) cannot accumulate in it but passes through it to accumulate over the surface coat in the urinary space and outline it like a negative stain

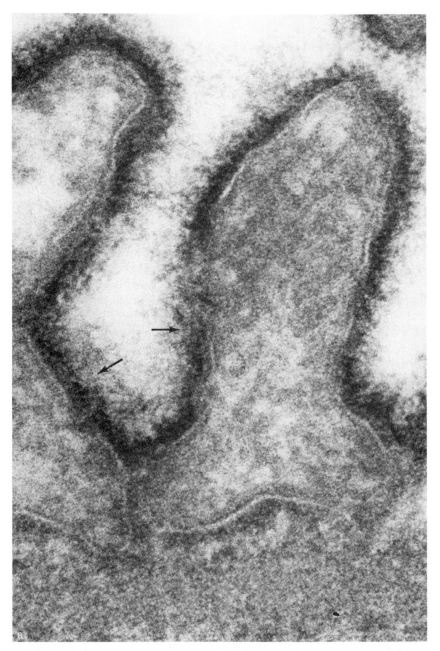

FIG. 8. *The free surface coat has a filamentous structure which is particularly evident in the regions marked by arrows. The two foot processes here are unusually close. The fibrillar lamina densa occupies the lowest 2 cm of the figure.* (*From Latta* et al. (*1975*).) × 312000.

(Fig. 2) (Latta, 1970, 1973). Horseradish peroxidase ($a_e = 30$ Å) can accumulate in the surface coat (Graham and Karnovsky, 1966) possibly because of its neutral isoelectric point ($pI = 7.2–7.4$).

The free surface coat completely covers the outer surface of the slit diaphragm (Fig. 7) (Latta et al., 1975). At present there is no evidence separating the barrier functions of the two structures and they should be considered together to account for the restrictions observed at this level. Tracers restricted are listed in Table IV. They include myeloperoxidase ($a_e = 44$ Å) (Graham and Karnovsky, 1966), catalase ($a_e = 52$ Å) (Venkatachalam et al., 1970), polycationic ferritin ($a_e = 61$ Å) in perfused kidneys (Rennke et al., 1975) and in Munich-Wistar rat kidneys fixed in vivo (Rennke

TABLE IV

The slit diaphragm and free surface coat as an apparent filtration barrier

Tracer	Molecular weight (daltons)	Effective radius, a_e (Å)	Shape or dimensions (Å)	pI	Charge[a]	References[a]
Myeloperoxidase	160 000	44		> 10	+	Graham and Karnovsky (1966)
Catalase	240 000	52	70 × 80 × 95	5.7	–	Venkatachalam et al. (1970)
IgG	150 000	55	Y-shaped	6.7–7.3	–	Ryan et al. (1976)
Cationic ferritin	480 000	61	Globular	8–9	+	Rennke et al. (1975)

[a] See footnotes to Table I.

and Venkatachalam, 1977a), and endogenous immunoglobin G (IgG) ($a_e = 55$ Å) when the blood flow stops (Ryan et al., 1976). Although earlier work favored the structures at this level as a barrier to serum albumin, the studies of Ryan and Karnovsky (1976) showed that stopping the circulation allowed serum albumin to pass through the entire capillary wall to the urinary space without apparent hinderance. Hence, the slit diaphragm–surface coat barrier permits serum albumin ($a_e = 36$ Å) and hemoglobin ($a_e = 32$ Å) to pass easily but restricts catalase ($a_e = 52$ Å) and larger protein molecules. Based on hydrodynamic radii, this would put the pore width of this barrier between 72 and 104 Å. However, we should consider the smallest dimensions of the molecules concerned, which are for serum albumin about 40 Å, for hemoglobin 50 Å, and for catalase 70 Å. In this case the effective width of the pores in the combined slit diaphragm–surface coat barrier would be between 50 and 70 Å.

Molecular Charge and Flexibility Related to Barrier Structure

The importance of molecular charge on glomerular permeability to proteins has long been known (Latta *et al.*, 1951). More recently it has been shown that native anionic ferritin penetrates the lamina rara interna with some difficulty and is generally excluded by the lamina densa, while cationic ferritin penetrates the lamina densa and concentrates in the lamina rara externa and in the filtration slits beneath the slit diaphragms (Rennke *et al.*, 1975; Rennke and Venkatachalam, 1977*a*). The relative clearance of cationic horse-radish peroxidase is larger than that of the neutral protein enzyme, and the clearance of the neutral molecules is much greater than that of an anionic derivitive (Rennke *et al.*, 1978). Fractional clearances of cationic dextrans are greater than neutral dextrans and these are greater than anionic dextrans of similar size (Brenner *et al.*, 1978). All the evidence points to the conclusion that the permeability barrier has a negative charge. The location of negative charges in the various layers of the glomerular capillary wall has been discussed above.

Dextrans have larger effective radii than protein molecules of similar weight, but they pass through the capillary wall more easily, possibly because they are more flexible (Farquhar, 1975). Rod-like or flexible molecules migrate through solutions of polymers faster than globular molecules of equivalent radii (Laurent *et al.*, 1975). Elongated molecules seem to move through polymeric networks end on. If they are flexible they may do it with worm-like movements. The different glycoprotein layers in the glomerular capillary wall probably resemble polymeric networks. Hence, much evidence contributes to the conclusion that molecular size, shape, flexibility, and charge are important in glomerular permeability.

Large masses of aggregated globin can work their way through the basement membrane, suggesting that the membrane acts as a thixotropic gel that liquifies under pressure (Menefee and Mueller, 1967). Another possibility is that the fibrils are displaced by large molecules moving under the pressure of the filtrate. Immune complexes seem to move through the basement membrane, but it is probably abnormal when this occurs. This is additional evidence that the permeability barriers are not fixed but are very labile structures.

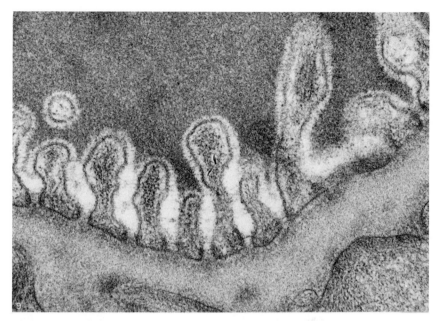

FIG. 9. *Hemoglobin concentrated in dark masses in the mesangium (in the lower part of the figure), in the lamina rara externa, and in the urinary space. The close resemblance to hemoglobin in peripheral glomerular capillary wall shown in Fig. 2 suggests that the mesangium can produce glomerular filtrate also. (From Latta (1970).) × 68000.*

Mesangial Region and Filtration

The appearance of hemoglobin in the mesangium, in the outer layer of the basement membrane, and over foot processes covering the mesangial region (Fig. 9) resembled closely the appearance of the peripheral glomerular capillary wall during hemoglobin filtration (Fig. 2) (Latta, 1970). This indicated that this part of the mesangial region was also involved in glomerular filtration (Fig. 10). The accumulation of ferritin and larger dextrans against the basement membrane in the mesangial region (Farquhar, 1975) is also suggestive. The localization of plasma proteins in the basement membrane and on foot processes over the mesangial area was also interpreted as indicating that the mesangial region has a filtration role (Laliberté *et al.*, 1978).

The mesangial region may affect glomerular filtration in other ways. Earlier a number of differences were found between mesangial cells and endothelial cells which led to the conclusion that mesangial cells are modified smooth muscle cells that could control capillary blood flow by contracting (Latta *et al.*, 1960). The blood plasma carries foreign substances

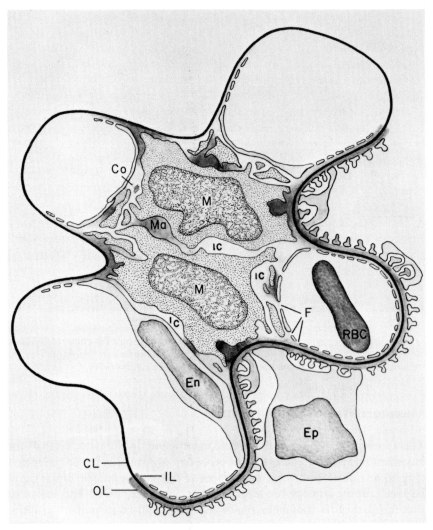

FIG. 10. *Diagram of the mesangial region in a glomerular lobule. Blood plasma and tracers pass through fenestrations (F) into mesangial or intercapillary channels (IC) where tracers can be filtered out by the mesangial matrix (Ma). The aqueous portion of the blood plasma has only to pass through the central (CL) and outer (OL) layers of the basement membrane and between foot processes to become glomerular filtrate. Epithelial (Ep), endothelial (En) and mesangial (M) nuclei are labeled. Occasional collagen (Co) fibers can be found in normal animals. The number of foot processes covered by epithelial cytoplasm is always odd, because adjacent foot processes come from different cells. (Modified from Latta et al. (1960).)*

into the mesangium (Latta *et al.*, 1960) where they are filtered out by the mesangial matrix and phagocytosed by mesangial cells (Latta *et al.*, 1962). Their remarkable phagocytic ability in contrast to adjacent endothelial cells suggested special and important functions. This has been confirmed by Farquhar and Palade (1962) and others (see Latta, 1973). Mesangial cells swell readily (Cook *et al.*, 1965), often during fixation by immersion (Latta, 1973) and sometimes during imperfect perfusion fixation (Johnston *et al.*, 1973). Swelling of mesangial and endothelial cells seems to be responsible for cessation of glomerular blood flow following temporary renal ischemia (Johnston and Latta, 1977). Mesangial cells are associated with increases in mesangial matrix and abnormal deposits (Latta *et al.*, 1962). They proliferate rapidly in glomerular disease (Johnston and Latta, 1973) and they seem to control accumulation of foreign substances in the mesangium (Schneeberger *et al.*, 1977). In summary, the mesangial region seems to contribute to glomerular filtration and the mesangial cells seem to be important in controlling blood flow, in phagocytosing foreign substances, in reacting to stress, and in repairing glomerular damage.

Proteinuria and Changes in the Glomerular Capillary Wall

In aminonucleoside nephrosis, there is a focal loss or detachment of epithelial processes covering the basement membrane, with passage of ferritin through the basement membrane at these foci into the urinary space (Ryan and Karnovsky, 1975). Excess slit diaphragm becomes folded into highly stacked aggregates (Ryan *et al.*, 1975). There is a loss of glomerular surface coat polyanionic charge (Blau and Michael, 1971) and the formation focally of occluding junctions in the residual filtration slits (Ryan *et al.*, 1975; Caulfield *et al.*, 1976). Aminonucleoside is thought to interfere with the metabolism of the glomerular epithelial cells (Caulfield *et al.*, 1976), but which part of the extracellular filtration barriers is primarily altered to produce proteinuria is unknown. We (H. Latta and W. H. Johnston, unpublished) have studied aminonucleoside nephrosis with ruthenium red staining for anionic glycoproteins without finding any readily apparent changes in the staining intensity, thickness, or fibrillar structure of the basement membrane layers where epithelium was detached. The density of staining, thickness, and fibrillar structure of the polyanionic free surface coat seen did not seem greatly changed. This suggests that the loss of polyanion found by others must be due in large part to the greatly decreased surface area of epithelial cells that have lost many foot processes. However, there may be a more subtle loss of charge that our studies could not detect in the focal areas of increased permeability. This would be particularly true if the critical charge were in the lamina rara interna. Absence of subepithelial immune complex deposits in kidneys treated with aminonucleoside has been correlated with reduced polyanionic staining (Couser et al., 1978). Nephrotoxic serum nephritis also shows focal changes (Kühn et al., 1977). Reduced polyanion and fractional clearances suggest that the loss of negative charge is responsible for the increased filtration of anionic molecules like serum albumin (Brenner et al., 1978).

Proteinuria has long been associated with loss of foot processes. This has been called fusion, but without good evidence. The processes seem to become lost by retraction into the cell body, with the remaining processes spreading out as if to maintain a cover over the basement membrane (Latta, 1973; Seiler et al., 1977; Andrews, 1977). The final stage seems to be a mosaic of polygonal cells with few or no foot processes covering the glomerular capillaries. Perfusing kidneys with polycations (protamine sulfate, poly-L-lysine) produced changes similar to those in aminonucleoside nephrosis (Seiler et al., 1977). These changes, including the loss of foot processes, were attributed to neutralization of the charge in the epithelial surface coat. A remarkable feature was the rapidity with which the foot processes retracted and then reformed after the polycation was removed: 10 min sufficed for each step. Proteinuria itself, induced by intraperitoneal injection of serum albumin, does not cause loss of foot processes (Andrews, 1977). The role of the glomerular epithelial cells in taking up proteins and foreign particles passing across the basement membrane is discussed by Caulfield et al. (1976).

Summary

Three different barriers to glomerular filtration of macromolecules have been found under different circumstances in the glomerular capillary wall. During good blood flow the glomerular filtration barrier to serum albumin and larger protein molecules seems to be the lamina rara interna of the basement membrane beneath the endothelial fenestrations. This barrier breaks down with cessation of blood flow or brief ischemia and probably with other mild stress. Serum albumin is an anionic protein of 36 Å effective hydrodynamic radius (Einstein–Stokes radius or a_e). Smaller molecules pass through glomerular capillary walls in the living animal and appear in the urine. With immersion fixation the lamina densa is seen as a second barrier which largely blocks passage of thorotrast particles 90–100 Å in diameter, of native anionic (negatively charged) ferritin molecules ($a_e = 61$ Å), and of neutral dextrans with an effective radius of 78 Å. Catalase, an anionic protein ($a_e = 52$ Å), shows a concentration gradient across the lamina densa. A third barrier is found in the filtration slits and should be considered to consist of the slit diaphragm together with the free epithelial surface coat which covers it, so that both probably act together. Catalase and cationic (positively charged) ferritin stop at this barrier, which also largely blocks cationic myeloperoxidase ($a_e = 44$ Å). Clearance studies and other work indicate that molecular size, shape, flexibility, and charge are important in the selective permeability of the glomerulus. For molecules of the same size, those with a negative charge are restricted more than neutral molecules, and these are restricted more than molecules with a positive charge. The three permeability barriers may be regarded as consisting largely of hydrated polyanionic glycoprotein gels composed of roughly parallel but crossing fibrils with unknown degrees of cross-linkage and acting like a three-dimensional network. The negative charge is moderate in the lamina rara interna and externa, low in the lamina densa, and very high in the free epithelial surface coat after immersion fixation. The lability of the barrier structures should be emphasized. The free epithelial surface coat is compressible and expansile. Perfusion fixation removes large portions of it and the glycoproteins in the three layers of the basement membrane, and also stretches the slit diaphragm considerably. The ease with which the lamina rara interna loses its impermeability makes the outer barriers important in stress and disease, probably in restricting larger molecules because the outer barriers seem unable to prevent the loss of albumin.

The mesangial region probably contributes to the production of glomerular filtrate, in addition to mesangial cell functions which include control of blood flow, phagocytosis, and reaction to and repair of glomerular damage. Experimental proteinuria is associated with focal loss of epithelial cells or loosening from the basement membrane, and it is these focal areas that show increased permeability. The loss of foot processes that accompanies proteinuria is not a fusion but a spreading and retraction of the interdigitating processes into the cell bodies. This is associated with loss of the polyanionic surface coat, piling up of excess slit diaphragm, and formation of occluding junctions between epithelial cells.

Conclusion

Perhaps the most important concluding comment is that the permeability barriers in the glomerulus are complex and labile structures. Their characteristics and impermeability are easily changed by the conditions of observation and mild physiologic stress.

Acknowledgements

The investigations in the author's laboratories discussed in this chapter have been supported by Research Grant AM 06074 from the National Institute of Arthritis, Metabolism and Digestive Diseases, United States Public Health Service.

The assistance of Lya Cordova, Mark Glyman, and Kathleen Copeland is gratefully acknowledged.

References

Andrews, P. M. (1977). A scanning and transmission electron microscopic comparison of puromycin aminonucleoside-induced nephrosis to hyperalbuminemia-induced proteinuria with emphasis on kidney podocyte pedicel loss. *Lab. Invest.* **36**, 182–197.

Blau, E. and Michael, A. F. (1971). Rat glomerular basement membrane compposition and metabolism in aminonucleoside nephrosis. *J. Lab. clin. Med.* **77**, 97–109.

Brenner, B. M. and Humes, H. D. (1977). Mechanics of glomerular ultrafiltration. *New Engl. J. Med.* **297**, 148–154.

Brenner, B. M., Hostetter, T. H. and Humes, H. D. (1978). Molecular basis of proteinuria of glomerular origin. *New Engl. J. Med.* **298**, 826–833.

Carlson, E. C., Brendel, K., Hjelle, J. T. and Meezan, E. (1978). Ultrastructural and biochemical analyses of isolated basement membranes from kidney glomeruli and tubules and brain and retinal microvessels. *J. Ultrastruct. Res.* **62**, 26–53.

Caulfield, J. P. and Farquhar, M. G. (1974). The permeability of glomerular capillaries to graded dextrans. *J. Cell Biol.* **63**, 883–903.

Caulfield, J. P., Reid, J. J. and Farquhar, M. G. (1976). Alterations of the glomerular epithelium in acute aminonucleoside nephrosis. *Lab. Invest.* **34**, 43–59.

Cook, M. L., Osvaldo, L., Jackson, J. D. and Latta, H. (1965). Changes in renal glomeruli during autolysis. *Lab. Invest.* **14**, 623–634.

Couser, W. G., Jermanovich, N. B., Belok, S., Stilmant, M. D. and Hoyer, J. R. (1978). Effect of aminonucleoside nephrosis on immune complex localization in autologous immune complex nephropathy in rats. *J. clin. Invest.* **61**, 561–572.

Farquhar, M. G. (1975). The primary glomerular filtration barrier—basement membrane or epithelial slits? Editorial Review. *Kidney Int.* **8**, 197–211.

Farquhar, M. G. and Palade, G. E. (1961). Glomerular permeability. II. Ferritin transfer across the glomerular capillary wall in nephrotic rats. *J. exp. Med.* **114**, 699–715.

Farquhar, M. G. and Palade, G. E. (1962). Functional evidence for the existence of a third cell type in the renal glomerulus. Phagocytosis of filtration residues by a distinctive "third" cell. *J. Cell Biol.* **13**, 55–87.

Farquhar, M. G., Wissig, S. L. and Palade, G. E. (1961). Glomerular permeability. I. Ferritin transfer across the normal glomerular capillary wall. *J. exp. Med.* **113**, 47–66.

Graham, R. C. and Karnovsky, M. J. (1966). Glomerular permeability. Ultrastructural cytochemical studies using peroxidases as protein tracers. *J. exp. Med.* **124**, 1123–1134.

Groniowski, J., Biczyskowa, W. and Walski, M. (1969). Electron microscope studies on the surface coat of the nephron. *J. Cell Biol.* **40**, 585–601.

Johnston, W. H. and Latta, H. (1973). Acute hematogenous pyelonephritis induced in the rabbit with *Saccharomyces cerevisiae*. An electron microscopic study. *Lab. Invest.* **29**, 495–505.

Johnston, W. H. and Latta, H. (1977). Glomerular mesangial and endothelial cell swelling following temporary renal ischemia and its role in the no-reflow phenomenon. *Am. J. Path.* **89**, 153–166.

Johnston, W. H., Latta, H. and Osvaldo, L. (1973). Variations in glomerular ultrastructure in rat kidneys fixed by perfusion. *J. Ultrastruct. Res.* **45**, 149–167.

Jones, D. B. (1969). Mucosubstances of the glomerulus. *Lab. Invest.* **21**, 119–125.

Karnovsky, M. J. (1979). The structural bases for glomerular filtration. In *Kidney Disease: Present Status*, (J. Churg, B. H. Spargo, F. K. Mostofi and M. R. Abell, eds), International Academy of Pathology, Washington, DC, pp. 1–41.

Karnovsky, M. J. and Ainsworth, S. K. (1972). The structural basis of glomerular filtration. In *Advances in Nephrology*, Vol. II (J. Hamburger, J. Crosnier and M. H. Maxwell, eds), Yearbook Medical Publishers, Chicago, pp. 35–60.

Kefalides, N. A. (1973). Structure and biosynthesis of basement membranes. In *International Review of Connective Tissue Research*, Vol. II (D.A. Hall and D. S. Jackson, eds), Yearbook Medical Publishers, Chicago, pp. 63–104.

Kühn, K., Ryan, G. B., Hein, S. J., Galaske, R. G. and Karnovsky, M. J. (1977). An ultrastructural study of the mechanisms of proteinuria in rat nephrotoxic nephritis. *Lab. Invest.* **36**, 375–387.

Laliberté, F., Sapin, C., Belair, M. F., Druet, P. and Bariéty, J. (1978). The localization of the filtration barrier in normal rat glomeruli by ultrastructual immunoperoxidase techniques. *Biologie cellul.* **31**, 15–26.

Latta, H. (1970). The glomerular capillary wall. *J. Ultrastruct. Res.* **32**, 526–544.

Latta, H. (1973). Ultrastructure of the glomerulus and the juxtaglomerular apparatus. In *Handbook of Physiology*, Sect. 8, *Renal Physiology* (J. Orloff, R. W. Berliner, and S. R. Geiger, eds), American Physiological Society, Washington, DC, pp. 1–29.

Latta, H. and Cook, M. L. (1962). The plasma membrane of glomerular epithelium. *J. Ultrastruct. Res.* **6**, 407–412.

Latta, H. and Johnston, W. H. (1976). The glycoprotein inner layer of glomerular capillary basement membrane as a filtration barrier. *J. Ultrastruct. Res.* **57**, 65–67.

Latta, H., Gitlin, D. and Janeway, C. A. (1951). Experimental hypersensitivity in the rabbit. The cellular localization of soluble azoproteins (dye-azo-human serum albumins) injected intravenously. *J. Immunol.* **66**, 635–652.

Latta, H., Maunsbach, A. B. and Madden, S. C. (1960). The centrolobular region of the renal glomerulus studied by electron microscopy. *J. Ultrastruct. Res.* **4**, 455–472.

Latta, H., Maunsbach, A. B. and Cook, M. L. (1962). Relations of the centrolobular region of the glomerulus to the juxtaglomerular apparatus. *J. Ultrastruct. Res.* **6**, 562–578.

Latta, H., Johnston, W. H. and Stanley, T. M. (1975). Sialoglycoproteins and filtration barriers in the glomerular capillary wall. *J. Ultrastruct. Res.* **51**, 354–376.

Laurent, T. C., Preston, B. N., Pertoft, H., Gustafsson, B. and McCabe, M. (1975). Diffusion of linear polymers in hyaluronate solutions. *Eur. J. Biochem.* **53**, 129–136.

Leltman, H. and Huntsman, R. G. (1974). *Man's Hemoglobin*, J. B. Lippincott, Philadelphia, pp. 341–342.

Luft, J. H. (1976). The structure and properties of the cell surface coat. *Int. Rev. Cytol.* **45**, 291–382.

Menefee, M. G. and Mueller, C. B. (1967). Some morphological considerations of transport in the glomerulus. In *Ultrastructure of the Kidney* (A. J. Dalton and F. Haguenau, eds), Academic Press, New York, pp. 57–72.

Misra, R. P. and Berman, L. B. (1966). Studies on glomerular basement membrane. I. Isolation and chemical analysis of normal glomerular basement membrane. *Proc. Soc. exp. Biol. Med.* **122**, 705–710.

Pollak, V. E. and Pesce, A. J. (1972). Maintenance of body protein homeostasis. In *Pathophysiology. Altered Regulatory Mechanisms in Disease* (E. D. Frohlich, ed.), J. B. Lippincott, Philadelphia, pp. 195–214.

Renkin, E. M. and Gilmore, J. P. (1973). Glomerular filtration. In *Handbook of Physiology*, Sect. 8, *Renal Physiology* (J. Orloff, R. W. Berliner, and S. R. Geiger, eds), American Physiological Society, Washington, DC, pp. 185–248.

Rennke, H. G. and Venkatachalam, M. A. (1977*a*). Glomerular permeability: *in vivo* tracer studies with polyanionic and polycationic ferritins. *Kidney Int.* **11**, 44–53.

Rennke, H. G. and Venkatachalam, M. A. (1977*b*). Structural determinants of glomerular permselectivity. *Fedn. Proc. Fedn Am. Socs exp. Biol.* **36**, 2619–2626.

Rennke, H. G., Cotran, R. S. and Venkatachalam, M. A. (1975). Role of molecular charge in glomerular permeability. Tracer studies with cationized ferritins. *J. Cell Biol.* **67**, 638–646.

Rennke, H. G., Patel, Y. and Venkatachalam, M. A. (1978). Glomerular filtration of proteins. Clearance of anionic, neutral, and cationic horseradish peroxidase in the rat. *Kidney Int.* **13**, 278–288.

Rodewald, R. and Karnovsky, M. J. (1974). Porous substructure of the glomerular slit diaphragm in the rat and mouse. *J. Cell Biol.* **60**, 423–433.

Ryan, G. B. and Karnovsky, M. J. (1975). An ultrastructural study of the mechanisms of proteinuria in aminonucleoside nephrosis. *Kidney Int.* **8**, 219–232.

Ryan, G. B. and Karnovsky, M. J. (1976). Distribution of endogenous albumin in the rat glomerulus. Role of hemodynamic factors in glomerular barrier function. *Kidney Int.* **9**, 36–45.

Ryan, G. B., Rodewald, R. and Karnovsky, M. J. (1975). An ultrastructural study of the glomerular slip diaphragm in aminonucleoside nephrosis. *Lab. Invest.* **33**, 461–468.

Ryan, G. B., Hein, S. J. and Karnovsky, M. J. (1976). Glomerular permeability to proteins. Effect of hemodynamic factors on the distribution of endogenous immunoglobulin and exogenous catalase in the rat glomerulus. *Lab. Invest.* **34**, 415–427.

Ryan, G. B., Hein, S. J., Kreisberg, J. I. and Karnovsky, M. J. (1978). Effect of hemodynamic factors on the distribution of anionic groups in the glomerular capillary wall. *J. Ultrastruct. Res.* **65**, 227–233.

Sato, T. and Spiro. R. G. (1976). Studies on the subunit composition of the renal glomerular basement membrane. *J. biol. Chem.* **251**, 4062–4070.

Schneeberger, E. E. (1974). Glomerular permeability to protein molecules—its possible structural basis. *Nephron* **13**, 7–21.

Schneeberger, E. E., Levey, R. H., McCluskey, R. T. and Karnovsky, M. J. (1975). The isoporous substructure of the human glomerular slit diaphragm. *Kidney Int.* **8**, 48–52.

Schneeberger, E. E., Collins, A. B., Latta, H. and McCluskey, R. T. (1977). Diminished glomerular accumulation of colloidal carbon in autologous immune complex nephritis. *Lab. Invest.* **37**, 9–19.

Seiler, M. W., Rennke, H. G., Venkatachalam, M. A. and Cotran, R. S. (1977). Pathogenesis of polycation induced alterations ("fusion") of glomerular epithelium. *Lab. Invest.* **36**, 48–61.

Squire, P. G., Moser, P. and O'Konski, C. T. (1968). The hydrodynamic properties of bovine serum albumin. *Biochemistry* **7**, 4261–4272.

Venkatachalam, M. A., Karnovsky, M. J., Fahimi, H. D. and Cotran, R. S. (1970). An ultrastructural study of glomerular permeability using catalase and peroxidase as tracer proteins. *J. exp. Med.* **132**, 1153–1167.

Addendum

Since this review was written the following pertinent papers have been published.

Andrews, P. M. (1979). Glomerular epithelial alterations resulting from sialic acid surface coat removal. *Kidney Int.* **15**, 376–385.

Caulfield, J. P. and Farquhar, M. G. (1978). Loss of anionic sites from the glomerular basement membrane in aminonucleoside nephrosis. *Lab. Invest.* **39**, 505–512.

Druet, P., Bariéty, J., Laliberté, F., Bellon, B., Belair, M. and Paing, M. (1978). Distribution of heterologous antiperoxidase antibodies and their fragments in the superficial renal cortex of normal Wistar-Munich rat. *Lab. Invest.* **39**, 623–631,

Farquhar, M. G. and Kanwar, Y. S. (1980). Characterization of anionic sites in the glomerular basement membranes of normal and nephrotic rats. In *Renal Pathophysiology*, (A. Leaf, G. Giebisch, L. Bolis, and S. Gorini, eds), Raven Press, New York, pp. 57–74.

Haddad, A., Lachat, J. J., and Gonçalves, R. P. (1978). Electron microscopic radioautographic study of glycoprotein biosynthesis and renewal in renal glomeruli of the rat. 9th int. Congr. Electron Microsc., Toronto, Vol. II, p. 476 (abstract).

Kanwar, Y. S. and Farquhar, M. G. (1979a). Anionic sites in the glomerular basement membrane. *J. Cell Biol.* **81**, 137–153.

Kanwar, Y. S. and Farquhar, M. G. (1979b). Presence of heparan sulfate in the glomerular basement membrane. *Proc. nat. Acad. Sci. U.S.A.* **76**, 1303–1307.

Kanwar, Y. S. and Farquhar, M. G. (1979c). Isolation of glycosaminoglycans (heparan sulfate) from glomerular basement membranes. *Proc. Natl. Acad. Sci. U.S.A.* **76**, 4493–4497.

Kanwar, Y. S. and Farquhar, M. G. (1980). Detachment of endothelium and epithelium from the glomerular basement membrane produced by kidney perfusion with neuraminidase. *Lab. Invest.* **42**, 375–384.

Kelley, V. E. and Cavallo, T. (1980). Glomerular permeability: focal loss of anionic sites in glomeruli of proteinuric mice with lupus nephritis. *Lab. Invest.* **42**, 59–64.

Kerjaschki, D. (1978). Polycation-induced dislocation of slit diaphragms and formation of cell junctions in rat kidney glomeruli. The effects of low temperature, divalent cations, colchicine, and cytochalasin B. *Lab. Invest.* **39**, 420–440.

Latta, H. (1979). Filtration barriers in glomerular capillaries. *Proc. 3rd Asian Colloq. Nephrol.*, in press.

Nörgaard, J. O. R. (1979). Experimentally induced ultrastructural changes in epithelial cells of isolated glomeruli. *Lab. Invest.* **41**, 224–236.

2
Role of the Basement Membrane in Glomerular Filtration: Results Obtained with Electron-dense Tracers

Marilyn G. Farquhar

Introduction

There is now an extensive literature in which various tracers have been used to investigate glomerular filtration at the electron microscope level. It is not our intention in this presentation to review all this work since comprehensive reviews have already been published elsewhere (Farquhar, 1975, 1978). Rather, this presentation will consist of a brief personal account of the results obtained on this topic by our group, indicating stepwise developments in the evolvement of our current concepts, and how results of our work, as well as those obtained by others, have directed our experimental course.

Early Work with Ferritin, Colloidal Gold, and Thorotrast

My own interest in glomerular research began in the 1950s when I had the opportunity to study first at the light microscope level, and later at the electron microscope level, kidney tissues obtained at autopsy or biopsy from patients with various renal diseases. It became clear that there were characteristic pathological alterations in glomerular structure associated with each of the common glomerular diseases (Farquhar *et al.*, 1957, 1959); however, it was frustrating that little or no understanding of the significance of these changes in functional terms was possible because, at the time, we had no idea what role the various layers of the glomerular capillary wall played in the filtration process.

Accordingly, we decided to take advantage of the availability of several electron-opaque, particulate tracers which had just been introduced and to study glomerular permeability at the electron microscope level in experimental animals (Farquhar *et al.*, 1961). The main question to which we were seeking the answer was, "Which layer of the capillary wall acts as the main barrier which retains albumin in the circulation?" The approach used was the same as that used in all such tracer studies—namely, to inject the tracers intravenously, to fix the kidney tissue, and to identify directly the layer that prevented the tracer's passage. Our results clearly demonstrated that the glomerular basement membrane (GBM) acts as the main filter preventing the passage of ferritin (and the other particulate tracers used) since the

TABLE I

Function of glomerular structures[a]

The *basement membrane* as the main filter
The *endothelium* as a valve, which, by the number and size of its fenestrae, controls access to the filter
The *epithelium* as a monitor which partially recovers (by pinocytosis) proteins that leak through the filter
The *mesangium*, which serves to recondition and unclog the filter by phagocytosing and disposing of filtration residues which accumulate against it

[a]From Farquhar *et al.* (1961).

tracer molecules failed to penetrate the GBM to any great extent, and with time they accumulated against the GBM, especially in the mesangial regions. Additional findings were that the residues which accumulated against the GBM were phagocytosed and disposed of by the mesangium (Farquhar and Palade, 1962), and most of the few tracer molecules which did penetrate the GBM were taken up by the epithelial cells (by pinocytosis). Based on these results we developed a functional model for the glomerulus and defined a role for each of its components in the filtration process (Table I). Since then this has been—and still is—our working model for glomerular filtration.

In the later 1960s, this model was challenged by Karnovsky, Venkatachalam, and Cotran and their associates (for a review, see Karnovsky and Ainsworth, 1973), who used peroxidatic tracers to investigate the same problem. They concluded that the GBM represents a crude prefilter and the slits, rather than the GBM, represent the main barrier because these tracers penetrated the GBM and appeared to be restricted by the slits. They explained the discrepancy with our ferritin results on the grounds that ferritin is too large to serve as a marker for plasma proteins even though we and others (see Farquhar, 1975) had obtained similar results with a number of other tracers of widely varying sizes (20–110 Å).

Work with Dextrans

Be that as it may, in the early 1970s, in an attempt to resolve the issue, we set out to test the concept of the two barriers in series by preparing a single tracer of varying size. For this purpose we turned to neutral dextran as the tracer of choice because dextrans were available in a wide range of sizes (10 000–500 000 daltons molecular weight), and their filtration behavior was known. It had been shown that they behave like plasma proteins in the sense that there is increased resistance to glomerular passage with increasing size (molecular weight and effective molecular radius). We prepared a number of such fractions, but the two of greatest usefulness were one which was about the same size as albumin ($\sim 62\,000$ daltons molecular weight) and one which was considerably larger (125 000 daltons molecular weight). Our reasoning was that if there were indeed two barriers in series, then the larger particles in the latter fraction should accumulate against the GBM like the ferritin, whereas the smaller particles in the 62 000 dalton fraction should accumulate against the slits. However, it turned out that the findings were exactly the same with both dextran fractions (Figs 1 and 2). Both accumulated against the GBM, and there was no accumulation with either one in the slits or against the slit membrane (Caulfield and Farquhar, 1974). The only difference in the results with the two fractions was in the amount filtered, which, as might be anticipated, was greater with the smaller molecular weight fraction. In essence the findings were the same as those obtained with ferritin: most of the dextran was retained in the capillary lumen, there was a sharp drop in concentration along the inner surface of the GBM, and none in the lamina densa and beyond.

The main question that arose in the use of dextrans stemmed from the fact that the dextran particles were visualized in the capillary lumen, the urinary spaces, and within the inner, looser, subendothelial portions (lamina rara interna) of the GBM, where they occurred as aggregates of varying size (Figs 1 and 2). However, they were not often seen within the denser portions of the basement membrane (lamina densa). We reasoned that the failure to see many particles in this location was due to their low frequency

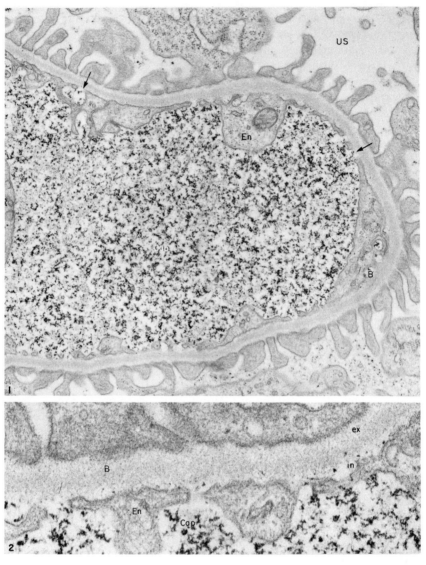

FIGS 1 and 2. *Portions of a glomerulus from a normal rat killed 3·5 h after the injection of 125 000 dalton molecular weight dextran. The capillary lumina (Cap) are filled with dense-staining dextran particles which appear irregularly aggegated. Particles appear to penetrate the fenestrae of the endothelium (En) (arrows) and can be seen in the lamina rara interna (in) of the GBM. No dextran is seen in the lamina rara externa (ex) or in the epithelial slits. (Fig. 2 is from Caulfield and Farquhar (1974).) Fig. 1, × 18 000; Fig. 2, × 71 000.*

(and, therefore, little opportunity for aggregation) and to the high background created by the density of the lamina densa which rendered their staining and therefore their visualization difficult in this layer. However, the possibility existed that their absence from the lamina rara externa (LRE) or slits could be due to some problem in detecting them at this level, rather than due to their low concentration or absence. This seemed unlikely from the beginning because if any significant accumulation occurred in the LRE or against the slits, the particles should be detectable there as well as in other locations. Moreover, subsequent work on aminonucleoside-nephrotic rats (Caulfield and Farquhar, 1975) has effectively ruled out local difficulties in detection, by showing that in these animals, where many more dextran particles do penetrate the GBM, the particles can be visualized in the lamina densa and are often detected in the LRE. Yet no accumulation of dextran particles occurs against the slits. This fact and the general consistency of the results obtained with all the particulate tracers attested to the validity of the results. The net effect of the dextran results on our thinking was to rule out the "two barriers in series" hypothesis because they showed that the GBM serves as the main barrier to molecules over a wide size range (30 000–125 000 daltons molecular weight). Since the dextrans used as probes were neutral molecules of identical composition, varying only in size, variations in behavior of probe molecules based on other properties (differences in molecular charge, shape, or chemical composition) were eliminated. Moreover, these results showed that all the particulate tracers used—native ferritin (an anionic protein), colloidal tracers (gold, thorotrast), and neutral (uncharged) dextrans of varying size—behave similarly in that they all fail to penetrate beyond the LRI to any great extent.

Results Obtained with Lysozyme in Normal Rats

The unresolved question which remained was, "How could one explain the findings obtained by the Harvard group with peroxidatic proteins which appeared to point to the slits as the main barrier for these tracers?" We considered a number of possibilities (cf. Farquhar, 1975), but the explanation that seemed most plausible was the possibility that the peroxidatic tracers, most of which *were* basic proteins with isoelectric points above 7·0, might bind to the highly negatively charged, sialic acid-rich, cell coat material of the epithelial cells, and the images obtained could reflect that binding. The cell coat material had already been shown to bind colloidal iron at acid ph (Fig. 3) and basic dyes such as alcian blue and ruthenium red (Jones, 1969; Mohos and Skoza, 1970; Michael *et al.*, 1970; Latta *et al.*, 1975).

We decided to test directly the idea that cationic proteins can bind to the

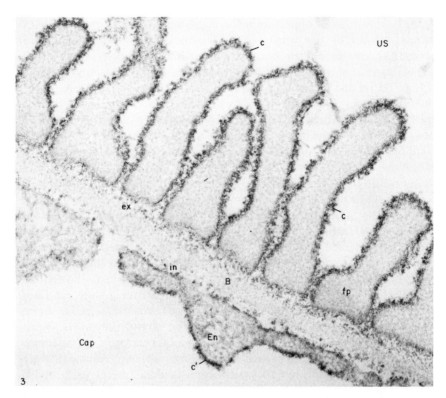

FIG. 3. *Glomerular capillary stained with colloidal iron (at pH 2·0) to demonstrate the existence of a thick, colloidal iron-stainable cell coat along the epithelial cell membrane (c) lining the foot processes (fp). A similar but thinner cell coat is also present along the endothelial surface (c'). These surface coats are known to be rich in sialic acid (presumably present in sialoproteins) because they are removed by neuraminidase treatment. Note also the presence of colloidal iron staining in the lamina rara interna (in) and externa (ex) of the GBM. The GBM sites are not removed by neuraminidase. Cap = capillary lumen; US = urinary spaces. (Y. S. Kanwar and M. G. Farquhar, unpublished observations.) × 49 000.*

epithelium by isolating the kidney from the circulation and infusing a basic protein. Toward this end we searched for a cationic protein which was well characterized and small enough to be freely filtered. A large protein (> 70 000 daltons molecular weight) would not do because it would not be freely filtered and therefore might not reach all the glomerular layers. Initially, we selected lysozyme to work with because it fulfilled these criteria: it is a small protein (14 000 daltons molecular weight) which is well characterized with a high net positive charge (pI = 11). When lysozyme was infused it proved to bind avidly to the epithelium which became completely "stained"

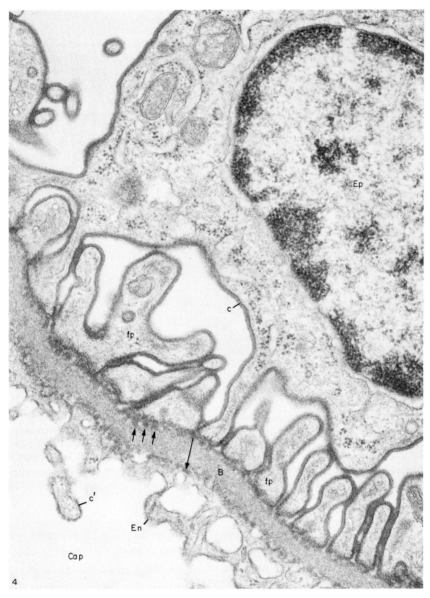

4

FIG. 4. *Field from the glomerulus of a normal rat perfused with lysozyme, a highly cationic protein* ($pI = 11 \cdot 0$). *The membrane of the epithelial cell* (*Ep*) *is outlined by a thick, dense-staining layer of bound lysozyme. Both those portions of the cell membrane surrounding the epithelial cell body* (*c*) *and those surrounding the foot processes* (*fp*) *are outlined. The staining results from the binding of this basic protein to the highly negatively charged epithelial cell coat. Binding also occurs to the endothelial cell coat* (*c′*) *and to the lamina rara interna* (*long arrow*) *and externa* (*short arrows*) *of the GBM which appear denser than the lamina densa* (*B*). *In a few places the binding sites in the LRE* (*arrows*) *show a regular repeating pattern.* (*From Caulfield and Farquhar* (*1978*).) × 41 000.

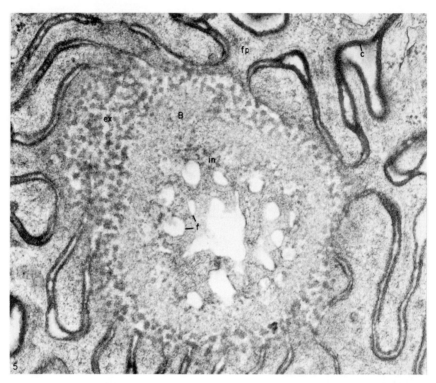

FIG. 5. *Tangential section through a normal glomerular capillary perfused with lysozyme. The section grazes through the GBM and shows to better advantage the reticular pattern created by the binding of lysozyme to anionic sites in the lamina rara interna (in) and externa (ex). Lysozyme binding to the epithelial cell membrane (c) lining the foot processes (fp) is also seen. f = endothelial fenestrae; B = lamina densa. (From Caulfield and Farquhar (1978).) × 41 000.*

by a thick (300–400 Å) dense layer of bound lysozyme (Caulfield and Farquhar, 1976*a*). Binding occurred all along the epithelial cell surface—both along the cell body and outlining the foot process (Figs 4 and 5). In short, images were produced which looked very much like those obtained with peroxidatic tracers, especially myeloperoxidase, the most basic ($pI = 10$) of the peroxidatic tracers used. A new and unexpected finding was that, in addition to binding to the epithelium, lysozyme also bound to sites in the GBM, particularly to those in the lamina rara interna (LRI) and LRE (Figs 4–5). In normal section (Fig. 4) the binding sites in the laminae rarae showed a regular periodic distribution in places, and in grazing section they were seen to be distributed in a reticular pattern (Fig. 5).

We concluded that basic proteins *can* and *do* bind to negatively charged glomerular components. Hence, they are not satisfactory to use as tracers in studies of glomerular permeability since when they are used one cannot distinguish between retention due to ionic interaction with anionic sites and retention due to their size being larger than that of the pores. However, we decided that, due to their ability to bind to negatively charged structures, basic proteins could be useful as "stains" for investigating the distribution of anionic sites in the glomerulus, especially those in the GBM, and later we decided to used them for this purpose, as will be related below.

With these results in hand, we were satisfied that the original purpose of the lysozyme experiments had been accomplished because they provided a satisfactory explanation for the difference between the results obtained with peroxidatic tracers, all of which (with the exception of catalase) are basic proteins, and the results obtained with particulate tracers which are anionic or neutral.

Concurrent Work by Others

Meanwhile, other groups were producing important and convergent results. Ryan and Karnovsky (1976), using immunocytochemistry, localized endogenous albumin in rat glomeruli and obtained findings very similar to those obtained with particulate tracers: they found that under normal flow conditions albumin could not be demonstrated beyond the LRI, indicating that albumin does not penetrate the lamina densa to any great extent. These results showed that endogenous albumin, the macromolecule of greatest physiological interest, behaved exactly the same as the exogenous, adminstered tracers. These experiments served to eliminate any objections that could be raised that the injected tracers behaved different from endogenous proteins.

This meant that if the results obtained with cationic peroxidatic tracers were set aside, those obtained with neutral tracers (dextrans) and anionic proteins (native ferritin, endogenous albumin, catalase and IgG (Ryan *et al.*, 1976), were remarkably consistent—all these tracers failed to penetrate beyond the LRI, indicating clearly that the GBM represents the main glomerular filter and the epithelial slits normally do not function in this capacity.

Work from still other laboratories was clarifying the importance of charge in the filtration behavior of macromolecules. Brenner *et al.* (1977, 1978) showed that negatively charged dextrans (dextran sulfate) have a much more restricted glomerular clearance than neutral dextrans of the same size. From the work of this group the concept emerged of the glomerulus as a "charge-selective filter" which contains fixed negative charges and sorts molecules to be filtered not only on the basis of size, but also on the basis of charge. Moreover, they went on to show that there is a loss of this charge selectivity in several experimental glomerular diseases (nephrotoxic serum nephritis and aminonucleoside nephrosis), and suggested that loss of fixed negative charges from the glomerulus was responsible for the proteinuria which occurs in these diseases. A problem then arose in regard to where in the glomerulus the charge barrier was located. Based on results of colloidal iron staining and influenced, no doubt, by the preoccupation with the filtration slits that existed at that time, Brenner and his associates concluded initially that the epithelial slits must constitute the charge barrier because of the high concentration of anionic sites provided by the close apposition of the sialoprotein-rich, epithelial cell membranes at this level. Moreover, the association between the epithelial cell coat material (epithelial polyanion) and the charge barrier function appeared to be strengthened by the finding that colloidal iron staining is lost in both aminonucleoside nephrosis (Michael et al., 1970) and in nephrotoxic serum nephritis (Brenner et al., 1977, 1978). However, this assumption did not jibe with the results of tracer studies, all of which pointed to the GBM as the main filter, since, as already mentioned, all neutral and anionic macromolecules tested failed to penetrate beyond the LRI, suggesting that the GBM represents both the size-selective and charge-selective barrier. It was difficult to visualize how changes in the epithelial cell coat material could influence the GBM's charge-selective properties. Evidence obtained in the meantime (or concurrently) by Seiler et al. (1977) has clarified the issue and has demonstrated that the main function of the epithelial polyanion or cell coat material is to maintain the normal foot process and slit arrangement (since the latter is disturbed by perfusion with polyanions).

The role of the GBM as the charge-selective barrier was demonstrated directly by the important (and concurrent) experiments of Rennke, Cotran and Venkatachalam (1975) with differently charged ferritins. These workers prepared cationized ferritins with isoelectric points up to 9·0 and found that the permeability of the GBM to the ferritin increases the greater the net charge of the ferritin. Whereas native anionic ferritin fails to penetrate beyond the LRI, the cationic molecules penetrate the GBM in greatly increased amounts. These experiments demonstrated directly that the charge of a molecule affects its filtration behavior and that the GBM represents the charge-selective barrier.

By implication it could be concluded that the GBM is a negatively charged structure, but their experiments did not serve to localize the sites in the GBM. Direct information on the distribution of negatively charged sites in the GBM was provided by our experiments with lysozyme, already mentioned (Caulfield and Farquhar, 1976*a*). This tracer bound to the GBM (as well as to the epithelium), and revealed the existence of a reticular arrangement of anionic sites in the laminae rarae (Figs 4 and 5).

Results Obtained with Lysozyme in Aminonucleoside-nephrotic Rats

The situation at this point in time (1976) could be summarized as follows: The tracer data clearly pointed to the GBM as the morphological equivalent of both the size and the charge barrier in the glomerulus, and clearance studies had demonstrated a partial loss of the glomerular charge barrier function in several experimental diseases associated with proteinuria. It follows that one would expect a loss of charged sites from the GBM to occur in such diseases. The results obtained on nephrotic animals with native (anionic) ferritin (Farquhar and Palade, 1961) had already pointed to a partial loss of the charge barrier function of the GBM by demonstrating penetration of increasing amounts of this negatively charged tracer into the lamina densa and beyond. As previously mentioned, loss of charged sites from the epithelium had been demonstrated in several disease states, but the distribution of anionic sites in the GBM in proteinuric states had not been rigorously investigated.

This being the situation, we decided that a detailed study of the distribution of anionic sites in glomeruli from animals with diseases in which there is proteinuria associated with a loss of charge selectivity was warranted. Hence we used lysozyme to investigate the distribution of anionic sites in the GBM of nephrotic rats, as we had done previously in normals. The specific question to which we were seeking the answer was, "Is the distribution of anionic sites in the GBM altered?" The answer was, "Yes", because the results of these experiments showed that there was a progressive loss of anionic sites from the GBM in this disease to the extent that lysozyme will no longer bind in most animals (Caulfield and Farquhar, 1976*b*, 1978). Early in the course of the disease (after 6–8 daily injections) when the epithelium has a reduced numbers of foot processes and the LRE is widened (Caulfield *et al.*, 1976), binding to the GBM (as well as the epithelium) is reduced, and the discrete sites in the laminae rarae are less regular (Figs 6–8). Later (after 9–11 daily injections) lysozyme no longer binds to the GBM in most animals (Fig. 9). The new finding was the demonstration of a loss of anionic sites from the GBM (as well as the epithelium) in this disease. Thus, the results are in keeping with the role of the GBM as the charge-selective barrier.

The fact that the anionic sites are partially but not completely lost in the disease is indicated by the fact that most of the anionic ferritin is still

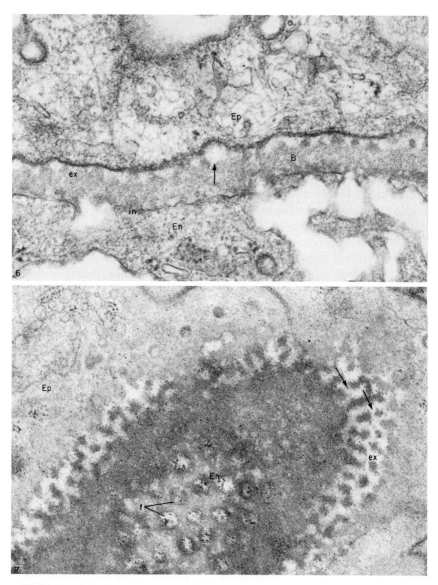

FIGS 6 and 7. *Fig. 6 is a normal section and Fig. 7 is a tangential section of a glomerular capillary from an 8-day nephrotic rat perfused with lysozyme. The pattern of binding to the lamina rara interna (in) and lamina rara externa (ex) is altered in that the frequency and number of dense deposits appears decreased and more irregular. In Fig. 7, it can be seen that the usual reticular pattern in the lamina rara externa (ex) is disturbed since more of the sites of heavy binding are unconnected (arrows). (From Caulfield and Farquhar (1978).) × 62000.*

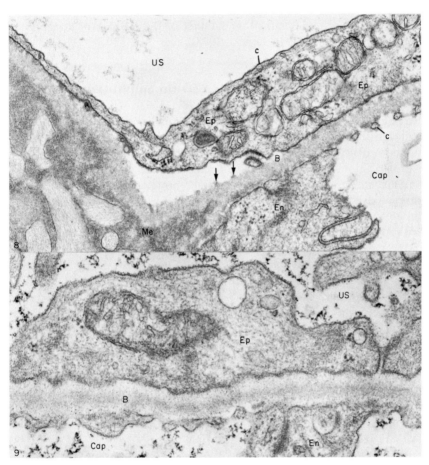

FIGS 8 and 9. *Fig. 8 is another field from the glomerulus of an 8-day nephrotic rat perfused with lysozyme showing a region where the epithelium (Ep) has become detached from the GBM. There is still some binding of lysozyme to the anionic sites in the lamina rara interna and externa of the GBM, but it is more irregular than in normals. In places where the epithelium has become partially detached, the lysozyme binding sites remain associated with the GBM (arrows). Some binding to the epithelial and endothelial cell coats (c) and to the mesangial matrix (Me) is still seen. Fig. 9 is from another nephrotic rat later in the disease (10 daily injections). There is a total lack of binding of lysozyme to any of the layers of the capillary wall. The presence of dextran in the capillary lumen (Cap) and the urinary spaces (US) indicates that the perfusate (which contained both lysozyme and dextran) reached the vessel. En = endothelium; B = lamina densa. (From Caulfield and Farquhar (1978).) Fig. 8, × 33 000; Fig. 9, × 49 000.*

restricted from passing beyond the LRI (Farquhar and Palade, 1961), the physiological data on clearance of dextran sulfate (Brenner *et al.*, 1977, 1978), and by results obtained on staining of the GBM sites in nephrotic animals with alcian blue (Caulfield, 1978).

Recent Studies with Cationized Ferritin and Ruthenium Red

Having established to our satisfaction that anionic sites exist in the GBM and that these sites undergo alterations in glomerular disease, we recently turned our attention to attempting to characterize the sites further using various cationic probes. We have found that we can stain or label the anionic sites using practically any cationic protein administered *in vivo* or cationic dye infused *in vitro*. The two probes which have proved most useful are cationized ferritin (CF), administered intravenously, and ruthenium red (RR), perfused *in vitro* (Kanwar and Farquhar, 1979a, 1979b).

We have prepared a number of cationized ferritin fractions of narrow range. The most useful fractions were those with a p*I* of 7·3–7·5, because these molecules bind only to discrete sites in the GBM; they do not bind to the endothelium or epithelium. Ferritin fractions with a p*I* of >7·5 bind not only to sites in the GBM, but to those on the endothelial and epithelial cell surfaces as well. Thus, the former fractions (p*I* of 7·3–7·5) which bound only to the GBM proved to be very useful for distinguishing between sites in the GBM and those on the closely associated cell coats. When this fraction is given intravenously (0·25 mg/g body weight), CF molecules are found in clusters distributed at regular (∼600 Å) intervals throughout the LRI, the LRE, and the mesangial matrix (Figs 10 and 13). In grazing section, the cationized ferritin deposits take on a regular reticular pattern, very similar to that observed previously with lysozyme.

We assumed that the binding of CF to the GBM sites is ionic in nature— i.e. due to charge interaction between the positively charged CF and concentrations of anionic sites in the GBM. To test this assumption we injected CF *in vivo* and then isolated the kidney and perfused it with buffers of increasing ionic strength. Prolonged perfusion with 0·1–0·2 M KCl resulted in little or no displacement of the tracer, and the CF molecules remained firmly bound to the GBM sites. However, at higher salt concentrations (0·3–0·4 M KCl) the molecules were displaced. These findings indicate that, as expected, the binding of CF to anionic sites in the GBM is by electrostatic interaction because CF was displaced when the ionic strength (or pH) of the perfusate was raised.

When the same kind of experiments were carried out on isolated GBMs, CF proved to bind (clustered at 600 Å intervals) to isolated GBMs, and,

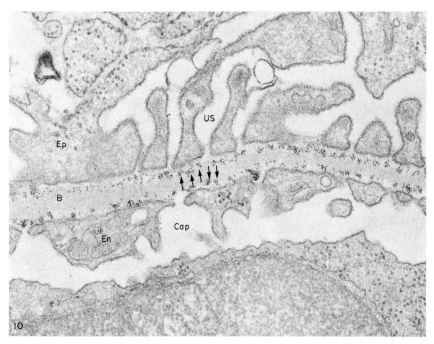

FIG. 10. *Portion of a peripheral region of glomerular capillary from a rat given cationized ferritin (pI = 7·3–7·5) by intravenous injection, after which the kidney was briefly flushed with Hank's balanced salt solution and fixed by aldehyde perfusion. The distribution of CF is restricted primarily to the lamina rara interna (↓) and externa (↑) of the GBM where it occurs in discrete clusters located at regular ~600 Å intervals (arrows). A few molecules are seen scattered in the lamina densa (B). No CF binding to the endothelium (En) or epithelium (Ep) is seen. US = urinary space; Cap = capillary lumen. (From Kanwar and Farquhar (1979a).) × 49 000.*

similarly, binding was lost when such isolated GBMs were treated with buffers of high ionic strength or pH (Kanwar and Farquhar, 1979a).

The most detailed information on the organization of the anionic sites was obtained with ruthenium red (RR), a cationic dye of high charge density and distinct electron opacity, which has been extensively used as a stain to characterize negatively charged cell coats and proteoglycan particles in connective tissues (see Hay et al., 1978). When kidneys were infused with aldehyde fixative containing this dye, small (20 nm) RR-stained particles were seen in the same locations (LRI, LRE, and mesangial matrix) as the CF molecules and they were distributed with the same ~600 Å repeating pattern (Figs 11 and 12). In places the sites appeared to have a quasi-regular, lattice-like arrangement. At higher magnification in favorable micrographs, it could be seen that fine (~2 nm) filaments radiated from the tips

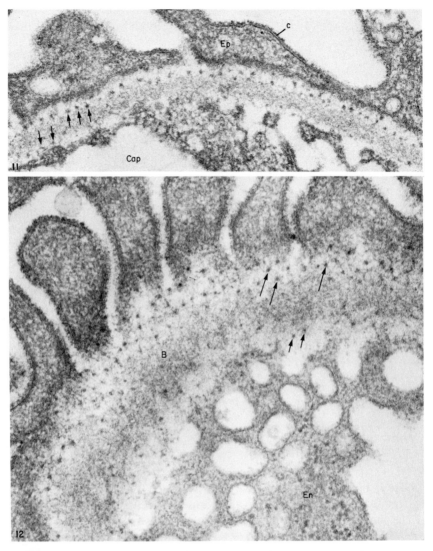

FIGS 11 and 12. *Portions of glomerular capillaries from a kidney perfused with aldehyde fixative containing ruthenium red (RR), a basic dye. Fig. 11 is a cross-section and Fig. 12 is a partially grazing section, illustrating the presence of a network of polygonal, RR-stained particles in the laminae rarae of the GBM. In Fig. 11, the particles are seen to occur in rows distributed at regular (~600 Å) intervals in both the lamina rara interna (↓) and externa (↑). Fine filaments connect the particles to the adjoining cell membranes of the epithelium (Ep) and endothelium. The epithelial cell coat (c) is also stained by the dye. In Fig. 12, a meshwork of particles is seen in the lamina rara externa (long arrows) at the base of the foot processes (fp) and in the lamina rara interna (short arrows) adjoining the endothelium (En). × 90 000.*

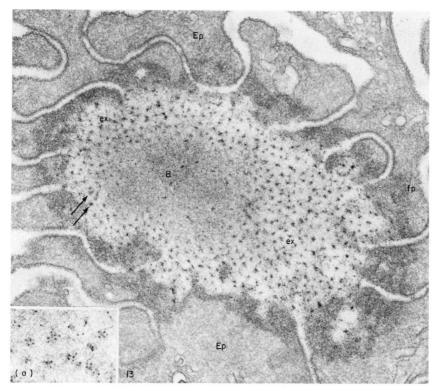

FIG. 13. *Grazing section of a glomerular capillary from the kidney of a rat which had been given CF in* vivo *followed by kidney perfusion with RR. Note that the distribution of the clusters of CF molecules and the RR-positive sites in the lamina rara externa (ex) coincide (arrows). The inset (a) is an enlargement of a portion of the LRE showing CF molecules clustered on the RR-stained particles. B = lamina densa; Ep = epithelium; fp = foot process. (From Kanwar and Farquhar (1979a).) Fig. 13, × 49 000; inset, × 86 000.*

of the polygonal-shaped particles connecting one site to another and extending to the adjoining epithelial and endothelial cell membranes.

Thus the anionic sites in the GBM are demonstrable by labeling *in vivo* (by CF binding), in unfixed kidneys perfused *in vitro* (by lysozyme or CF binding), in fixed kidneys perfused *in vitro* (by RR staining), and in isolated GBMs (by CF binding). It is also clear that RR and CF reveal the same sites, because if both procedures are carried out on the same kidney the two tracers coincide in distribution (Fig. 13). The fact that the anionic sites in the GBM can be demonstrated using several different cationic probes in tissues prepared in many different ways attests to their reality and effectively rules out their being some sort of preparative or technical artifact.

Work in Progress

The delineation of anionic sites in the GBM immediately raises several questions: "What is the nature of the sites?" "Do they resemble any other structure of known composition?" The answer is that the GBM sites bear a striking resemblance to proteoglycan "granules" or particles found in various connective tissues matrices (e.g. cartilage, aorta) stained with ruthenium red (for a review, see Hay *et al.*, 1978). Moreover, proteoglycan granules, consisting in part of chondroitin sulfate, have been described in association with basement membranes in several other locations, including embryonic basement membranes (Hay *et al.*, 1978) and those of aortic smooth muscle (Wight and Ross, 1975). Quite recently we have carried out enzyme digestion experiments (using highly purified enzymes free of proteolytic activity) designed to shed light on the chemical composition of these sites. The results we have obtained so far (Kanwar and Farquhar, 1979*b* show that the particles are not removed by neuraminidase treatment (under conditions in which the sialoglycoprotein of the epithelial cell coat is removed), or by collagenase, chondroitinase ABC, or testicular and leech hyaluronidase; however, they could not be demonstrated after treatment with pronase, heparinase[a] or heparatinase.[a] Thus, these results suggest that the concentration of negatively charged sites in the GBM do not consist of carboxyl groups of either sialic acid or the collagenous peptides, but rather they contain glycosaminoglycans (GAGs) which consist in part of heparin sulfate.

The two outstanding points which remain to be established and occupy us at present are, first, to obtain biochemical confirmation (by analysis of GBM fractions) of the presence of GAGs in the GBM, and second, to obtain direct information on the functional role of the sites in glomerular filtration[b]. In regard to the last point it should be added that the meshwork formed by clusters of anionic sites in the LRI and their fibrillar connections could provide a lattice which would interfere with the penetration of anionic macromolecules into the lamina densa. Thus it is tempting to suggest that the anionic sites in the LRI constitute the main elements responsible for establishing the charge barrier function of the GBM. This idea is attractive because the presence of polysaccharide polymers of proteoglycans have already been shown to limit the transport of macromolecules through connective tissue matrices. However, we hasten to add that at the moment it has not been established whether anionic groups in the LRI or those in the lamina densa (sialoglycoprotein? collagenous peptides? others?) are more

[a] Kindly provided by Dr A. Linker and P. Hovingh (1972).
[b] See note added in proof, p. 51.

important in the creation and maintenance of the charge barrier properties of the GBM. Furthermore, the fact that even more highly developed polyanionic networks exist in the LRE of the GBM and in the laminae rarae of other basement membranes (Bowman's capsule, kidney tubule, endothelium) suggest that they have more than one function.

Acknowledgements

The author gratefully acknowledges the collaboration of Drs John Caulfield and Yashpal Kanwar in recent studies of anionic sites in the glomerular basement membrane; the expert technical assistance of Bonnie Peng, Nancy Bull and Barbara Dannacher; and the excellent editorial assistance of Lynne Wootton. The original research reported in this paper has been supported (since 1974) by grant number AM 17724 from the National Institute of Arthritis, Metabolism and Digestive Disease, United States Public Health Service.

References

Brenner, B. M., Bohrer, M. P. and Baylis, C. (1977). Determinants of glomerular permselectivity: insights derived from observations *in vivo*. *Kidney Int.* **12**, 229–237.

Brenner, B. M., Hostetter, T. H. and Humes, H. D. (1978). Molecular basis of proteinuria of glomerular origin. *New Engl. J. Med.* **298**, 826–833.

Caulfield, J. P. (1978). The distribution of anionic sites in the glomerular basement membrane of normal and nephrotic rats. In *Biology and Chemistry of Basement Membranes* (N. A. Kefalides, ed.), Academic Press, New York and London, pp. 81–98.

Caulfield, J. P. and Farquhar, M. G. (1974). The permeability of glomerular capillaries to graded dextrans. Identification of the basement membrane as the primary filtration barrier. *J. Cell Biol.* **63**, 883–903.

Caulfield, J. P. and Farquhar, M. G. (1975). The permeability of glomerular capillaries of aminonucleoside nephrotic rats to graded dextrans. *J. exp. Med.* **142**, 61–83.

Caulfield, J. P. and Farquhar, M. G. (1976a). Distribution of anionic sites in glomerular basement membranes. Their possible role in filtration and attachment. *Proc. natn. Acad. Sci. U.S.A.* **73**, 1646–1650.

Caulfield, J. P. and Farquhar, M. G. (1976b). Distribution of anionic sites in normal and nephrotic glomerular basement membranes. *J. Cell. Biol.* **70**, 92a (abstract).

Caulfield, J. P. and Farquhar, M. G. (1978). Loss of anionic sites from the glomerular basement membrane in aminonucleoside nephrosis. *Lab. Invest.* **39**, 505–512.

Caulfield, J. P., Reid, J. A. and Farquhar, M. G. (1976). Alterations of the glomerular epithelium in aminonucleoside nephrosis. Evidence for formation of occluding junctions and epithelial cell detachment. *Lab. Invest.* **34**, 43–59.

Farquhar, M. G. (1975). The primary glomerular filtration barrier—basement membrane or epithelial slits? *Kidney Int.* **8**, 197–211.

Farquhar, M. G. (1978). Structure and function in glomerular capillaries. Role of the basement membrane in glomerular filtration. In *Biology and Chemistry of Basement Membranes* (N. A. Kefalides, ed.), Academic Press, New York and London, pp. 43–80.

Farquhar, M. G. and Palade, G. E. (1961). Glomerular permeability. II. Ferritin transfer across the glomerular capillary wall in nephrotic rats. *J. exp. Med.* **114**, 699–716.

Farquhar, M. G. and Palade, G. E. (1962). Functional evidence for the existence of a third cell type in the renal glomerulus. Phagocytosis of filtration residues by a distinctive "third" cell. *J. Cell Biol.* **13**, 55–87.

Farquhar, M. G., Hopper, J., Jr and Moon, H. D. (1959). Diabetic glomerulosclerosis: electron and light microscopic studies. *Am. J. Path.* **35**, 721–755.

Farquhar, M. G., Vernier, R. L. and Good, R. A. (1957). An electron microscope study of the glomerulus in nephrosis, glomerulonephritis and lupuserythematosus. *J. exp. Med.* **106**, 649–660.

Farquhar, M. G., Wissig, S. L. and Palade, G. E. (1961). Glomerular permeability. I. Ferritin transfer across the normal glomerular capillary wall. *J. exp. Med.* **113**, 47–66.

Hay, E. D., Hasty, D. L. and Kiehnau, K. L. (1978). Morphological investigations of fibers derived from various types. Fine structure of collagens and their relation to glucosaminoglycans (GAG). In *Collagen–Platelet Interaction* (H. Gastpar, K. Kuhn and R. Marx, eds), F. K. Schattauer Verlag, Stuttgart and New York, pp. 129–151.

Jones, D. B. (1969). Mucosubstances of the glomerulus. *Lab. Invest.* **21**, 119–125.

Kanwar, Y. S. and Farquhar, M. G. (1979a). Anionic sites in the glomerular basement membrane. *In vivo* and *in vitro* localization to the laminae rarae by cationic probes. *J. Cell Biol.* **81**, 137–153.

Kanwar, Y. S. and Farquhar, M. G. (1979b). Presence of heparan sulfate in the glomerular basement membrane *Proc. natn. Acad. Sci. U.S.A.* **76**, 1303–1307.

Karnovsky, M. J. and Ainsworth, S. K. (1973). The structural basis of glomerular filtration. *Adv. Nephrol.* **2**, 35–60.

Latta, H., Johnston, W. H. and Stanley, T. M. (1975). Sialoglycoproteins and filtration barriers in the glomerular capillary wall. *J. Ultrastruct. Res.* **51**, 354–376.

Linker, A. and Hovingh, P. (1972). Heparinase and heparatinase from flavobacterium. *Methods Enzymol.* **28**, 902–911.

Michael, A. F., Blau, E. and Vernier, R. L. (1970). Glomerular polyanion. Alteration in aminonucleoside nephrosis. *Lab. Invest.* **23**, 649–657.

Mohos, S. C. and Skoza, L. (1970). Histochemical demonstration and localization of sialoproteins in the glomerulus. *Exp. molec. Path.* **12**, 316–323.

Rennke, H. G., Cotran, R. S. and Venkatachalam, M. A. (1975). Role of molecular charge in glomerular permeability. Tracer studies with cationized ferritin. *J. Cell Biol.* **67**, 638–646.

Ryan, G. B. and Karnovsky, M. J. (1976). Distribution of endogenous albumin in the rat glomerulus: role of hemodynamic factors in glomerular barrier function. *Kidney Int.* **9**, 36–45.

Ryan, G. B., Hein, S. J. and Karnovsky, M. J. (1976). Glomerular permeability to proteins. Effects of hemodynamic factors on the distribution of endogenous immunoglobulin G and exogenous catalase in the rat glomerulus. *Lab. Invest.* **34**, 415–427.

Seiler, M. W., Rennke, H. G., Venkatachalam, M. A. and Cotran, R. S. (1977). Pathogenesis of polycation-induced alterations ("fusion") of glomerular epithelium. *Lab. Invest.* **36**, 48–61.

Wight, T. N. and Ross, R. (1975). Proteoglycans in primate arteries. I. Ultrastructural localization and distribution in the intima. *J. Cell Biol.* **67**, 660–674.

Note Added In Proof:

Since submission of this manuscript, we have obtained additional new information on both these points as follows:

1. We have isolated GAG from purified fractions of GBM and have partially characterized them by chemical analysis and cellulose acetate electrophoresis (Kanwar and Farquhar, 1979). The results support and confirm the cytochemical data by demonstrating that heparan sulfate is the only sulfated GAG present in the GBM. In addition, our results suggest that a small amount of non-sulfated GAG (hyaluronic acid) is present.

2. We have obtained evidence (Kanwar *et al.*, 1980) that removal of heparan sulfate by digestion with heparinase) leads to a dramatic increase in the permeability of the GBM to native ferritin. These results provide direct evidence that heparan sulfate plays a role in creating the normal restrictive permeability properties of the GBM.

Kanwar, Y. S., and Farquhar, M. G. (1979). Isolation of glycosaminoglycans (heparan sulfate) from glomerular basement membranes. *Proc. natn. Acad. Sci. U.S.A.* **76**, 4493–4497.

Kanwar, Y. S., Linker, A. and Farquhar, M. G. (1980). Increased permeability of the glomerular basement membrane to ferritin after removal of glycosaminoglycans (heparan sulfate) by enzyme digestion. *J. Cell Biol.* **86**, 688–693.

3
Study of the Glomerular Filtration Barrier by Detection of Circulating Anti-peroxidase Antibodies and their Fragments

Jean Bariéty, Philippe Druet, Catherine Sapin, Marie-France Belair and Michel Paing

Introduction

The localization of the glomerular filtration barrier for circulating proteins is still much debated. As further discussed below, the results and conclusions have varied depending upon the method used and the proteins studied. Recently, considerable importance has been attributed to the haemodynamic conditions (Ryan and Karnovsky, 1976; Ryan *et al.*, 1976) and to the electric charges of the proteins (Caulfield and Farquhar, 1976; Chang *et al.*, 1975; Rennke *et al.*, 1975; Rennke and Venkatachalem, 1977).

The aim of this experimental study was to use anti-peroxidase antibodies and their fragments to investigate the glomerular filtration barrier for IgG (160 000 daltons), $F(ab')_2$ (100 000 daltons) and Fab (50 000 daltons) in normal Munich-Wistar rats.

Materials and Methods

Animals
Male Munich-Wistar rats weighing 200–250 g were used in this study.

Antisera
A rat anti-peroxidase antiserum (containing isologous anti-peroxidase IgG)

was obtained by immunizing Munich-Wistar rats with horse-radish peroxidase (Boehringer Grade I) mixed with Freund's adjuvant. A sheep anti-peroxidase antiserum (containing heterologous anti-peroxidase IgG) was raised in the same way. The sheep anti-peroxidase IgG were isolated using an immunoadsorbent made of an activated peroxidase–bovine serum albumin conjugate (Avrameas and Ternynck, 1969) insolubilized with glutaraldehyde (Avrameas and Ternynck, 1971). The anti-peroxidase activity of the rat anti-peroxidase antiserum and the sheep anti-peroxidase IgG was demonstrated by immunodiffusion in agarose using peroxidase as antigen. The peroxidase activity of the precipitation line was then revealed (Avrameas and Uriel, 1966).

Antibody fragments
Pepsin (Nisonoff *et al.*, 1960) and papain fragments (Porter, 1959) were obtained from a solution of purified sheep anti-peroxidase antibodies according to published procedures.

Separation of fragments and molecular weight estimation
F(ab')$_2$ and Fab fragments were separated from undigested IgG by gel filtration through a G-200 Sephadex column (2·9 cm × 95 cm). Similarly, IgG anti-peroxidase antibodies were separated from aggregated IgG. The gel was equilibrated with phosphate-buffered saline (PBS). The column was then calibrated with lysozyme (15 000 daltons), peroxidase grade I (45 000 daltons), bovine serum albumin (69 000 daltons) and 7 s human IgG (160 000 daltons). The exclusion volume was given by the elution volume of dextran blue. The calculated molecular weights were 50 000 daltons for the papain fragments, 100 000 for the pepsin fragments, and 160 000 for the monomeric undigested IgG. Except when high concentrations were required, the IgG, or the fragments, were used without further concentration.

Detection of anti-peroxidase antibodies and their fragments
  (a) *Autologous antibodies.* Autologous antibodies were detected in three rats immunized with peroxidase.
  (b) *Isologous antibodies.* Three rats were intravenously injected with 1 ml of rat anti-peroxidase antiserum. *In situ* fixation was performed 60 min after the beginning of the injection of the antiserum.
  (c) *Heterologous antibodies and their fragments.* Twenty-one rats were injected intravenously with sheep anti-peroxidase IgG or their fragments. The amount of protein injected was from 1·5 to 20 mg per 100 g body weight for Fab and from 0·1 to 11 mg per 100 g body weight for F(ab')$_2$. *In situ* fixation was performed 5 or 20 min after the beginning of injection.

Immunohistochemical procedure
Kidneys were fixed *in situ* according to Ryan and Karnovsky (1976). Briefly, after decapsulation, the kidney surface was fixed for 1 h by dripping a solution of 2 per cent glutaraldehyde in 0·1 M potassium phosphate buffer, pH 7·35. Sections of superficial cortex, of maximal thickness 1 mm, were cut and immersed in the same fixative for 1 h at 4 °C. Kidney samples were washed for 16 h with three changes of buffer. Thick sections (40 μm) were then obtained with a Smith and Farquhar tissue sectioner. After incubation with peroxidase (Leduc *et al.*, 1968) in phosphate buffer saline, the sections were washed and the peroxidase activity was revealed as described by Graham and Karnovsky (1966*b*). Finally, the sections were processed for electron microscopy as described elsewhere (Laliberté *et al.*, 1978).

Controls
On all kidney samples, the detection of endogenous peroxidase activity was

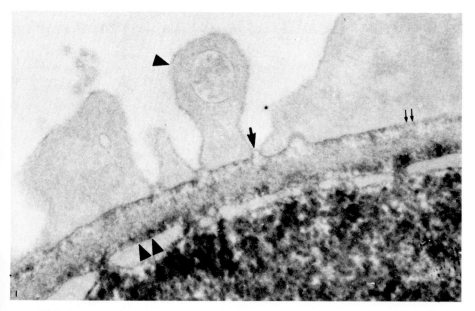

FIG. 1. *Glomerular capillary wall. Fixation was started 5 min after injection of sheep anti-peroxidase IgG. The basement membrane is stained, but the lamina rara interna (double arrowheads) is more strongly stained than the lamina densa. In the lamina rara externa the staining is heterogeneous. The embedded cell coat (double arrows) of the foot processes is stained, but the free cell coat (arrowhead) of the foot processes is unstained. No accumulation of the reaction product is visibile under the slit diaphragm (single arrow). × 40 000.*

performed using the incubation medium for peroxidase only, as described by Graham and Karnovsky (1966*b*) Kidneys from two Munich-Wistar rats fixed *in situ* were incubated with peroxidase-labelled normal sheep IgG. Then the peroxidase activity was revealed as above. In addition, kidneys from four Munich-Wistar rats were fixed *in situ* and kidney samples were incubated with sheep anti-peroxidase IgG or their (Fab')$_2$ or Fab fragments in a concentration of 0·2 mg/ml in phosphate buffer. After washing, the peroxidase activity was revealed as above.

Results

The present observations apply only to the superficial renal cortex, in areas where glomeruli were homogeneously filled with plasma and where the lumens of the tubules were opened. In most cases, the antibodies or their fragments were uniformly revealed by peroxidase in these superficial areas.

Anti-peroxidase IgG
The results were the same with heterologous, isologous or autologous anti-

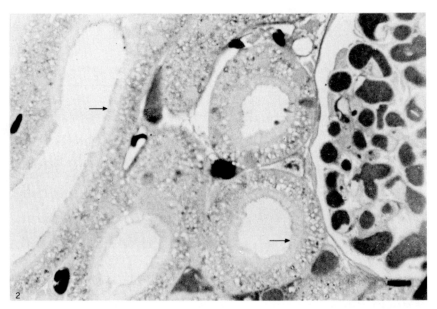

FIG. 2. *Same specimen as shown in Fig. 1. The plasma in glomerular and interstitial capillaries is stained. The brush borders (arrows) and the cytoplasm of the tubular cells are negative.* × 700.

peroxidase antibodies. In the glomerular capillary wall, the lamina rara interna was intensely stained. The lamina densa was generally much less labelled than the lamina rara interna. A heterogeneous staining was observed in the lamina rara externa essentially on the tracts connecting the embedded cell coat of foot processes to the lamina densa. The embedded cell coat of foot processes was stained. No accumulation of the reaction product was seen under the slit diaphragm. The free cell coat of the foot processes were not (or were very slightly) labelled. No evidence for an endocytotic process was seen in the visceral epithelial cells (Fig. 1). The brush border of proximal tubules and the cytoplasm of tubular cells was never stained (Fig. 2).

Fab fragments
Results were similar whatever the amount of Fab injected. In the glomerular

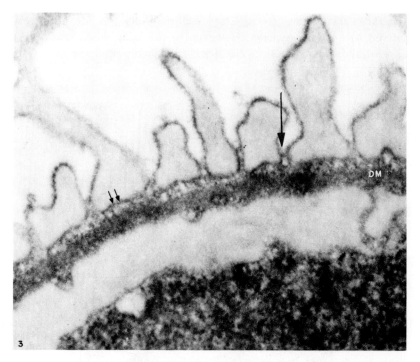

FIG. 3. *Glomerular capillary wall. Fixation was initiated 5 min after injection of sheep anti-peroxidase Fab. The basement membrane (BM) is strongly stained, but the staining in the lamina rara externa is heterogeneous, essentially on the tract connecting the embedded cell coat of the foot processes (double arrows) and the lamina densa. No accumulation of reaction products was seen under the slit diaphragm (single arrow). The free cell coat of the foot processes is stained. × 40 000.*

capillary wall, staining was observed in the basement membrane. When the kidney was fixed, 5 or 20 min after the injection, the lamina rara interna and the lamina densa were homogeneously stained. Only the vertical tracts joining the lamina densa to the embedded cell coat of foot processes were stained. Usually, no accumulation of the reaction product was observed under the slit diaphragm. The whole of the cell coat of foot processes was diffusely stained along the capillary loops and the mesangial areas. No reaction product was seen in the cytoplasm of podocytes (Fig. 3). In the proximal tubules, diffuse staining occurred at 5 min within the cell coat of the brush borders and on the membrane of numerous apical vacuoles (Fig. 4). At 20 min numerous lysosomes appeared to be stained throughout the cytoplasm.

$F(ab')_2$ fragments

The results differed little whether 11 mg or 0·25 mg $F(ab')_2$ fragments were injected. In the glomerular capillary wall, staining was identical to that observed with Fab fragments. However, in the same glomerular tuft, the free cell coat of foot processes was negative in some capillaries and positive

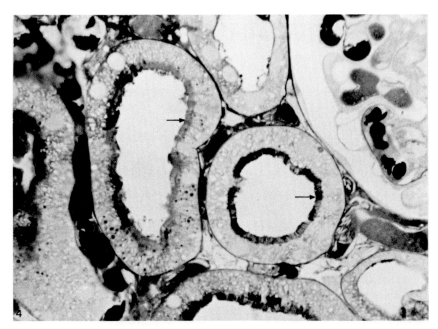

FIG. 4. *Same specimen as shown in Fig. 3. The brush borders (arrows) are stained in the proximal tubules.* × *800.*

in others. In some sections of proximal tubules, staining similar to that described for Fab fragments at 5 min and 20 min was found (Fig. 4). Nevertheless some proximal tubules had unstained brush borders, apical vacuoles and lysosome-like structures. No significant staining was observed after injection of 0·1 mg of F(ab′)$_2$ fragments.

Identical staining was observed with the anti-peroxidase antibodies or their fragments. In the mesangial areas, diffuse and intense staining was observed in the mesangial matrix and in the intercellular channels. In the juxta-glomerular apparatus, staining occurred in the matrix between the cells and in the intercellular spaces of the macula densa. The basement membrane of the Bowman's capsule, the basement membrane of interstitial capillaries, the interstitial tissue and the tubular basement membrane were stained heterogeneously. Staining was also observed in the extracellular spaces between the tubular cells up the tight junctions and in the basal invaginations.

Controls
All the controls were negative except for the well known endogenous activity of red blood cells, polymorphonuclear cells, and, occasionally, microbodies and mitochondrial cristae.

Discussion

The technique used in this study offers several advantages:

(1) It is very sensitive.

(2) It is specific and all controls gave negative results except for endogenous peroxidase-like activity.

(3) The proteins used are serum proteins with well defined molecular weights.

(4) The proteins were easily detected after incubation with free peroxidase, a low molecular weight reagent that penetrates easily and deeply into tissues well fixed with glutaraldehyde (Leduc *et al.*, 1968).

Several findings emerged from this study:

(1) All of the proteins studied penetrated the glomerular basement membrane.

(2) All the proteins studied penetrated diffusely into the mesangial matrix and channels and even into the juxtaglomerular apparatus.

(3) The glomerular filtration barrier appeared to be complete for IgG (160 000 daltons). Indeed, no anti-peroxidase antibodies were detected on

the free cell coat of foot processes. Moreover, a pattern suggestive of tubular reabsorption was never observed. In the capillary wall, the lamina rara interna was more heavily stained than the lamina densa. This suggests that the lamina densa is a barrier for IgG. The staining observed in the lamina rara externa and the embedded cell coat of foot processes is poorly understood, but no evidence for the existence of a second filtration barrier was found at the slit diaphragm level as no clear accumulation of the reaction product was seen under it.

(4) The glomerular filtration barrier appeared to be incomplete for Fab fragments (50 000 daltons). Indeed, these fragments were found on the free cell coat of foot processes. Moreover, there was morphological evidence of tubular reabsorption as described by others in other experimental systems (Bariéty et al., 1978; Ericsson, 1964; Graham and Karnovsky, 1966a, b; Graham and Kellermeyer, 1968; Horster and Larsson, 1976; Karnovsky and Rice, 1969; Maunsbach, 1966a, b; Miller and Palade, 1964; Oliver and Essner, 1972).

(5) The filtration barrier for F(ab')$_2$ fragments in a given glomerular tuft appeared to complete in some capillary loops and incomplete in others.

The role of electrostatic charges was not evaluated in the present study but the serum proteins studied had a broad spectrum of electrophoretic mobility.

Studies using neutral graded dextrans (Caulfield and Farquhar, 1974), native ferritin (Farquhar et al., 1961) and other particulate tracers (Deodhar et al., 1964; Farquhar and Palade, 1959; Farquhar et al., 1961; Farquhar and Palade, 1962; Latta et al., 1960; Pessina et al., 1972) showed that the basement membrane appeared to be the only filtration barrier. These results have been confirmed in the mouse using cationized ferritin derivatives, after different types of fixation (Rennke et al., 1975; Rennke and Venkatachalam, 1977). In this situation, the degree of permeability of the basement membrane is greater for the more cationized derivatives.

Studies using enzymes as tracers and immersion fixation first indicated that there was a first coarse filter in the basement membrane and a finer one at the slit diaphragm level (Karnovsky and Ainsworth, 1973). Subsequently, it was claimed that these results were mainly due to the fixation procedure (Ryan and Karnovsky, 1976). In fact, after in situ fixation, where blood flow conditions are presumably better, autologous rat albumin (Ryan and Karnovsky, 1976) and IgG (Ryan et al., 1976), detected by immunoenzyme techniques, were found neither in the basement membrane nor in the urinary space. However, different results have been presented using similar immunoenzyme techniques and in situ fixation (Laliberté et al., 1978). These conflicting observations using similar techniques are difficult to explain. Technical problems, mainly due to the penetration of the conjugate, may account for the differences. The technique used here overcomes these problems at least partially, and strengthens our previous results (Laliberté *et al.*, 1978). Moreover, the results reported by Ryan and Karnovsky (Ryan and Karnovsky, 1976; Ryan *et al.*, 1976) are difficult to reconcile with the following facts:

(a) albumin has been detected in the rat glomerular ultrafiltrate by micropuncture (Cortney *et al.*, 1970; Eisenbach *et al.*, 1975; Gaizutis *et al.*, 1972; Leber and Marsh, 1970; Oken and Flamenbaum, 1971; Oken *et al.*, 1972; Van Liew *et al.*, 1970).

(b) Ultrastructural evidence for proximal tubular reabsorption has been reported for rat albumin (Bariéty *et al.*, 1978) and in this study for Fab and F(ab')$_2$ anti-peroxidase IgG fragments.

(c) Heterologous anti-GBM antibodies injected intravenously bind to the glomerular capillary wall after a few minutes (Unanue and Dixon, 1965).

Conclusions

Circulating anti-peroxidase antibodies (160 000 daltons) and their F(ab')$_2$ (100 000 daltons) and Fab (50 000 daltons) fragments were demonstrated by incubation with free peroxidase, after *in situ* fixation, in the superficial renal cortex of normal Munich-Wistar rats. The glomerular filtration barrier was found to be complete for IgG and a barrier for IgG was localized in the lamina densa. The glomerular filtration barrier was found to be incomplete for F(ab')$_2$ and Fab fragments. These filtered proteins were found to be reabsorbed in the proximal tubule.

References

Avrameas, S. and Ternynck, T. (1969). The cross-linking of proteins with glutaraldehyde and its use for the preparation of immunoadsorbents. *Immunochemistry* **6**, 53–66.

Avrameas, S. and Ternynck, T. (1971). Peroxidase labeled-antibody and Fab conjugates with enhanced intercellular penetration. *Immunochemistry* **8**, 1175–1179.

Avrameas, S. and Uriel, J. (1966). Methode de marquage d'antigènes et d'anticorps avec des enzymes et son emploi en immunodiffusion. *C.r. hebd. Séanc. Acad. Sci., Paris* **262**, 2543–2551.

Bariéty, J., Druet, P., Laliberté, F., Sapin, C., Belair, M. F. and Paing, M. (1978). Ultrastructural evidence, by immunoperoxidase technique, for a tubular reabsorption of endogenous albumin in normal rat. *Lab. Invest.* **38**, 175–180.

Caulfield, J. P. and Farquhar, M. G. (1974). The permeability of glomerular capillaries to graded dextrans. Identification of the basement membrane as the primary filtration barrier. *J. Cell Biol.* **63**, 883–903.

Caulfield, J. P. and Farquhar, M. G. (1976). Distribution of anionic sites in glomerular basement membranes: their possible role in filtration and attachment. *Proc. natn. Acad. Sci. U.S.A.* **73**, 1646–1650.

Chang, R. L. S., Deen, W. M., Robertson, C. R. and Brenner, B. M. (1975). Permselectivity of the glomerular capillary wall. III. Restricted transport of polyanions. *Kidney Int.* **8**, 212–218.

Cortney, M. A., Sawin, L. L. and Weiss, D. D. (1970). Renal tubular protein absorption in the rat. *J. clin. Invest.* **49**, 1–4.

Deodhar, S. D., Cuppage, F. E. and Gableman, E. (1964). Studies on the mechanism of experimental proteinuria induced by renin. *J. exp. Med.* **120**, 677–690.

Druet, P., Bariéty, J., Laliberté, F., Belton, B., Belair, M. F. and Paing, M. (1978). Distribution of heterologous anti-peroxidase antibodies and their fragments in the superficial renal cortex of normal Wistar-Munich rats. An ultrastructural study. *Lab. Invest.* **39**, 623–631.

Eisenbach, G. M., Van Liew, J. B. and Boylan, J. W. (1975). Effect of angiotensin on the filtration of protein in the rat kidney: A micropuncture study. *Kidney Int.* **8**, 80–87.

Ericsson, J. L. E. (1964). Absorption and decomposition of homologous hemoglobin in renal proximal tubular cells. An experimental light and electron microscopic study. *Acta path. microbiol. scand.* Suppl. 168, 1–121.

Ericsson, J. L. E. (1968). Fine structural basis for hemoglobin filtration by glomerular capillaries. *Nephron* **5**, 7–23.

Farquhar, M. G. and Palade, G. E. (1959). Behaviour of colloidal particles in the glomerulus. *Anat. Rec.* **133**, 378–389.

Farquhar, M. G. and Palade, G. E. (1962). Functional evidence for the existence of a third cell type in the renal glomerulus. Phagocytosis of filtration residues by a distinctive "third" cell. *J. Cell Biol.* **13**, 55–87.

Farquhar, M. G., Wissig, S. L. and Palade, G. E. (1961). Glomerular permeability. I. Ferritin transfer across the normal glomerular capillary wall. *J. exp. Med.* **113**, 47–66.

Gaizutis, M., Pesce, A. J. and Lewy, J. E. (1972). Determination of nanogram amounts of albumin by radioimmunoassay. *Microchem. J.* **17**, 327–334.

Graham, R. C. and Karnovsky, M. J. (1966a). Glomerular permeability: ultrastructural cytochemical studies using peroxidase as protein tracers. *J. exp. Med.* **124**, 1123–1134.

Graham, R. C. and Karnovsky, M. J. (1966b). The early stages of absorption of injected horseradish peroxidase in the proximal tubules of mouse kidney: ultrastructural cytochemistry by a new technique. *J. Histochem. Cytochem.* **14**, 291–302.

Graham, R. C. and Kellermeyer, R. W. (1968). Bovine lactoperoxidase as a cytochemical protein tracer of electron microscopy. *J. Histochem. Cytochem.* **16**, 275–278.

Horster, M. and Larsson, L. (1976). Mechanism of fluid absorption during proximal tubule development. *Kidney Int.* **10**, 348–363.

Karnovsky, M. J. and Ainsworth, S. K. (1973). The structural basis of glomerular filtration. In *Advances in Nephrology*, Vol. 2 (J. Hamburger, J. Crosnier and M. H. Maxwell, eds), Year Book Medical Publishers, Chicago, pp. 35–60.

Karnovsky, M. J. and Rice, D. F. (1969). Exogenous cytochrome *c* as an ultrastructural tracer. *J. Histochem. Cytochem.* **17**, 751–753.

Laliberté, F., Sapin, C., Belair, M. F., Druet, P. and Bariéty, J. (1978). The localization of the filtration barrier in normal rat glomeruli by ultrastructural immunoperoxidase techniques. *Biologie cellul.* **31**, 15–26.

Laliberté, F., Sapin, C., Bellon, B., Druet, P. and Bariéty, J. (1975). Study of experimental glomerulonephritis and of normal glomerular protein filtration by immunoperoxidase. In *Immunoenzymatic Techniques* (G. Feldman *et al.*, eds), North Holland/Elsevier, Amsterdam and New York, pp. 409–423.

Latta, H., Maunsbach, A. B. and Madden, S. C. (1960). The centrolobular region of the renal glomerulus studied by electron microscopy. *J. Ultrastruct. Res.* **4**, 455–472.

Leber, P. D. and Marsh, D. J. (1970). Micropuncture study of concentration and fate of albumin in rat nephron. *Am. J. Physiol.* **219**, 358–363.

Leduc, E. H., Avrameas, S. and Bouteille, M. (1968). Ultrastructural localization of antibody in differentiating plasma cells. *J. exp. Med.* **127**, 109–118.

Maunsbach, A. B. (1966a). Absorption of ^{125}I-labeled homologous albumin by rat kidney proximal tubule cells. A study of microperfused single proximal tubules by electron microscopic autoradiography and histochemistry. *J. Ultrastruct. Res.* **15**, 197–241.

Maunsbach, A. B. (1966b). Absorption of ferritin by rat kidney proximal tubule cells. Electron microscopic observations of the initial uptake phase in cells of microperfused single proximal tubules. *J. Ulstrastruct. Res.* **16**, 1–12.

Miller, F. (1960). Hemoglobin absorption by the cells of the proximal convoluted tubule in mouse kidney. *J. biophys. biochem. Cytol.* **8**, 689–718.

Miller, F. and Palade, G. E. (1964). Lytic activities in renal protein absorption droplets. An electron microscopical cytochemical study. *J. Cell Biol.* **23**, 519–552.

Nisonoff, A., Wissler, F. C., Lipman, L. N. and Woernley, D. L. (1960). Separation of univalent fragments from the bivalent rabbit antibody molecule by reduction of disulfide bonds. *Archs Biochem. Biophys.* **89**, 230–238.

Oliver, C. and Essner, E. (1972). Protein transport in mouse kidney utilizing tyrosinase as an ultrastructural tracer. *J. exp. Med.* **136**, 291–304.

Oken, D. E. and Flamenbaum, W. (1971). Micropuncture studies of proximal tubule albumin concentrations in normal and nephrotic rats. *J. clin. Invest.* **50**, 1498–1505.

Oken, D. E., Cotes, S. C. and Mende, C. W. (1972). Micropuncture study of tubular transport of albumin in rats with aminonucleoside nephrosis. *Kidney Int.* **1**, 3–11.

Pessina, A. C., Hulme, B. and Peart, W. S. (1972). Renin induced proteinuria and the effects of adrenalectomy. II. Morphology in relation to function. *Proc. R. Soc. B.* **180**, 61–71.

Porter, R. R. (1959). The hydrolysis of rabbit gamma globulin and antibodies with crystalline papain. *Biochem. J.* **73**, 119–126.

Rennke, H. G. and Venkatachalam, M. A. (1977). Glomerular permeability: *in vivo* tracer studies with polyanionic and polycationic ferritins. *Kidney Int.* **11**, 44–53.

Rennke, H. G., Cotran, R. S. and Venkatachalam, M. A. (1975). Role of molecular charge in glomerular permeability. Tracer studies with cationized ferritins. *J. Cell Biol.* **67**, 638–646.

Ryan, G. B. and Karnovsky, M. J. (1976). Distribution of endogenous albumin in the rat glomerulus: role of hemodynamic factors in glomerular barrier function. *Kidney Int.* **9**, 36–45.

Ryan, G. B., Hein, S. J. and Karnovsky, M. J. (1976). Glomerular permeability to proteins. Effects of hemodynamic factors on the distribution of endogenous immunoglobulin G and exogenous catalase in the rat glomerulus. *Lab. Invest.* **34**, 415–427.

Unanue, E. R. and Dixon, F. J. (1965). Experimental glomerulonephritis. V. Studies on the interaction of nephrotoxic antibodies with tissues of the rat. *J. exp. Med.* **121**, 697–714.

Ventakachalam, M. A., Karnovsky, M. J., Fahimi, H. D. and Cotran, R. S. (1970). An ultrastructural study of glomerular permeability using catalase peroxidase as tracer proteins. *J. exp. Med.* **132**, 1153–1167.

Van Liew, J. B., Buenting, W., Stolte, H. and Boylan, J. W. (1970). Protein excretion: micropuncture study of rat capsular and proximal tubule fluid. *Am. J. Physiol.* **219**, 299–305.

4
The Glomerular Ultrafiltration Process

Mats Wolgast, Karin Hermansson, Karin Nygren,
Mikael Larson and Mats Sjöquist

Introduction

The glomerular ultrafiltration process is of fundamental importance in the control of the extracellular fluid volume and thereby the control of the plasma volume, cardiac output and systemic blood pressure. It is also the target process in a variety of clinical disorders known as renal failure. An evaluation of this process and the properties of the glomerular membrane requires different modes of attack with different technical and methodological approaches. The present paper is primarily an evaluation of the hydrostatic and colloidal osmotic pressure differences across the glomerular membrane and the hydraulic conductivity, but it will also deal with the control of the most important determinants of the driving forces.

Determinations of Glomerular Pressures

The pressure measurements in all modern studies are carried out with the servo-nulling pressure measurement device described by Wiederhielm et al. (1964) in a successful modification developed by Intaglietta et al. (1970). For direct punctures of superficial glomeruli the pressure measuring device is attached to sharpened glass pipettes with outer diameters of 1–2 μm. The punctures are blind, but the location of the tip can be verified by the injection of Lissamin green. An intracapillary location of the tip will then be followed by a rapid passage of the dye through the glomerular tuft emptying into the efferent arteriole, which can be readily identified on the kidney surface. Some dyed fluid, in principle equal to the part filtered, will pass out into the Bowman's space. In some cases the tip can be obliterated by coagulated blood or due to hitting of the capillary wall, in which case any pressure can be recorded. In these cases, the counter-pressure from the pump will not balance with the intracapillary pressure and the pressure will depend on the current to the pump. Because of these phenomena such erroneous recordings can be identified and eliminated. If the tip is located partly in the capillary and partly in the Bowman's space, the pressure will fluctuate, and thereby indicate an inappropriate puncture. However, the technique remains much more difficult than conventional micropuncture, and especially so if the kidney volume changes, e.g. during sympathetic nerve stimulation.

An indirect technique for the determination of hydrostatic pressure has also been applied (Gertz *et al.*, 1966) in which an oil block is injected into the early part of the proximal tubule. The pressure recorded proximal to the oil blockade will then amount to the glomerular capillary pressure minus the systemic colloid osmotic pressure when the filtration has ceased. Several comparisons between the results from direct punctures and the indirect stop-flow technique in the same nephron have shown identical pressures.

The colloid osmotic pressure in the proximal end of the glomerular capillaries is calculated from the systemic plasma protein concentration. The corresponding pressure in the distal end is obtained from the protein concentration in efferent arteriolar blood as punctured in the "star vessels" which are easily identified on the kidney surface and which represent the distal end of the efferent arterioles. The sampling pipettes have to be fairly large, with an outer diameter of 12–15 μm. Even the haematocrit can be accurately determined. The evaluation of the ultrafiltration process is then completed by determination of the single nephron glomerular filtration rate (SNGFR). The single nephron plasma flow (SNPF) is simply calculated from the SNGFR and the filtration fraction, the latter being obtained from the protein concentration in efferent arteriolar blood. An alternative method is to determine the single nephron clearance of *p*-aminohippurate (PAH) from punctures in the distal tubules, as PAH will be selectively secreted in the proximal tubules. However, the extraction fraction has to be taken into account, but it can be obtained from micro-injections into the peritubular capillary network and the subsequent sampling of urine from the two kidneys (Larsson *et al.*, 1979). The relation between the amounts of PAH secreted in the unilateral and contralateral kidneys allows the calculation of the extraction of PAH. The pressures recorded in glomerular capillaries will show astonishingly small variation, whereas SNGFR and the plasma flow show a larger scattering, which is due largely to methodological errors. Finally it should be noted that, with respect to the driving forces for the ultrafiltration process, the measurement of pressure and plasma flow and blood flow allows for the analysis of the resistances in the efferent and afferent arteriole.

Driving Forces for Glomerular Filtration

Two opinions prevail with respect to the driving forces for the ultrafiltration process. Studies carried out on Munich-Wistar rats, a mutant Wistar strain, by Brenner and coworkers (Brenner and Deen, 1974; Deen *et al.*, 1974) show a filtration equilibrium at the distal end of the glomerular capillaries. This means that there is a balance between the net hydrostatic and net colloid osmotic forces. In the Sprague-Dawley rat (Källskog *et al.*, 1975*a*, *b*) the net hydrostatic pressure difference in the distal end of the glomerular capillaries is 5–10 mm Hg above the corresponding colloid osmotic pressure

TABLE I

Determinants of glomerular ultrafiltration in Munich-Wistar and Sprague-Dawley rats

Condition	Glomerular capillary pressure (mmHg)	Single nephron plasma flow (nl/min)	SNGFR (nl/min)	Filtration fraction	Total blood flow (ml/min)
Munich-Wistar[a]					
Control	45	70	26	0·38	4·2
Noradrenalin injection	58	50	26	0·49	3·0
Sprague-Dawley[b]					
Control	58	164	54	0·28	9·8
2 Hz stimulation	56	138	46	0·29	8·2

[a] From Deen *et al.* (1974).
[a] From Hermansson *et al.* (1980).

difference. Table I shows that this is due to the fact that the Munich-Wistar rat has a glomerular capillary pressure substantially lower than that in the Sprague-Dawley rat. Moreover SNGFR and plasma flows is much higher in the Sprague-Dawley rat, which is also reflected in differences in the total renal blood flow. It is of great importance that the filtration fraction in the Munich-Wistar rat is close to 0·4, whereas in the Sprague-Dawley rat it approaches 0·3. With the lower glomerular capillary pressure for the Munich-Wistar rat and the higher filtration fraction (with concomittant steep

increase in the protein concentration) the above mentioned filtration equilibrium will occur. This means that the amount of fluid filtered is fairly insensitive to changes in the hydrostatic pressure and also insensitive to changes
in the hydraulic conductivity of the glomerular capillary membrane. Instead,
the filtration will be highly dependent on the plasma flow, i.e. dependent
on the resistance in the efferent *or* afferent arteriole. In the Sprague-Dawley
rat the filtration will be more dependent on the hydrostatic pressure, which
is determined by the *relation* between afferent and efferent resistance. Also

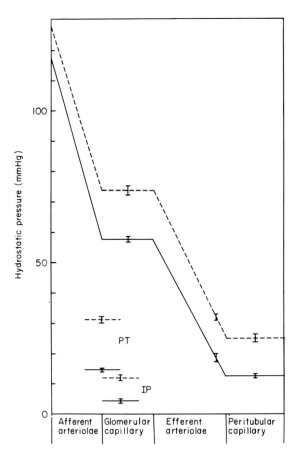

FIG. 1. *Hydrostatic pressure (means ± S.D.) within the superficial structures during
control (———) and extracellular volume expansion (– – – –). PT denotes proximal
tubular pressure and IP interstitial pressure. The decreased resistance over the afferent
arteriolae leads to an increased glomerular capillary pressure and increased blood
flow.*

the permeability of the glomerular capillary membrane will be of major importance. Figure 1 shows typical pressures and flows underlying the evaluation of the dynamics of glomerular ultrafiltration.

During disequilibrium conditions the net driving force along the glomerular capillary or the mean net driving force can be calculated as shown in Fig. 2. Under control conditions the curve for the net driving force decreases almost linearly, from about 20 to about 10 mmHg. A 2 Hz sympathetic nerve stimulation is followed by a depression of the net driving force. The

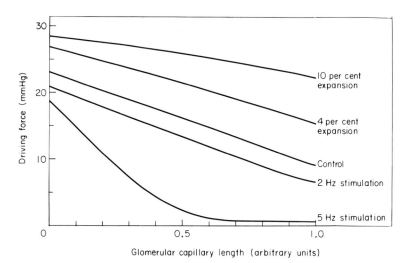

FIG. 2. *The net driving force along the glomerular capillary during control 2 Hz sympathetic nerve stimulation and after extracellular volume expansion with saline of 4 and 10 per cent of the body weight. During 5 Hz stimulation a filtration equilibrium condition is obtained, which does not allow for a true calculation. The curve shown is obtained by artificially increasing the hydrostatic pressure with 2 mmHg and then (after calculation of the profile) reducing it with the same figure. The figure shows how such a profile could both be and not be the true curve. The hydraulic conductivity is about 0·9 nl min⁻¹ per 100 g rat in all instances.*

hydraulic permeability remains essentially unchanged at about 1 nl min⁻¹ mmHg⁻¹ per 100 g rat. Extracellular volume expansion of 4 and 10 per cent is followed by an increase in the net driving force along the whole of the glomerular capillaries, and this is simply the consequence of the dilution of the plasma proteins. In all the instances shown the SNGFR change in proportion to the change in net driving force. This means that the hydraulic conductivity remains fairly unchanged. The equilibrium conditions found on the Munich-Wistar strain do not allow the calculation of the hydraulic conductivity. In the Sprague-Dawley rat a typical value of the hydraulic conductivity on a 300 g rat is 2·7 nl min^{-1} mmHg^{-1}. Assuming a viscosity of the ultrafiltrate of 0·01 P (Landis and Pappenheimer, 1963), a relation between assumed pore radius and the permeability factor $A_p/\Delta x$ (pore area divided with the pore length) can be obtained (Fig. 3). The scales to the right in the figure gives the total pore area, A_p, assuming a pore length of 150 mm (Majno, 1965). Assuming a total surface of the glomerular filtration

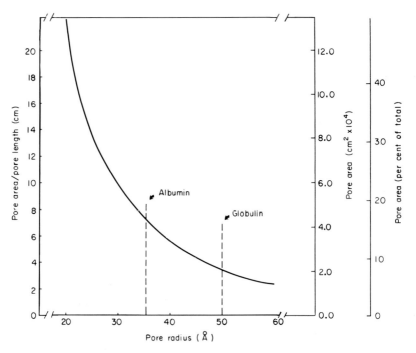

Fig. 3. *The permeability factor "pore area/pore length"* ($A_p/\Delta x$) *as a function of the radius of functional channels through the membrane. The scale to the right gives the pore area for a pore length of 150 nm and the scale to the extreme right the fractional area for an assumed total area of 2·6 × 10^{-3} cm^2.*

barrier of 2·6 × 10^{-3} cm^2 per glomerulus recently found by L. Larsson and A. B. Maunsbach (unpublished observations), the fractional pore area could be calculated (scale to the right). It is evident that the permeability of the glomerular capillary wall is extremely high and that the pore area available for filtration is as high as about 10 per cent, i.e. much higher than in other capillary beds generally assumed to be about 0·1 per cent (Landis and Pappenheimer, 1963).

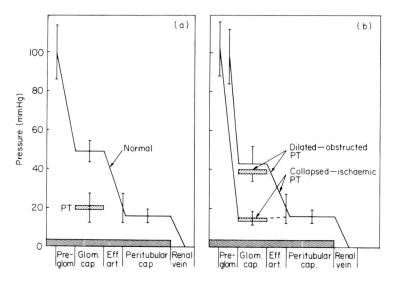

FIG. 4. *Vascular and proximal tubular hydrostatic pressure (means ± s.d.) in three different nephron populations in transplanted kidney graft exposed to 12 h of cold ischemia before the transplantation. About 5 per cent of the nephrons illustrated in (a) belonged to the "normal" type with a filtration about half the normal (SNGFR 7·3 ±s.d. 2·0 nl). The rest of the nephrons shown in (b) have no filtration due to either obstruction or glomerular ischaemia. (From Norlén (1978).)*

Pathophysiology of Glomerular Ultrafiltration

Of particular interest is the function of the glomerular membrane during conditions of renal failure where GFR is known to be greatly reduced. Figure 4 shows the pressure conditions within superficial structures in acute renal failure, here caused by 12 h of cold ischaemia on a kidney transplant (Norlén, 1978). The damage is of intermediate severity with 50 per cent mortality in survival experiments. The same pattern of response is found for renal failure caused by warm ischaemia of 45 min duration. The nephrons can be classified into three types. A few of the nephrons (type 1) have a "normal" gross appearance and the glomerular capillaries have fairly normal pressures. Proximal tubular pressure is, however, elevated to about twice the normal values. The net driving force is calculated to about half the normal value and so is the SNGFR, which means that the hydraulic conductivity remains essentially unchanged. These nephrons are the ones responsible for the filtrate and the urine volumes produced. The majority of the nephrons are either heavily dilated (type 2) or completely collapsed (type 3) and the glomerular ultrafiltration is zero (see Fig. 4(b)). In the collapsed nephrons this is due to the fact that the glomerular capillary pressure approaches the pressure in Bowman's space. In the dilated nephrons the glomerular capillary pressure remains fairly intact, but here the pressure in the Bowman's space is greatly increased, which is almost certainly due to obstruction of the nephron. The obstructions are located in the loop of Henle and the collecting duct in the inner parts of the outer medulla and the outer parts of the inner medulla. They are formed by epithelial cells and cell debris released into the tubular lumen in combination with filtered plasma proteins (Harvig, 1979). The cause of the cell necrosis in these central parts of the renal medulla is an impaired medullary blood flow even after recirculation, i.e. a continuing warm ischaemia with a blood flow reduced from about $1 \cdot 0$ ml min^{-1} g^{-1} to about $0 \cdot 09$ ml min^{-1} g^{-1}. In the normal tubules, the obstruction is only partial. An important part of the formation of these plugs and the subsequent depression of the glomerular filtration is that the glomerular capillary membrane becomes permeable for the plasma proteins. By comparison, it can be mentioned that the peritubular capillary membrane will show the same changes with leakage of the plasma proteins. At present it is not known why the protein permeability increases, but at least one part of the increased leakage seem to be due to a loss of negative charge in the membrane. In the intact membrane neutralized albumin will penetrate, whereas the normal negatively charged albumin is restricted. During renal failure the two proteins permeate at the same rate (unpublished observations). It should be added that the isostenuria and the depressed potassium secretion typical of acute renal failure is directly due to the medullary ischaemia.

Conclusions

It can be concluded that the hydrostatic pressure within the glomerular capillaries is the major determinant of the glomerular ultrafiltration, and that there is a pressure disequilibrium at the distal end of the glomerular capillaries. This means that the glomerular ultrafiltration is dependent on the *relation* between afferent and efferent arteriolar resistance. The hydraulic conductivity of the glomerular capillary membrane will remain unchanged during extracellular volume expansion and during influence of sympathetic nerve activity. Also, during conditions of acute renal failure caused by ischaemic damage, the hydraulic permeability will remain unchanged, although there will be leakage of plasma proteins into the tubular lumen. These proteins will, together with necrotic cells from the loop of Henle and the collecting ducts in the central portions of the renal medulla, provide the basis for tubular obstructions with subsequent increase in the proximal tubular pressure and thereby a reduction of the net driving force and the glomerular fluid filtration. The isostenuria and deficient potassium secretion are caused directly by the impaired medullary circulation with damage of the cell function.

References

Brenner, B. M. and Deen, W. M. (1974). The physiological basis of glomerular ultrafiltration. In *Kidney and Urinary Tract Physiology* (K. Thurau, ed.), Butterworth, London and University Park Press, Baltimore, pp. 335–357.

Deen, W. M., Myers, B. D., Troy, J. L and Brenner, B. M. (1974). Effects of vasoactive substances on the preglomerular, glomerular and postglomerular microcirculation. *Kidney Int.* 6, 35A.

Gertz, K., Brandis, M., Braun-Schubert, G. and Boylan, J. W. (1966). The effect of saline infusion and single nephron filtration rate. *Pflügers Arch. ges. Physiol.* 310, 193–205.

Harvig, B. (1979). Effects of cold ischemia on the preserved and transplanted rat kidney. *Acta Univ. upsal.* 324, 1–22.

Hermansson, K., Källskog, Ö., Larson, M. and Wolgast, M. (1980). Influence of renal nerve activity on arteriolar resistance, ultrafiltration dynamics, and fluid reabsorption. *Pflügers Arch. ges. Physiol.* In press.

Intaglietta, M., Pawula, R. F. and Tompkins, W. R. (1978). Pressure measurements in the mammalian microvasculature. *Microvasc. Res.* 2, 212–220.

Källskog, Ö., Lindbom, L. O., Ulfendahl, H. R. and Wolgast, M. (1975a). Kinetics of the glomerular ultrafiltration in the rat kidney. A theoretical study. *Acta physiol. scand.* 95, 191–200.

Källskog, Ö., Lindbom, L. O., Ulfendahl, H. R. and Wolgast, M. (1975b). Kinetics of the glomerular ultrafiltration in the rat kidney. An experimental study. *Acta physiol. scand.* 95, 293–300.

Landis, M. and Pappenheimer, J. R. (1963). Exchange of substances through the capillary wall. In *Handbook of Physiology*, Sect. 6, *Circulation II* (W. F. Hamilton and P. Dow, eds), American Physiological Society, Washington, DC, pp. 961–1034.

Larson, M., Hermansson, K. and Wolgast, M. (1980). Functional characteristics of the peritubular capillary membrane in the rat kidney. *Acta physiol. Scand.* In press.

Larsson, L. and Maunsbach, A. B. (1980). The ultrastructural development of the glomerular filtration barrier in the rat kidney: a morphometric analysis. *Ultrastruct. Res.* In press.

Majno, G. (1964). Ultrastructure of the vascular membrane. In *Handbook of Physiology*, Sect. 7, *Circulation III* (W. F. Hamilton and P. Dow, eds), American Physiological Society, Washington, DC, pp. 2293–2375.

Norlén, B. J. (1978). Nephron function of the preserved and transplanted rat kidney. *Kidney Int.* 14, 10–20.

Wiederheilm, C. A., Woodbury, J. W., Kirk, S. and Rushmer, R. F. (1964). Pulsatile pressures in the microcirculation of frog's mesentary. *Am. J. Physiol.* 297, 173–176.

5
Concentration Polarization: A Determining Factor in Filtration across Basement Membranes?

Garth B. Robinson and Thomas G. Cotter

Introduction

Ultrafiltration in the glomerulus is remarkably effective in that the ultra-filtrate is virtually free from protein although derived from plasma which is protein-rich. This filtration process has elicited much interest: it has been intensively studied, and these studies have led to elegant mathematical descriptions of the filtration process (Renkin and Gilmore, 1973; Chang et al., 1975; Dubois et al., 1975). The process presents some enigmas. For instance, the rejection of protein may diminish transiently as in postural proteinuria and proteinuria induced by exercise. Administration of renin rapidly elicits proteinuria, apparently as a result of changes in renal haemodynamics (Pessina and Peart, 1972; Bohrer et al., 1977). In all these examples the lowered protein rejection could result from a physical altera-tion of the filtration barrier, but there seems to be no strong evidence for this proposition. Intuitively it is difficult to believe that a very stable con-nective tissue such as basement membrane can undergo rapid, reversible, structural changes.

Almost all the studies of filtration have been conducted *in vivo* using clearance methods, micropuncture or morphological techniques. While yield-ing valuable information, these studies are inevitably limited, since experi-mental manipulation is circumscribed by the necessity of maintaining the integrity of the preparation. For example, in studying filtration, much information can be gained from examining the filtration of simple solu-tions under conditions where filtration pressures can be readily altered, and such investigations cannot be undertaken in the living animal.

The development of methods for isolating renal basement membranes using detergents rather than ultrasonication (Ligler and Robinson, 1977) has made it possible to prepare these membranes as large intact segments rather than as tiny fragments. These large segments can be compacted into thin coherent layers on filter supports (Fig. 1) and the filtration properties of these films studied using conventional filtration methods (Robinson and Brown, 1977; Cotter and Robinson, 1978). This approach provides a model far removed from the *in vivo* situation, but nonetheless it does permit filtration across basement membranes to be studied under conditions unattainable *in vivo*, so providing insights which may be relevant in considering glomerular filtration.

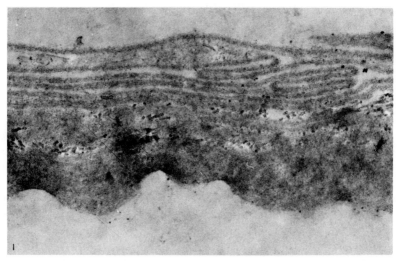

FIG. 1. *Electron micrograph of a transverse section of a basement membrane film lying on a Millipore membrane. The film is prepared from 1·5 mg of basement membrane protein and covers a surface area of 13·8 cm².* (*From Robinson and Cotter* (*1979*).) × 18 000.

The Filtration Process

The theoretical basis of filtration has been described in detail elsewhere (Michaels, 1968; Hwang and Kammermeyer, 1975), but in following the subsequent discussion it will be helpful to reiterate some of the basic ideas here. Flux of solvent, commonly water, across a filter barrier, can be expressed approximately as follows:

$$J_w = (K_w(\Delta P - \Delta\pi))/t, \tag{1}$$

where J_w is the flux per unit area, K_w is the mean permeability co-efficient of the membrane for water, ΔP is the hydrostatic pressure difference, $\Delta\pi$ is the osmotic pressure difference between the filtrate and the bulk (overstanding) solution which applies when solute in the bulk solution is rejected by the filter, and t is the membrane thickness.

In the case of solute transport, this can be mediated in two ways, either by diffusion, or by convective flow. Diffusional movement occurs by the random thermal movement of solute molecules between the chains comprising the polymeric net of the filter; flexible segments of the polymer will be oscillating to create transient channels. Convective movement occurs when there are discrete channels through the filter matrix which are large enough to permit flow of bulk solution; the channels must be sufficiently large to offer no resistance to the passage of solute molecules. It should be added that water movement through convective channels is expressed somewhat differently from the approximation shown in equation (1), but this difference is not critically relevant to the present discussion.

For diffusion the movement of solute can be approximated as

$$J_s = (\bar{D}_s(C_b - C_f))/t, \tag{2}$$

where J_s is the flux of solute per unit area, $\bar{D}_s$ is the mean diffusion co-efficient for solute in the membrane, C_b is the solute concentration in bulk solution and C_f that in the filtrate. Since, for mass conservation,

$$J_s = J_w C_f, \tag{3}$$

equations (1), (2) and (3) can be combined to give

$$1 - \frac{C_f}{C_b} = \frac{(K_w/\bar{D}_s)(\Delta P - \Delta\pi)}{1 + (K_w/\bar{D}_s)(\Delta P - \Delta\pi)}. \tag{4}$$

The term $1 - C_f/C_b$ expresses the rejection (σ) of solute by the filter, i.e. it is the fraction of solute which does not pass through. In physiological studies the term "permeability" is frequently used, which is C_f/C_b or $(1 - \sigma)$. Equation (4) demonstrates that rejection (or permeability) is not an absolute value but is dependent on filtration pressure, rejection increasing hyperbolically with pressure.

For convective movement the situation is different. If the filter is comprised of channels, some of which permit the flow of bulk solution while the remainder occlude solute but permit water flow, the flux of solute may be approximated as

$$J_s = aJ_w C_b, \tag{5}$$

where α is the fraction of solvent flow passing through the larger channels. Solution of equations (1), (3) and (5) gives

$$1 - (C_f/C_b) = 1 - \alpha. \tag{6}$$

For these membranes solute flux is pressure dependent, whereas rejection is independent of pressure.

Concentration Polarization

Studies of the filtration of solutions of macromolecules across synthetic membranes have demonstrated that filtration does not proceed according to theory. Blatt *et al.* (1970) have proposed that this anomalous behaviour results from the effects of concentration polarization, that is, from the build-up of rejected macromolecules to form a boundary layer on the filter surface: the layer acts as an additional barrier to filtration, reducing water flux. Accumulation of solute in the boundary layer will depend upon the rate at which solute is carried to the filter surface by solvent flowing through the filter, and dispersal of the layer on the rate at which solute diffuses from the layer into bulk solution, which will be assisted by stirring, together with loss of solute through the filter. For a wholly rejected solute these relationships have been formalized (Blatt *et al.*, 1970) as

$$(C_w/C_b) = \exp{(J_w/k_s^\circ)}, \tag{7}$$

where C_w is the wall concentration of solute and k_s° is a mass transfer coefficient defined by the diffusion coefficient of the solute and the stirring conditions. Increasing the water flux through the filter, by increasing ΔP, will increase C_w, while improving stirring will decrease the ratio. As will be described below, the consequences of polarization are complicated, particularly when complex solutions such as serum are filtered.

Studies with Basement Membranes

Before discussing the results obtained using filters constructed from isolated basement membranes, it is relevant to describe the methods used, as the *in vitro* model is very different from the glomerulus. Rabbit renal basement membranes, as prepared and used in these studies (Ligler and Robinson, 1977), consist of a mixture of glomerular and tubular membranes. Suspensions of these membrane fragments are placed in conventional pressure filtration cells which are fitted with cellulose acetate membranes (Millipore Ltd., 0·45 µm exclusion). The suspension is forced through the filter by applying pressure, so that the fragments are forced to form a thin coherent layer on the millipore support. Experiments are commonly conducted with 1·5 mg of basement membrane protein which cover a filtration area of 13·8 cm². The film of membranes is, on average, 30 layers of basement membrane thick, with an overall thickness of 1·5 μm.

When the films are formed they can be used for conventional filtration studies, and during experiments the contents of the filtration chambers are stirred magnetically at speeds of 1000–1200 r.p.m. Experiments are normally conducted at 20 °C at filtration pressures of 150 kPa, and protein solutions are made up in 0·15 M sodium chloride containing 10 mM Tris-HCl buffer, pH 7·4. Filtrate is collected over timed periods, and the protein concentration is measured either as absorbance (A_{280}) or by the Folin procedure (Lowry et al., 1951). With such films the rejection value for horse IgG is $\sigma = 0.985$, and for serum proteins $\sigma = 0.999$, which indicates that very little protein seeps through leakage channels.

The Effects of Filtration Pressure on the Filtration of Protein Solutions

Since diffusive solute flux is independent of filtration pressure (equation (2)) while convective flux is not (equation (4)), it is instructive to examine the results obtained when protein solutions are filtered at different pressures (Fig. 2). When sodium chloride solution is filtered, the flux of water increases linearly with pressure as predicted (equation (1)). Surprisingly, when this flux is extrapolated back to zero pressure it does not pass through the origin; the reason for this is not understood, but a similar phenomenon is seen in gas permeation across membranes, and has been termed "surface flow" (Bartholomew and Flood, 1965).

When cytochrome c is filtered the flux of protein increases with pressure, tending to plateau at pressures > 100 kPa; the flux of water also increases with pressure, but again tends to plateau at pressures > 100 kPa. When bovine serum albumin is filtered, the flux of protein is pressure independent, although the flux of water increases with pressure: again J_w tends to plateau.

The sensitivy of cytochrome c flux to pressure indicates that at least a part of this flux is due to convective flow, whereas the insensitivity of the albumin flux indicates that movement of this protein occurs by diffusion. The tendency of the water and cytochrome c fluxes to reach a plateau with increasing pressure could result from compression of the film altering its permeability characteristics. However, such an effect might be expected to change the flux of water when sodium chloride solution is filtered, and of

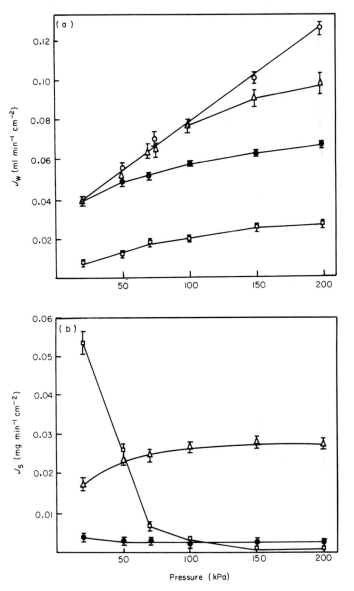

FIG. 2. *Filtration of solutions of different proteins through films of basement mem-brane (1·5 mg of basement membrane protein) at different applied pressures, in stirred filtration chambers. Each result is the mean of three observations on each of three films; the bars represent ± 1 S.D. (a) Water flux* J_w; *(b) protein flux* J_s. ○, *Buffered saline;* △, *cytochrome* c, *0·5 mg/ml;* ●, *bovine serum albumin;* □, *whole rabbit serum. (From Robinson and Cotter (1979).)*

albumin, but these effects are not seen. An alternative explanation is to propose that the effects are a consequence of concentration polarization. Increasing ΔP will increase J_w, resulting in an increase in C_w. The increase in C_w will tend to oppose the increase in J_w, since the layer of protein at the membrane surface will physically obstruct water flow and will also increase the osmotic pressure difference across the membrane. At the same time the increase in C_w will tend to be offset by increased diffusion of solute out of the layer and by the decrease in J_w. Hence with increasing ΔP, J_w and C_w will tend to plateau, that is, to reach an equilbrium. Since C_w, rather than C_b, determines J_s, this will also tend to plateau.

When serum is filtered at increasing pressures, the flux of protein decreases as the pressure increases, while water flux, though very low, tends to increase to a plateau. Similar results obtain with cytochome c when it is mixed with IgG and the mixture is filtered (Fig. 3); this result contrasts with the behaviour of cytochrome c when it is filtered alone (Fig. 2). The difference can again be explained in terms of concentration polarization. When IgG is present, this protein, which is almost entirely rejected, forms a polarization layer which tends to become more concentrated as pressure, and hence J_w, is increased. This layer then progressively prevents the passage of both

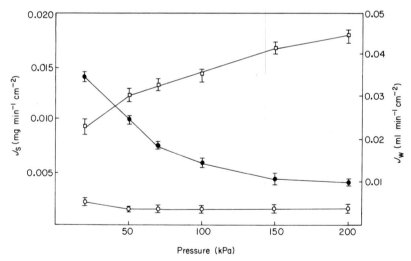

FIG. 3. *Filtration of a solution containing cytochrome* c *(0·5 mg/ml) and horse IgG (2·0 mg/ml) at different pressures through basement membrane films (1·5 mg) in stirred filtration chambers. Each result is the mean of three observations on three separate films; the bars represent ±1 S.D. Left ordinate, protein flux* J_s; *right ordinate water flux* J_w. □, *Water flux;* ●, *cytochrome* c *flux;* ○, *IgG flux. (From Robinson and Cotter (1979).)*

cytochrome c and water. A similar mechanism would explain the results obtained with serum.

An alternative explanation of these effects would be to argue that the films become plugged, which means that the larger proteins become trapped in channels and so occlude them. However, such trapped proteins could not be readily removed without backwashing the filter, whereas the effects seen at the higher pressures are readily reversed merely by reducing the filtration pressure. This finding supports the contention that a surface (polarization) layer is responsible for the changes in behaviour.

The Importance of Stirring during Filtration

Equation (7) predicts that stirring should affect C_w, and indeed changes in stirring markedly affect the filtration behaviour of basement membrane films (Cotter and Robinson, 1978). Ceasing stirring during the filtration of serum results in both a reduction in water flux and an increase in protein flux, the combined effects causing a fall in the protein rejection (Fig. 4). These changes are readily reversed, suggesting that they result from changes in the boundary conditions at the face of the membrane. When stirring ceases the polarization layer would be expected to become more concentrated, which will lead to a reduction in J_w. At the same time, the increased C_w will promote movement of more protein across the filter.

When these results are compared with those obtained when filtration pressure is changed, it is apparent that the effects of polarization are contradictory. In both cases polarization increases the impedance of the films to water, but when stirring is stopped, increased polarization leads to a higher protein flux through the films, whereas when pressure is increased, the protein flux is diminished. The reason for this difference in behaviour is obscure, but it seems reasonable to propose that it reflects a difference in the nature of the polarization layers created under the different conditions. Regardless of the size of the proteins, entry to the polarization layer will depend only on the concentration of the individual protein in the bulk solution and on the flux of water. Removal from the layer will, however, depend on the size of the protein. Small proteins will escape through the film more rapidly than large proteins, and they will also diffuse back into bulk solution more quickly. Hence the polarization layer will tend to become enriched with larger proteins. The degree of enrichment will depend upon the filtration condition prevailing; stirring will tend to accelerate movement of the smaller molecules back into bulk solution to a greater extent than for larger molecules, so that enrichment of the layer is likely to be more pronounced with stirring. The results in Fig. 3 show that large molecules

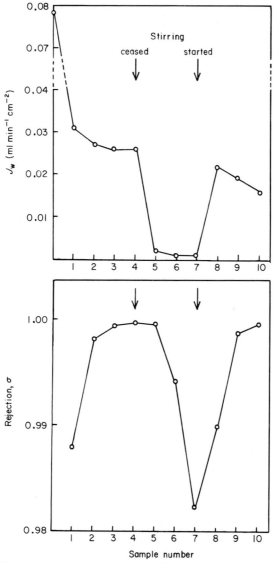

FIG. 4. *Effect of stirring on the filtration of rabbit serum through basement membrane films (1·5 mg). The serum was filtered initially with stirring; stirring was stopped at the point indicated (arrow) and then restarted. The lag in response of the rejection to the cessation of stirring results from the washout of previous filtrate from the apparatus. Initial flow rates were measured with buffer alone. The results shown represent one experiment only since the different time bases used in different experiments make it impossible to aggregate the results. Six experiments, each with three filters, showed essentially identical results. (From Cotter and Robinson (1978).)*

can effectively seal the films against smaller molecules, and thus this sealing effect will be more pronounced with stirring than without.

The Selectivity of the Films under Different Filtration Conditions

Filtrates of serum obtained under the different conditions of filtration were examined by polyacrylamide gel electrophoresis and by gel exclusion chromatography to establish the molecular size range of the proteins which passed through the filters. Filtrates obtained at low filtration pressures with stirring and at high pressures without stirring were compared with whole serum by gel chromatography (Fig. 5). The filtrates contained some high molecular weight material, but the proportion of this material was reduced as compared with serum. Thus, under these conditions of filtration, the films did show some selectivity for molecular size.

Filtrates obtained from serum at high filtration pressures with stirring, when rejection was high, contained too little protein for convenient analysis by gel chromatography, but polyacrylamide gel electrophoresis showed albumin as the predominant protein, although there were traces of other proteins in the filtrate.

The Significance of the Results

The relevance of the model
Since the model filtration system used in the experiments is very different from the glomerulus, it is important to attempt to evaluate the model with respect to glomerular filtration.

In the model experiments, basement membranes are employed as the filtration barrier, whereas in the glomerulus filtration occurs across a complex barrier of basement membranes and cells. However, serum filtration through the films under conditions of high protein rejection, at high pressure with stirring, shows that the films can function effectively as ultrafilters, and indeed they are as effective as the capillary wall. When serum is filtered through films under such conditions, the protein concentration in the filtrate is 7 ± 3 µg/ml and the hydraulic flux is 270 ± 50 nl min^{-1} mm^{-2}. These values are similar to those recorded for glomerular filtration where the filtrate protein concentration is $13 \cdot 5$ µg/ml (Eisenbach *et al.*, 1975) and the hydraulic flux is 70–170 nl min^{-1} mm^{-2} (Renkin and Gilmore, 1973). Thus there is no reason to assume that there need be filtration barriers other than basement membrane in the glomerulus, if filtration in the glomerulus occurs

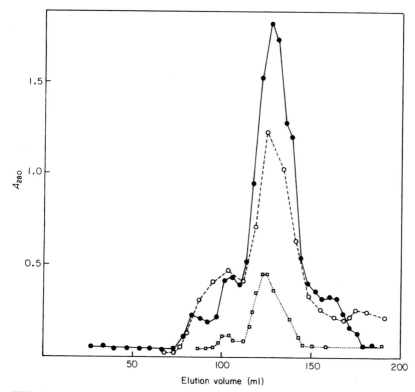

FIG. 5. *Comparison of the molecular weight range of proteins in whole serum and in filtrates from serum obtained using films prepared from 1·5 mg of basement membrane protein. Samples were separated on a column of Sephadex G–150, 1 cm × 100 cm eluted with buffered saline.* ○----○, *Serum;* ●———●, *filtrate of serum at 50 kPa with stirring;* □......□, *filtrate of serum at 150 kPa with no stirring. (From Robinson and Cotter (1979).)*

under conditions where concentration polarization occurs. Morphological studies support the view that the basement membranes are the principal filtration barrier *in vivo* (Caulfield and Farquhar, 1974). In the kidney the basement membrane is lined with fenestrated endothelial cells and the fenestrae could provide pockets where unstirred boundary layers would form. In the model the films are much thicker than the glomerular barrier, and they are operated at much higher filtration pressures (150 kPa as compared with 4–5 kPa in the glomerulus). The greater thickness of the films counteracts the higher pressures in that the pressure fall across each membrane will be 5 kPa if the film is 30 membrane layers thick and this is comparable with the physiological pressure. However, the thickness of the films has other consequences. Studies of the filtration of cytochrome *c* indicate that as film thickness is increased, the convective flux of this small protein is disproportionately reduced (Robinson and Cotter, 1979). For convective channels to remain patent when the membranes are layered one on another, requires that the layering is so arranged that the channels maintain their continuity. With haphazard layering such as occurs in forming the films, the channels will not always coincide and, as the number of layers increases, there will be a greater probability that continuity will diminish. Thus using multilayers will reduce convective flow, although this flow may be important physiologically.

In the model the films are composed of tubular as well as glomerular basement membrane, and the properties of the tubular membrane may be different from those of glomerular membrane. In terms of composition tubular membrane is not very different from glomerular membrane (Ligler and Robinson, 1977), but there could be subtle differences in structure which affect filtration behaviour. Studies of the permeability properties of tubular membranes using microperfusion indicate that this membrane has a high permeability towards albumin (Welling and Grantham, 1972). However, in these studies there is no effective stirring of the membrane surface, and when membrane films are used to filter albumin, albumin readily passes through them only when stirring is stopped (Cotter and Robinson, 1978). Hence the microperfusion experiments do not necessarily demonstrate that the properties of tubular membranes are different from glomerular membranes in terms of albumin permeability, since the apparent permeability is markedly influenced by the stirring conditions.

That polarization effects may be important *in vivo* as well as *in vitro* is suggested by the findings of Ryan and Karnovsky (1976), who demonstrated that albumin penetrated the glomerular filtration barrier when renal blood flow ceased, but not when flow was maintained. This result can be explained by the formation of a polarization barrier under *in vivo* filtration conditions, when filtration pressure is maintained. It is of interest to note here that attempts have been made to demonstrate that basement membranes exclude macromolecules on the basis of size by gel exclusion chromatography using basement membranes as the gel medium (Huang *et al.*, 1967; Igarashi *et al.*, 1976). These attempts have not met with marked success, and this is understandable if the membranes are not inherently impermeable to proteins except under conditions where polarization can be established, as in filtration.

The physiological relevance of concentration polarization
Basement membranes are found in most tissues, where they serve to separate cells of different functions. Not only do they provide mechanical support for the cells, but they serve to define the architecture of the tissue.

When isolated, the glomerular basement membranes retain their native shape (Ligler and Robinson, 1977), illustrating this idea. In some situations the membranes are permeable to proteins; for instance, plasma proteins can pass from the capillary lumen to interstitial fluid across the basement membrane, but this does not occur in the glomerulus. The differences in permeability might be the result of differences in the structures of the membranes in different locations, but it could equally well result from differences in the permeation conditions. When there is no effective stirring, and at low filtration pressure, proteins will readily cross the membranes, but under high pressures with stirring the membranes will be rendered impermeable. Thus the same membrane can be used to achieve different effects depending upon the local conditions, and this notion is attractive because of its simplicity.

If it is indeed true that concentration polarization effects render the glomerular capillaries impermeable to proteins, then changes in the polarization status, resulting from lowered filtration pressure or a reduced stirring efficiency, should cause proteinuria. Stirring in the capillaries is achieved mainly by the sweeping effects of the erythrocytes (Deen et al., 1974), so that a reduction in blood velocity should result in the changes seen in the experiment portrayed in Fig. 3, that is a reduced water flux and an increased protein flux. One experimental situation where such changes are seen is in renin- or angiotensin II-induced proteinuria. Here, proteinuria and a reduced filtration rate result from a constriction of the efferent arterioles induced by the hormone, and the changes are rapidly reversible, at least at low doses of hormone (Pessina and Peart, 1972; Pessina et al., 1972). In other experiments (Bohrer et al., 1977) similar results were observed, although in this study there was no reduction in filtration rate. However, filtration pressure was increased, which would tend to counteract a decrease in filtration. Bohrer et al. (1977) suggested that the proteinuria results from the haemodynamic changes induced by the hormones; resulting changes in the polarization layer may explain the mechanism of the proteinuria.

It is tempting to speculate that proteinuria in pathological conditions results from changes in haemodynamics and hence in the polarization status in the glomeruli, although there is little direct evidence for this idea. However, injection of nephritogenic antibody reduces renal plasma flow, and the glomerular filtration rate, within 60 min (Blantz and Wilson, 1976). Concentration polarization effects would be expected to lead to an increased leakage of protein across the capillary wall as a result of diminished stirring efficiency, and proteinuria has been observed within 4 h of antibody injection (Baldamus et al., 1975), so leakage of protein across the glomerular barrier is quickly established in this condition. Clearly, more experiments are needed with this model to establish whether polarization changes can explain the proteinuria.

Conclusions

The studies on the filtration of protein solutions across basement membranes *in vitro* have established that these membranes are not inherently impermeable to proteins, and they also demonstrate that under particular filtration conditions, at high pressure with efficient stirring, the membranes are rendered effectively impermeable. The most likely reason for this change in behaviour is that concentration polarization effects modify the permeability of the membranes. The formation of the concentration polarization layer is determined by the conditions of filtration and also by the composition of the solution being filtered. It appears that when proteins of different sizes are filtered together, the larger proteins tend to form a polarization layer which prevents smaller proteins escaping through the filter. The formation of the layer may be influenced by yet more subtle events than those outlined here. Some proteins may bind to the membranes by electrostatic or hydrophobic interactions, and the polarization layer would be enriched with these proteins: the theory on which this discussion is based has not taken such interactions into account. There is as yet no direct proof for this theory in the context of basement membrane filtration, nor is it known to what extent, if any, polarization effects might determine behaviour in glomerular ultrafiltration. Clearly, more experiments are needed both *in vitro* and *in vivo* if the arguments are to be substantiated, but the present results suggest that further experimentation would be fruitful in enlarging our understanding of the ultrafiltration process *in vivo*.

References

Baldamus, C. A., Galaske, R., Eisenbach, G. M., Krause, H. P. and Stolte, H. (1975). Glomerular protein filtration in normal and nephritic rats. *Contr. Nephrol.* **1**, 37–49.

Bartholomew, R. F. and Flood, E. A. (1965). The flow of gases through microporous carbon. *Can. J. Chem.* **43**, 1968–1972.

Blantz, R. C. and Wilson, C. B. (1976). Acute effects of anti-glomerular basement membrane antibody on the process of glomerular filtration in the rat. *J. clin. Invest.* **58**, 899–911.

Blatt, W. F., Dravid, A., Michaels, A. S. and Nelsen, L. (1970). In *Membrane Science and Technology* (J. E. Flynn, ed.), Plenum Press, New York, pp. 47–97.

Bohrer, M. P., Deen, W. M., Robertson, C. R. and Brenner, B. M. (1977). Mechanism of angiotensin II-induced proteinuria in the rat. *Am. J. Physiol.* **2**, F13–F21.

Caulfield, J. P. and Farquhar, M. G. (1974). The permeability of glomerular capillaries to graded dextrans: identification of the basement membrane as the primary filtration barrier. *J. Cell Biol.* **63**, 883–903.

Chang, R. L. S., Robertson, C. R., Deen, W. M. and Brenner, B. M. (1975). Permselectivity of the glomerular capillary wall to macromolecules: I. Theoretical considerations. *Biophys. J.* **15**, 861–886.

Cotter, T. G. and Robinson, G. B. (1978). Effects of concentration polarisation on the filtration of proteins through filters constructed from isolated renal basement membrane. *Clin. Sci. molec. Med.* **55**, 113–119.

Deen, W. M., Robertson, C. R. and Brenner, B. M. (1974). Concentration-polarisation in an ultrafiltering capillary. *Biophys. J.* **14**, 412–431.

Dubois, R., Decoodt, P., Gassee, J. P., Verniory, A. and Lambert, J. P. (1975). Determination of glomerular intracapillary and transcapillary pressure gradients from sieving data. I. A mathematical model. *Pflügers Arch. ges. Physiol.* **356**, 299–316.

Eisenbach, G. E., Van Liew, J. B. and Boylan, J. W. (1975). Effect of angiotension on the filtration of protein in the rat kidney: a micropuncture study. *Kidney Int.* **8**, 80–87.

Huang, F. Hutton, L. and Kalant, N. (1967). Molecular sieving by glomerular basement membrane. *Nature, Lond.* **216**, 87–88.

Hwang, T. and Kammermeyer, K. (1975). *Membranes in Separations*, John Wiley and Sons, New York.

Igarashi, S., Nagase, M., Oda, T. and Honda, N. (1976). Molecular sieving by glomerular basement membrane isolated from normal and nephrotic rabbits. *Clin. chim. Acta* **68**, 255–258.

Ligler, F. S. and Robinson, G. B. (1977). A new method for the isolation of renal basement membrane. *Biochim. biophys. Acta* **468**, 327–340.

Lowry, O. H., Rosebrough, N. J., Farr, A. L. and Randall, R. J. (1951). Protein measurement with the Folin phenol reagent. *J. biol. Chem.* **193**, 265–275.

Michaels, A. S. (1968). Ultrafiltration. *Prog. Separation Purification* **1**, 297–334.

Pessina, A. C. and Peart, W. S. (1972). Renin induced proteinuria and the effects of adrenalectomy. *Proc. R. Soc.* B **180**, 43–60.

Pessina, A. C., Hulme, B. and Peart, W. S. (1972). Renin induced proteinuria and the effects of adrenalectomy. II. Morphology in relation to function. *Proc. R. Soc.* B **180**, 61–71.

Renkin, E. M. and Gilmore, J. P. (1973). In *Handbook of Physiology*, Sect. 8, *Renal Physiology* (J. Orloff and R. W. Berliner, eds), American Physiological Society, Washington, DC, pp. 185–248.

Robinson, G. B. and Brown, R. J. (1977). A method for assessing the molecular sieving properties of renal basement membranes *in vitro*. *Fedn Eur. biol. Socs Letters* **78**, 189–193.

Robinson, G. B. and Cotter, T. G. (1979). Studies on the filtration properties of isolated renal basement membranes. *Biochim. biophys. Acta* **551**, 85–94.

Ryan, G. B. and Karnovsky, M. J. (1976). Distribution of endogenous albumin in the rat glomerulus; role of hemo-dynamic factors in glomerular barrier function. *Kidney Int.* **9**, 36–45.

Welling, L. W. and Grantham, D. J. (1972). Physical properties of isolated perfused renal tubules and tubular basement membranes. *J. clin. Invest.* **51**, 1063–1075.

6
Molecular Sieving Properties of Isolated Bovine Glomerular Basement Membrane

N. Gunnar Westberg

Introduction and Clinical Background

The problem of the permeability of the glomerular capillary filter (GCF) has first and most persistently been put to us in cases concerning children, and it is therefore timely to remind ourselves of this clinical origin of our study. Idiopathic nephrotic syndrome with minimal changes in the glomeruli is relatively rare in the adult, but common in childhood. In this peculiar disease, the child is well one day, with no albumin present in the urine. Suddenly, next day, 10–20 g of albumin, and to a smaller extent larger serum proteins, are excreted in the urine. The oncotic pressure of the blood decreases, the urinary output goes down, and after only a few days extensive oedema has developed. Almost as suddenly as it came, the proteinuria goes away, sometimes spontaneously, sometimes after the administration of large doses of corticosteroids. The child is then well again, and the glomerular filter functions perfectly, as far as we can measure. Commonly, the disease recurs, and the child may experience a dozen or so such periods of nephrotic syndrome. The disease, as a rule, disappears permanently before adulthood.

In this disease, the ultrastructure of the glomerular basement membrane (GBM) is often normal. In the epithelial cell layer the foot processes are fused (Farquhar *et al.*, 1957). The glycocalyx is lost, or can at least not be identified using colloidal iron (Blau and Haas, 1973). Whether this change is the result of the proteinuria or is related to its cause is not known, but it is not specific, and can be observed in every proteinuric state, regardless of its cause (Michael *et al.*, 1973).

It has been shown that, while the clearance of albumin is greatly increased in this disease, the clearance for uncharged polyvinyl pyrolidone (PVP) of the same molecular size, or even smaller, is decreased (Robson *et al.*, 1974). Thus, in this disease the ability of the filter to retain uncharged molecules is not decreased, the apparent pore size is not increased, but the ability to block the passage of charged protein is lost.

One important variant of the idiopathic nephrotic syndrome of childhood is unresponsive to steroid treatment. In the glomeruli, primarily in those of the juxtamedullary area, a focal and local sclerosis is seen. In this form of the syndrome progression to uraemia is common, while this does not occur in the "minimal lesion" form. When, finally, a transplant becomes necessary, and a graft is placed in the patient, the new kidney frequently contracts the same disease, often immediately. The profuse proteinuria may recur during the operation, and the new kidney may produce a urine with 20 g of albumin per litre or more (Raij *et al.*, 1972).

From the above clinical observations we can learn at least three things. Firstly, there is at least one component of the GCF which is indispensable for the retention of serum proteins, and which either has a very rapid turnover, or can loose and regain its function from one day to next. The GBM synthesis is likely to be too slow to explain this observation. Secondly, there is a serum factor that is important for the function of the filter. This factor may be a toxic substance, that disturbs the normal function of the filter. The serum factor could also be a serum constituent, present in normal serum, but absent in that of these patients, a factor necessary for the normal function of the GCF. There is at present no evidence for this hypothesis either. Thirdly, the charge of the serum proteins is important for their retention by the normal filter.

In addition to the idiopathic nephrotic syndrome, there is the much larger problem of secondary nephrotic syndrome, particularly secondary to malaria. In areas where malaria is endemic, the nephrotic syndrome is also endemic (Kibukamusoke, 1978). Thus, in countries such as Uganda, Nigeria and Yemen, the incidence of nephrotic syndrome may be as high as 2–3 per cent of the population, and even higher in children.

The problem of the permeability of the GCF is surprisingly complex in view of its deceptive appearance as a simple, passive filter. The permeability of the GCF may be influenced by the pore size and charge of its three layers, and by the haemodynamic situation. Because of the complex interrelationship between these factors, studies of the permeability of isolated GBM could simplify the interpretation of the results. The experimental system described in the following is not physiological, but allows the investigation of the influence of physical and chemical factors on the permeability and a comparison of the permeability of the GBM in health and disease.

Molecular Sieving of Isolated GBM

To study the apparent porosity of GBM, a column was packed with isolated bovine GBM. A sample containing serum proteins and smaller tracer substances was applied and the separation was studied.

When a matrix with a certain porosity is packed into a column, and a sample containing molecules of different sizes is applied, the molecules could theoretically be handled in several different ways:

(1) *Peribetes* (Fig. 1) ($\pi\epsilon\rho\iota$, *around* + $\beta\alpha\iota\nu\epsilon\iota\nu$, *to go; cf. diabetes*)   In this situation the molecules do not to any significant extent penetrate into the matrix, but pass around the particles. No separation will take place.

(2) *Filtration* (Fig. 2)   Pores in the GBM could provide "short-cuts" for molecules small enough to pass through them. If the pores are much bigger than the largest test molecule studied, no separation will take place. If the pores are smaller than the largest molecules, the latter will be delayed on the column, and smaller molecules will be eluted first.

(3) *Diffusion* (Fig. 3)   If the laws of diffusion are applicable to the movement of macromolecules in the GBM matrix, small molecules will travel faster than large molecules.

(4) *Gel filtration* (Fig. 4)   Here the GBM can be conceptualized as a mesh containing water spaces of different sizes. The available solute volume for smaller molecules will be larger than that for larger molecules. Thus, smaller molecules will be retarded compared to larger ones.

(5) *Binding*. In addition to the above mechanisms, bindings of various types could influence the elution pattern.

Materials and Methods

Isolation of GBM

Fresh bovine kidneys were obtained from the slaughterhouse and transported on ice. The preparation was started the same day and the tissue was never frozen. GBM was isolated using established methods (Spiro, 1967; Westberg and Michael, 1970) with the aid of steel screens and ultrasound (Table I). The purity of the preparations was repeatedly checked using phase contrast microscopy. Light microscopy of thin sections and electron microscopy confirmed the quality of the preparations (Figs 5 and 6). GBM can not be obtained in an absolutely pure state. Some tubular fragments, pieces of Bowman's capsule and presumably mesangial material are always present. As a rule, less than 5 per cent of the particles seen were clearly not of GBM

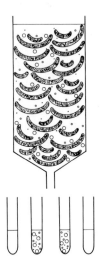

FIG. 1. *"Peribetes". (From Westberg (1978).)*

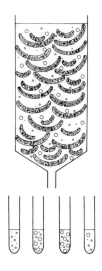

FIG. 2. *Filtration. (From Westberg (1978).)*

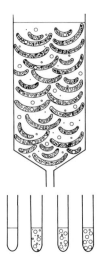

FIG. 3. *Diffusion. (From Westberg (1978).)*

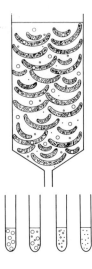

FIG. 4. *Gel filtration (From Westberg (1978).)*

TABLE I

Preparation of bovine glomerular basement membrane[a]

Cut cortex into small pieces
Squeeze through 100 mesh screen with 0·15 M NaCl
Filtrate through 60 mesh screen
Retain glomeruli on 150 mesh screen
Wash extensively with 0·15 M NaCl
Sediment retained glomeruli at 3000 r.p.m. (121 **g**)
Suspend glomeruli in 1 M NaCl
Sonicate for 3–6 min in 30 s bursts
Pass suspension through 250 mesh screen
Centrifuge filtrate four times at 1000 r.p.m. (121 **g**) for 15 min
Wash preparation repeatedly with buffer

[a] According to Westberg and Michael (1970).

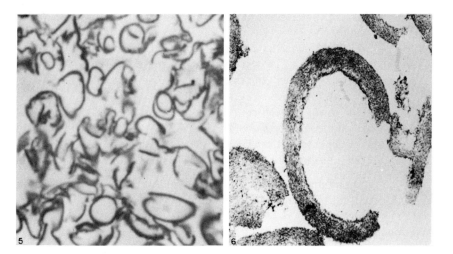

FIG. 5. *Light micrograph of GBM preparation.*

FIG. 6. *Electron micrograph of GBM preparation.*

nature. The amount of phospholipid phosphorus present provided a helpful index of the degree of contamination of the sample. Biochemical analyses for amino acids and carbohydrates in a large number of samples have given quite consistent results. It has not been possible to ascertain if the preparations are in any way denatured compared to native GBM. Other methods for GBM preparation, usually involving detergents, may give other types of changes in the GBM, and the mesangium is included with these preparations.

Columns

The GBM preparations were equilibrated with the appropriate buffers. The GBM was poured into glass columns, 8 mm × 300 mm, and allowed to pack under a low hydrostatic pressure, which later had to be increased to 100–200 cm of water to obtain a useful flow. The flow was usually 2–4 drops per hour during the first experiments, but decreased after several months to 1 drop per hour or even less. Each experiment usually took more than 1 month. It included equilibration of the column with at least two column volumes of buffer, followed by the sample application and the collection of approximately two column volumes of eluate. The test tubes were covered to prevent evaporation. The runs were performed in the cold room.

Buffers

The following buffers were used:

(1) Tris-HCl with 0·02 per cent sodium azide, pH 7·4, osmolality 300 mosmol/kg water.

(2) Tris-HCl–Ca^{2+}, same as above with 0·005 M $CaCl_2$ added.

(3) Tris-HCl–EDTA, as Tris-HCl with 0·005 M Na_2EDTA.

(4) Tris-HCl–Ca^{2+}, higher concentration: NaCl added to Tris-HCl–Ca^{2+} to an osmolality of 400 mosmol/kg water, pH 7·4.

(5) Tris-HCl, lower concentration, water was added to decrease the osmolality to 180 mosmol/kg water at pH 7·4.

(6) Acidic phosphate buffer, 0·05 M Na_2PO_4 with NaCl added to an osmolality of 280 mosmol/kg water, pH 5·6.

Bovine serum albumin (BSA) was added to all buffers at a concentration of 5 g/l, except in four runs using Tris-HCl.

Neuraminidase digestion

GBM was poured from the column and washed with the acidic phosphate buffer repeatedly. Neuraminidase (Sigma N-3001 Type VI) was added, four units, and the preparation incubated at 37 °C for 24 h. In samples of GBM subjected to this procedure, the sialic acid content (Warren, 1959) was decreased from 23·7 to 2·75 μM/g (average of two experiments). The GBM was again washed, and then packed into the glass column as before.

Samples

In 29 experiments 100 μl of the following mixture was applied to the column: frozen human serum from one donor, 35 μl; β_2-microglobulin, 10μl (concentration 1·5 g/l) (a gift from professor Göran Lindstedt); inulin-(methoxy-^{3}H), 35 μl; ^{51}Cr-EDTA (ethylenediaminetetraacetate), 25 μl; 1 M KCl, 10

µl. In five later runs 100 µl of this mixture was applied: human serum
albumin, 200 g/l, 10 µl; β_2-microglobulin, 10 µl; myoglobin, 1·34 g/l, 50 µl;
human immunoglobulin light chain type λ (lambda) isolated from the urine of
a patient with myeloma, 10 g/l, 10 µl; inulin-(methoxy-^{3}H), 15 µl; ^{51}Cr-
EDTA, 10 µl; 1 M KCl, 10 µl. In preliminary experiments, when tritiated
water was used (but not tritiated inulin), using Tris-HCl buffer at an
osmolality of 300 mosmol/kg water, potassium was found to elute in the same
place as THO.

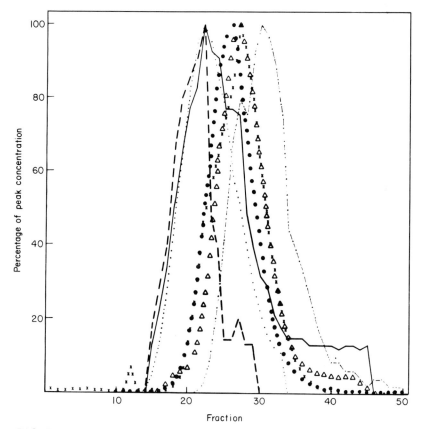

FIG. 7. *Experiment* V_3. *Tris buffer with 0·005 M Ca^{2+} without BSA, pH 7·4, 300
mosmol/kg H$_2$O. To facilitate comparison between different curves, the maximum value
for each tracer is set at 100 per cent. Two groups of peaks are seen, and in addition
β_2-microglobulin is retarded.* —─—, α_2-*macroglobulin;* ———, *immunoglobulin G;* ······,
albumin; ─·─·─, β_2-*microglobulin;* ●●●, *tritiated inulin;* △△△, ^{51}*Cr-EDTA;* × × ×,
K$^+$. (From Westberg (1978).)

Quantification of fraction constituents

α_2-Macroglobulin, immunoglobulin G, β_2-microglobulin, myoglobin and light chain were quantified using radial immunodiffusion (Mancini, 1965). Albumin was measured with the rocket immunoelectrophoresis (Laurell, 1966). Tritiated inulin radioactivity was measured in a Packard Tri-Carb liquid scintillation counter and ^{51}Cr-EDTA radioactivity was counted in a Selectronic gamma counter. Potassium was quantified in a flame photometer.

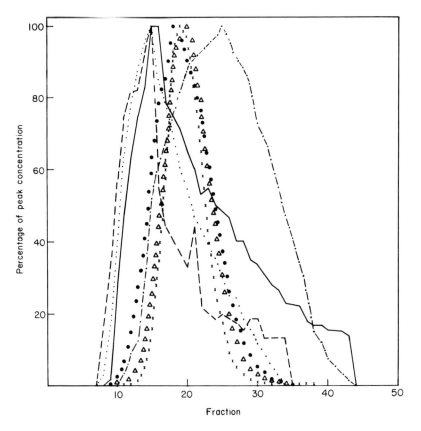

FIG. 8 *Experiment V—neuraminidase-2. Sodium phosphate buffer with 0·005 M Ca²⁺ without BSA, pH 5·6, 300 mosmol/kg H₂O. The GBM was removed from the column, treated with neuraminidase and again packed into the column. The separation is similar to that obtained before neuraminidase treatment. Symbols as in Fig. 7.*

Results

In the 29 runs in which human serum was included, a separation according to molecular size was obtained with the larger molecules eluting ahead of the smaller ones (Figs 7–9). β_2-Microglobulin, however, was eluted last, after the smaller tracers inulin, Cr-EDTA and potassium. There was a separation into three peaks, more or less clearly, with α_2-macroglobulin, immuno-

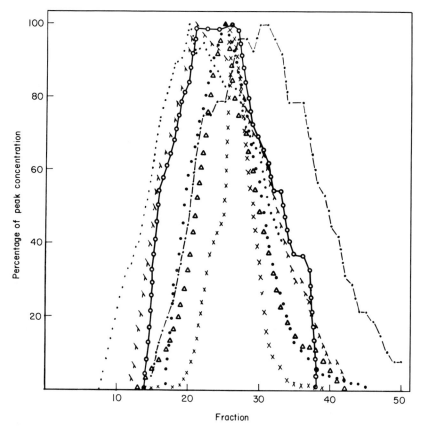

FIG. 9. *Experiment VIII—neuraminidase-1. Tris buffer with 0·005 M Ca²⁺ and 5g/l BSA, pH 7·4, 300 mosmol/kg H₂O. Here myoglobin and light chains are used as additional molecular size tracers instead of α₂-macroglobulin and immunoglobulin. The anomalous elution pattern of β₂-microglobulin compared to the two other molecules of similar size is evident. ○—○, Myoglobulin; λλλ, lambda light chains; remaining symbols as in Fig. 7.*

globulin G and albumin in the first peak. Often α_2-macroglobulin eluted slightly before the two other proteins, and never later. The second peak contained tritiated inulin, ^{51}Cr-EDTA and K^+. β_2-Microglobulin eluted in a third peak, often with a pronounced degree of trailing. The degree of the separation was not very great, and there was some variation from experiment to experiment, using the same buffer and the same column, but the general pattern was not changed. Most experiments were run in triplicate.

Because of the anomalous behaviour of β_2-microglobulin, new experiments were designed using proteins of similar size, myoglobin and immunoglobulin light chain. The light chains in particular are biochemically very similar to β_2-microglobulin. Two such runs were made using Tris-HCl–CaCl$_2$–BSA buffer, pH 7·4, osmolality 400 mosmol/kg, and three runs after neuraminidase treatment. Myoglobin and light chain were found to elute together, slightly after albumin and ahead of the smaller tracers, and in particular ahead of β_2-microglobulin (Fig. 8).

There was no influence on the separation by the presence or absence in the buffer of bovine serum albumin, calcium ions or EDTA, by pH or by ionic strength.

Discussion

Many reports have been published where the permeability of the GCF was studied *in vivo* using electron-dense tracers of known molecular size. Because of the interaction between the functions of the three different layers of the glomerular capillary wall and haemodynamic factors, it is in some respects difficult to interpret the results. The study of the physical chemistry of GBM in isolated form in a chromatography column is certainly not a very physiologic approach. There is no blood flow past the capillary fragments; the GBM may well be changed during the preparation procedure; and the pressure fall per unit path length is much lower than *in vivo*. The main value of the type of the experiment described here would be to compare the separation of macromolecules by isolated GBM under different physical conditions, and to compare GBM obtained from healthy kidneys and kidneys with, for example, diabetic nephropathy. This may provide some insight into the internal structure of GBM in health and disease.

Four theoretically possible methods of molecular sieving are described in this paper according to molecular size: "peribetes", filtration, diffusion and gel filtration. Of these four, only gel filtration would give a separation where the larger molecules are eluted ahead of the smaller tracers. It would thus seem that the molecular structure of the GBM is such as to provide solvent spaces of variable sizes, ranging from the size of inulin to that of albumin.

As α_2-macroglobulin tended to elute ahead of immunoglobulin G and albumin, there may exist a small compartment accessible to immunoglobulin G but not to α_2-macroglobulin. The solute concentration or the presence or absence of the chaotropic ion Ca^{2+} did not influence the elution pattern. This is in contrast to the effect of chaotropic ions on the water domain of, for example, hyaluronic acid. One interpretation would be that the GBM "mesh" is not maintained by the repulsion of negative charges.

The anomalous retardation of β_2-microglobulin on the column is un-explained. Some kind of binding to the GBM seems to be the most likely explanation. Binding could also occur *in vivo*, as β_2-microglobulin is seen in both glomerular and tubular basement membrane in the human kidney (Ooi *et al.*, 1977). This binding force could not be overcome by lowering the pH to 5·6 or by an increase of the osmolality to 400 mosmol/kg water. Immunoglobulin light chains, which are not delayed in the column, have a structure that is very similar to that of β_2-microglobulin, and no difference in electric charge, chemical composition or shape is known that could explain the retardation.

Studies of the separation of macromolecules on columns packed with GBM were first reported by Huang *et al.* (1967). They prepared GBM from rat kidneys and filled capillary tubes, only 5 mm in length. They obtained a very small degree of separation between ^{131}I-labelled albumin, eluting ahead of the other test substance, ^{14}C-labelled mannose. Separation was not obtained with GBM prepared from the kidneys of rats made nephrotic with puromycin aminonucleoside. This single experimental observation remains to be con-firmed.

Igarashi *et al.* (1968) reported on similar experiments using rabbit kidney. The degree of separation between one peak containing ^{131}I-labelled albumin and ^{125}I-labelled globulin and a second peak with ^{125}I-labelled insulin and tritiated water obtained by these authors was far greater than that obtained by me. Only one experiment using normal rabbit GBM was reported. Using GBM from rabbits made nephrotic with anti-rabbit GBM serum in a second experiment, ^{125}I-labelled globulin was found to elute slightly ahead of ^{131}I-labelled albumin.

Gekle *et al.* (1966) approached the problem of permeability of GBM *in vitro* in a study of the equilibrium partition coefficient of macromolecules in a mixture of GBM and buffer. I have tried to use this direct and fast method, but have been unable to get reproducible results.

Robinson and Brown (1977) recently described a novel approach for the study of the permeability of the basement membrane. They pack the isolated GBM on a filter into a very thin pad. The reflection of the test substances then indicates the permeability of the GBM preparation. This rapid and simple method should be further explored.

Conclusions

Under the experimental conditions described in this paper, there is no evidence for filtration through pores. The distribution space of the largest test substance used, α_2-macroglobulin, is slightly larger than that of immunoglobulin G and albumin, which in turn are substantially larger than that of the small test substances used, from inulin to potassium. The mesh structure of GBM is not dependent upon pH or the presence of chaotropic ions or sialic acid.

References

Blau, E. B. and Haas, J. E. (1973). Glomerular sialic acid and proteinuria in human renal disease. *Lab. Invest.* **28**, 477–481.

Farquhar, M. G., Vernier, R. L. and Good, R. A. (1957). An electron microscope study of the glomerulus in nephrosis, glomerulonephritis and lupus erythematosus. *J. exp. Med.* **106**, 649–660.

Gekle, D., Bruchhausen, F. von and Fuchs, G. (1966). Über die Grösse der Porenäquivalente in isolierten Basalmembranen der Rattennierenrinde. *Pflügers Arch. ges. Physiol.* **289**, 180–190.

Huang, F., Hutton, F. and Kalant, N. (1967). Molecular sieving by glomerular basement membrane. *Nature, Lond.* **216**, 87–88.

Igarashi, S., Nagase, M., Oda, T. and Honda, N. (1976) Molecular sieving by glomerular basement membrane from normal and nephrotic rabbits. *Clin. chim. Acta* **68**, 255–258.

Kibukamusoke, W. J. (1978). Quartan malaria nephropathy. In *Proceedings of the VIIth International Congress of Nephrology*, Les Presses de L'Université de Montréal, Montreal, pp. 69–75.

Laurell, C. B. (1966). Quantitative estimation of proteins by electrophoresis in agarose gel containing antibodies. *Analyt. Biochem.* **15**, 45–52.

Mancini, G., Carbonara, A. O. and Heremans, J. F. (1965). Immunochemical determination of antigens by single radial immunodiffusion. *Immunochemistry* **2**, 235–245.

Michael, A. F., Blau, E., Mauer, S. M. and Hoyer, J. (1973). Glomerular capillary permeability and experimental nephrotic syndrome. In *Membranes and Viruses in Immunopathology* (S. Day and R. Good, eds), Academic Press, New York and London, pp. 477–501.

Ooi, B. S., Rubin, S. C., Pesce, A. J. and Pollack, V. E. (1977). Immunofluorescent localization of beta$_2$-microglobulin in the human kidney. *Transplantation* **24**, 1–3.

Raij, L., Hoyer, J. R. and Michael, A. F. (1972). Steroid-resistant nephrotic syndrome. Recurrence after transplantation. *Annls intern. Med.* **77**, 581–586.

Robinson, G. B. and Brown, R. J. (1977). A method for assessing the molecular sieving properties of renal basement membranes *in vitro*. *Fedn Eur. biochem. Socs Letters* **78**, 189–193.

Robson, A. M., Giangiacomo, J., Kienstra, R. A., Naqvi, S. T. and Ingelfinger, J.

R. (1974). Normal glomerular permeability and its modification by minimal change nephrotic syndrome. *J.clin.Invest.* **54**, 1190–1199.

Spiro, R. G. (1967). Studies on the renal glomerular basement membrane. Preparation and chemical composition. *J. biol. Chem.* **242**, 1915–1922.

Warren, L. (1959). The thiobarbituric acid assay of sialic acid. *J. biol. Chem.* **234**, 1971–1982.

Westberg, N. (1978). Molecular sieving properties of isolated glomerular basement membrane. In *Biology and Chemistry of Basement Membranes* (N.A. Keflaides, ed.), Academic Press, New York and London, pp. 205–214.

Westberg, N. G. and Michael, A. F. (1970). Human glomerular basement membrane. Preparation and composition. *Biochemistry* **9**, 3837–3846.

7
A Macromolecular Model of the Glomerular Basement Membrane

Jacob W. Schurer, Gert-Jan Fleuren,
Philip J. Hoedemaeker and Izaäk Molenaar

Introduction

In the glomerular basement membrane (GBM), anionic sites with a regular spacing can be detected with cationic tracers (Rennke *et al.*, 1975; Caulfield and Farquhar, 1976; Seiler *et al.*, 1977; Schurer *et al.*, 1977). In other investigations, using polyethyleneimine (PEI) as cationic tracer, anionic sites were also found to be regularly distributed on basement membrane material of other sources and on collagen fibrils (Schurer *et al.*, 1978). The similarity between the localization in basement membrane and collagen is strikingly illustrated in Fig. 1 for the choroid plexus. In the glomerulus, PEI was localized in both laminae rarae of the GBM (Fig. 2) with a spacing identical to that found on collagen fibrils. Therefore structural similarities between the material of the laminae of the GBM and of collagen were supposed.

This idea led us to develop a new model for the GBM, being speculative in some respects, but which is consistent with the available chemical, physical and ultrastructural information.

The Model

Structure
It has been assessed by chemical analyses, immunological methods and physical techniques that the GBM contains collagen, most probably type IV (Kefalides, 1977, 1978). The GBM material, including tropocollagen

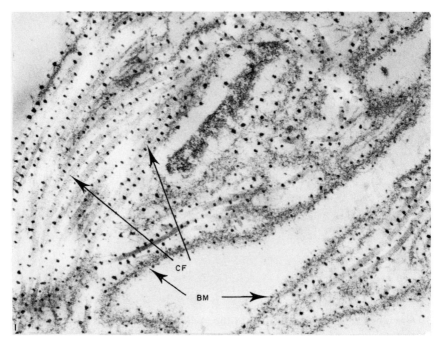

FIG. 1. *Rat choroid plexus immersed with PEI 1800. PEI is localized on collagen fibrils (CF) and on basement membrane material (BM) with an identical distribution.* × 48 000.

molecules, is secreted by the glomerular epithelial and the endothelial cells as a layer on the surface of their plasma membranes.

Our model (Fig. 5) is based on the following assumptions:

(1) The presence of the cationic tracer PEI in our experiments depicts the localization of the three carboxylic groups of the tropocollagen molecule, because PEI can be expected to be bound much more strongly through the tricarboxyl groups of the tropocollagen molecules than through isolated carboxyl groups. Furthermore, anionic sites with a regular spacing are more to be expected in collagen than in non-collageneous substances.

(2) The assembling of tropocollagen molecules into collagen fibrils on the surface of the plasma membranes of the epithelial and endothelial cells is hampered by steric hindrance, caused by the known high content of the disaccharide glucosylgalactose, bound to the hydroxylysine molecules of the polypeptide chain (Kefalides, 1978).

These assumptions would result in a layer composed of tropocollagen molecules, arranged as a "sheet" instead of as collagen fibrils. These

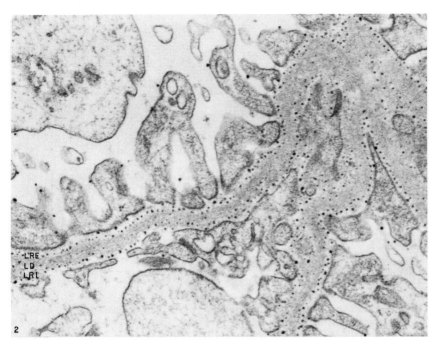

FIG. 2. *Rat GBM immersed with PEI 1800. A regular PEI distribution is present at the interface between LRE and LD, and somewhat less regular in the LRI. Occasionally a particle is found close to the cell membrane of the epithelial foot processes.* × 38 000.

molecules contain anionic and cationic end-groups. It is known that in fibrillar collagen the distance between these groups is 40 nm (Gallop and Paz, 1976; Grant and Jackson, 1976).

The arrangement of tropocollagen molecules in a sheet (Fig. 3(a)) with a basic collagen structure results in longitudinal "pores", having a length of 40 nm, as already mentioned. In Fig. 3(b) it is demonstrated that the width of such a pore is derived from the diameter of one tropocollagen molecule (1·2 nm) added to twice the length of a cross-link (about 1·0 nm), resulting in a width of about 3·2 nm. This means that these pores occupy 17 per cent of the total surface. At the short sides the pores are bordered by amino (cationic) and acid (anionic) end-groups. At the longitudinal sides the pores are lined by the rigid helical tropocollagen molecules.

The polypeptide chains of the collagenic sheet function as carriers for adhering carbohydrates. These carbohydrates, bound to the hydroxylysine of the tropocollagen (Grant and Jackson, 1976), together with the glyco-proteins of the glycocalyx of the epithelial and endothelial cell (Jones, 1969; Bruchhausen and Merker, 1967), cover the sheet as a gel, exerting a stabilizing

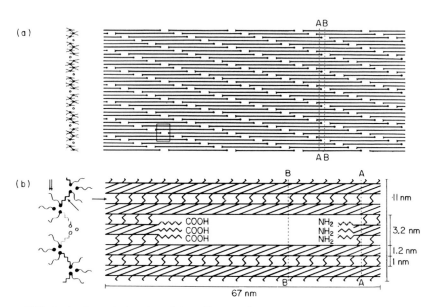

FIG. 3. *A schematic drawing of the collagenic sheet.* (*a*) *Arrangement of tropocollagen molecules in a sheet results in a regular pore distribution. At left the sheet is seen in cross-section.* (*b*) *Higher magnification of a repetative collagenic pore unit. At left the pore is drawn in cross-section.*

effect on the sheet structure. Since the epithelial (and endothelial) cell will produce new layers of collagen-like material, there will be a continuous movement of this material, leaving the sphere of influence of the cell. This leads to a loss of stabilizing effect on the newly produced sheet material. Consequently the collagenic sheet will change into a more stable filamentous structure, which remains embedded in a carbohydrate matrix (Bruchhausen and Merker, 1967; Latta *et al.*, 1975), rendering mechanical support to the GBM and being known as the lamina densa (LD). Moreover, the sheet may undergo regressive changes by neutralization of anionic and cationic groups in the pores. These alterations in structure and composition cause a morphological transition in the GBM which can be observed with the electron microscope as the difference between the lamina rara and the LD.

In spite of the continuous production of material of the GBM, this structure remains equally thick, indicating the existence of a breakdown process. This will occur through depolymerization, probably by enzymic degradation, and results in small fragments which leave the GBM and can be excreted into the urinary space. They may also be re-used for synthesis of new GBM material, especially by the epithelial cell, because of the direction of flow of the filtrate. The production of sheet material by the epithelial

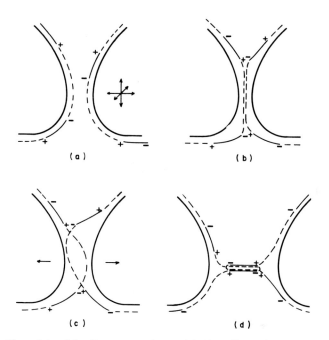

FIG. 4. *The origin of the slit pore membrane. (a) The cell membranes of two adjacent epithelial foot processes are covered by charged collagenic sheets. The solid parts of the lines represent a cross-section, as indicated by AA in Fig. 3. The dotted lines in the sheet represent a cross-section through the pores, as indicated by BB in Fig. 3. (b) Moving and orientation of the foot processes result in binding between the charges of the two sheets as indicated. The rigid parts of one sheet penetrate the collagenic pores of the contralateral sheet. (c) Subsequently an increase of the filtration pressure leads to widening of the slit pore and a sharp bending of the rigid parts. (d) The resulting collagenous SPM is stabilized by extra hydrogen bonds.*

and endothelial cells will probably be proportional to their cell volume and consequently the movement of the material produced by the thin and fenestrated endothelial cell will be relatively slow. Therefore the degradation of the material of the GBM in the LD will occur mainly at the side of the lamina rara interna (LRI).

The slit pore membrane (SPM) originates in our model during development from a contact between the collagenic sheets covering two adjacent epithelial foot processes. At first newly formed sheets on the cell membranes will repel each other because of an overall anionic charge (Fig. 4(a)). However, by a movement of epithelial foot processes the regularly distributed bipolarities in the collagenic sheets will orient themselves until a binding occurs which is shown schematically in Fig. 4(b). This closing effect will cause the hydrodynamic pressure to rise. Consequently the epithelial foot processes will be forced apart, causing four rigid parts of the tropocollagen molecules to bend and together to penetrate the opposite longitudinal pore of the contralateral sheet (Fig. 4(c)). With rising hydrodynamic pressure both sheets will disengage themselves from the cell surfaces, giving rise to a rigid and thin SPM (Fig. 4(b)).

Function

In principle the proposed GBM model (Fig. 5) offers three different filtration modes:

(1) A "mechanical" filtration through the "collagenic pores" (excluding molecules exceeding a diameter of 3·2 nm) and closely adherent collagenic filaments.

(2) An ion exchange function by means of the charged end-groups of the tropocollagen molecules bordering the pores. The amino groups lend anion exchange properties to the GBM, while the acid groups are responsible for cation exchange properties.

(3) A mechanism of molecular sieving through the carbohydrate gel. It is interesting to note that, although these carbohydrates make up only 10 per cent of the weight of the GBM collagen, their volume is (in the case of a 1 per cent gel) 10 times the volume of the collagen sheets, lending the GBM high and laminar flow properties.

In filtration the first barrier is encountered in the LRI. Because of the relatively small production of tropocollagen by the endothelial cells as compared to the epithelial cells, the presence of fenestrations in the endothelial cell, and the depolymerization of the filamentous material of the LD, the distribution of "collagenic pores" in the LRI, as reflected by the presence of PEI, is somewhat irregular. For this reason the LRI functions as preselector through mechanical filtration and ion exchange. The overall charge of the LRI is thought to be anionic. Therefore the passage of relatively large anionic molecules like serum albumins is blocked, while cationic molecules such as urea are attracted and pass the LRI. After the passage of the LRI the filtrate possesses a certain amount of turbulence.

The second barrier is the LD. Because of the tightly packed collagenic filaments, embedded in a carbohydrate gel, this layer acts as a coarse filter and blocks the passage of large molecules which escape the first barrier. The carbohydrate gel changes the turbulent flow into a laminar flow and distributes the pressure evenly.

The third barrier is formed by the lamina rara externa (LRE), including the SPM. Because in this layer the "collagenic pores" are more regularly distributed than in LRI, the LRE makes an important contribution through mechanical filtration and ion exchange. Because the collagenic sheet is

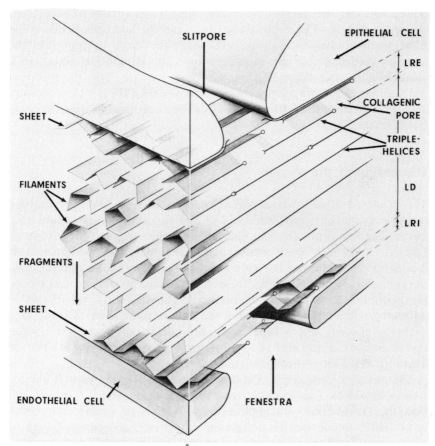

FIG. 5. *A model of the GBM. The thickness of the GBM, the size of the endothelial fenestra, and the size of the slit pore are drawn at the same scale; the material of the GBM is visualized at the macromolecular level. In the slit pore, between the epithelial foot processes, the slit pore membrane is not drawn. The sheet material, especially from the epithelial cell, is gradually changed into filaments, while the collagenic pores are being closed. Subsequently these filaments are degradated into fragments, close to the LRI. Sheet and filaments are embedded in a carbohydrate gel (not drawn).*

produced by—and is therefore in close approximation to—the cell membrane of the epithelial foot processes, the filtrate which passed the sheets is orientated along these cellular surfaces towards the slit pore.

The SPM exerts a final influence on the composition of the filtrate through both mechanical filtration and ion exchange. The supposed structure of the SPM is stabilized by electrostatic forces between opposite, counter-charged end-groups of the tropocollagen molecules and besides through hydrogen bonds between the parallel orientated rigid parts of the tropocollagen molecules (Fig. 4). The electrostatic forces and the hydrogen bonds in the SPM, the hydrodynamic pressure, and finally the forces determined by the adjacent epithelial cells are in equilibrium. This equilibrium results in a variable pore size, depending on the local pressure. This phenomenon provides the SPM with an auto-regulated control for the filtration pressure (Fig. 7). Therefore the GBM can fulfil its filtration function under optimal pressure conditions.

Discussion of the Model

The proposed model stresses the significance of both laminae rarae for monitoring the filtration process. The lamina densa serves mainly as a mechanical support, built from filaments (Bruchhausen and Merker, 1967; Latta *et al.*, 1975) of great tensile strength. Moreover, by its development it is not a separate layer, but intimately connected to and continuous with the laminae rarae at both sides. These three laminae together present a firm, but permeable basis for both epithelial and endothelial cell membranes to adhere to. Although the thickness of the laminae rarae of the GBM as seen with the electron microscope might be influenced by the preparation procedures for electron microscopy (e.g. shrinking of collagen due to aldehyde fixation), this does not invalidate our theory.

The model is provoked by the demonstration of the presence of anionic sites in the GBM. This was reported by several investigators. Caulfield and Farquhar (1976) demonstrated these sites with lysozyme, while recently Seiler *et al.* (1977) found that the polycation protamine sulphate was bound to similar sites. In addition to organized anionic groups in the GBM, "cationic sites" could also be demonstrated by staining with a positively charged molecule like methacrylic acid. This procedure resulted in an identical regular pattern in the laminae rarae (unpublished results).

The presence of collagen in the laminae rarae of the GBM as a sheet results in a structure rich in pores, having a width of 3·2 nm and a length of 40 nm. These pores bordered by the rigid tropocollagen molecules will permit the passage of molecules up to 3·2 nm in diameter. The passage of larger molecules will be blocked. Evidence for such a mechanical filter effect was demonstrated by several investigators using tracers of different size (for a review, see Farquhar, 1975).

In addition to this mechanical filter, the presence of anionic and cationic end-groups will supply the pore with the possibility of controlling the passage of molecules by means of charge. Molecules containing amino groups and/or other cations will be attracted to anionic end-groups, while metal ions with complexing properties and anions will be attracted to amino end-groups. Depending on the number of charged groups, these molecules, if smaller than 3·2 nm in diameter, will pass the GBM slowly or rapidly. This was indeed demonstrated by Rennke *et al.* (1975) and Rennke and Venkatachalam (1977), who showed that, although native ferritin molecules are not able to pass the GBM, passage of cationized ferritin is possible. Apparently the charged ferritin molecules are attracted by the overall anionic LRI and the overall anionic charges in the LRE. However, at the same time the passage of these molecules is blocked by their size. Once bound to the anionic pore-end, the molecules will be forced through the pores by the hydrodynamic pressure. Also the results from the investigations with neutral (Chang *et al.*, 1977), anionic (Chang *et al.*, 1975) and cationic (Bohrer *et al.*, 1977) dextran molecules, as reviewed recently by Brenner *et al.* (1978) are easily explained in our model through the pore size and the effect of the overall anionic charged LRI on the neutral or charged dextran molecules. The same results were recently obtained by Rennke *et al.* (1978) using charged or neutral horse-radish peroxidase molecules.

The binding of PEI particles in the laminae rarae of the GBM as demonstrated by Schurer *et al.* (1977) can also be explained by our model. Injection of PEI into normal rats results in a regular localization of PEI in the LRE and in a little less regular localization in the LRI. Larger PEI particles are also found in the LRI. Apparently these particles are blocked by the first barrier because they exceed the critical size of the pore. No PEI particles are seen in the lamina densa, because of the absence of anionic sites. After 2 h PEI starts to disappear from the LRE and LRI while the larger PEI particles remain present in the LRI. Apparently the small PEI particles pass the LD rapidly because of their size and because no charged sites are present in this layer. After passing the LD, PEI is again bound in the pores of the LRE. After some time this binding also loosens and the particles leave the LRE. The larger particles pass the GBM more slowly because of their size and are last seen in the SPM, until after 4 h they have passed through this structure.

The SPM plays an important role in the glomerular filtration process, as has been established by Karnovsky and his associates (Graham and Karnovsky, 1966; Graham and Kellermeyer, 1968; Venkatachalam *et al.*, 1970). In the proposed model this membrane is not a structure *per se* but is viewed as a specialized part of the lamina rara externa (LRE). It is interesting to note that the structure and dimensions of the slit pore membrane as proposed by us is in fact identical with the structure proposed previously by Rodewald and Karnovsky (1974) (Fig. 6). The structure of the SPM will be a dynamic one, which will be held in equilibrium by electrostatic forces and hydrodynamic pressure (Fig. 7).

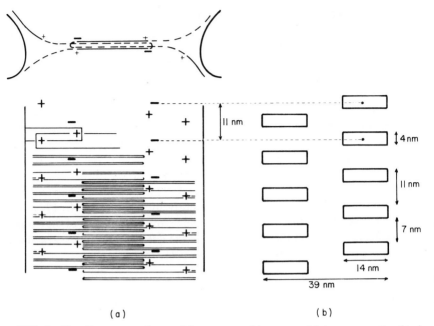

(a)   (b)

FIG. 6. *The slit pore membrane: (a) as proposed in our model, in cross-section (top) and viewed from above (bottom). (b) as proposed by Rodewald and Karnovsky. The dimensions in (a) and (b) are very much in accordance. The rectangles in (b), being electron-dense in the proposal of Rodewald and Karnovsky, are most likely stained anionic sites.*

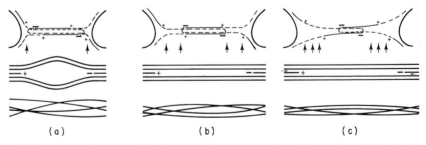

(a)   (b)   (c)

FIG. 7. *The behaviour of the SPM, "collagenic pores" and the packing of the lamina densa filaments at different filtration pressures. (a) Low pressure: the SPM is closed, the pores in the GBM are open. (b) Normal pressure: SPM and the pores in the GBM are open to a certain extent. (c) High pressure: the SPM opens, the pores in the GBM close.*

The proposed GBM model could also explain the effect of ischaemia on GBM filtration which was demonstrated by Ryan and Karnovsky (1976). They found that after ligation of the renal artery protein was found in the GBM. After restoring the blood pressure, the protein leaves the GBM. In our model the pressure in the glomerular capillaries will maintain tensile strain on the tropocollagen molecules of the GBM, keeping the sheets stretched and the filaments in the LD closely packed, preventing the approximation of the anionic and cationic groups in the collagen pores. Through a loss of this pressure in ischaemia, slackening of the tensile strain will occur, resulting in a loosening of the filaments of the LD. Also an approximation of the anionic and cationic groups will occur, resulting in a widening of the space between the two rigid bordering tropocollagen molecules (Fig. 7), and thus in an oval deformation and a larger width of the pore. At the same time, however, the pores in the SPM close, as was discussed before (Fig. 7), resulting in an accumulation of protein in the GBM, as described by Ryan and Karnovsky (1976).

Conclusion

Polymerization of tropocollagen on the surface of epithelial and endothelial cells into a sheet of collagen (type IV) results in longitudinal "collagenic pores" of 3.2 nm $\times$ 40 nm, bordered by anionic and cationic end-groups. These charged pores, lined by the rigid parts of tropocollagen molecules, have mechanical filtering properties and, because of the ion exchange capacity, a possibility for pH control. These properties, together with molecular sieving capacity attributed to the carbohydrates of the GBM, the packing of the filaments, and the pressure control of the slit pore membrane enable the GBM to fulfil its specific filtration function under optimal conditions. It is to be stressed that the properties of the GBM will have a relatively strong influence on the composition of the filtrate, because the total plasma volume will be subjected to the filtration process in the GBM many times a day.

This GBM model offers an explanation for the various aspects of glomerular filtration. In addition we believe that it may be used to understand many of the structural and functional disorders of the GBM encountered in renal disease.

Acknowledgements

The authors thank Mr C. Lingeman for drawing Fig. 5. This work was supported by the Netherlands Organization for the Advancement of Pure Research.

References

Bohrer, M. P., Humes, H. D., Baylis, C., Robertson, C. R. and Brenner, B. M. (1977). Facilitated transglomerular passage of circulating polycations. *Clin. Res.* **25**, 505.

Brenner, B. M., Hostetter, T. H. and Humes, H. D. (1978). Molecular basis of proteinuria of glomerular origin. *New Engl. J. Med.* **298**, 826–833.

Bruchhausen, F. von and Merker, H. J. (1967). Morphologischer und chemischer Aufbau isolierter Basalmembranen aus der Nierenrinde der Ratte. *Histochemie* **3**, 100–103.

Caulfield, J. P. and Farquhar, M. G. (1976). Distribution of anionic sites in glomerular basement membranes: their possible role in filtration and attachment. *Proc. natn. Acad. Sci. U.S.A.* **73**, 1646–1650.

Chang, R. L. S., Deen, W. M., Robertson, C. R. and Brenner, B. M. (1975). Permselectivity of the glomerular capillary wall: III. Restricted transport of polyanions. *Kidney Int.* **8**, 212–218.

Chang, R. L. S., Uehi, I. F., Troy, J. L., Deen, W. M., Robertson, C. R. and Brenner, B. M. (1977). Perselectivity of the glomerular capillary wall to macromolecules. II. Experimental studies in rats using neutral dextrin. *Biophys. J.* **15**, 887–906.

Farquhar, M. H. (1975). The primary glomerular filtration barrier—basement membrane or epithelial slits? *Kidney Int.* **8**, 197–211.

Gallop, P. M. and Paz, M. A. (1975). Post translational protein modifications, with special attention to collagen and elastin. *Physiol. Rev.* **55**, 413–437.

Graham, R. C., Jr and Karnovsky, M. J. (1966). Glomerular permeability: ultra-structural cytochemical studies using peroxidases as protein tracers. *J. exp. Med.* **124**, 1123–1134.

Graham, R. C., Jr and Kellermeyer, R. W. (1968). Bovine lactoperoxidase as a cytochemical protein tracer for electron microscopy. *J. Histochem. Cytochem.* **16**, 275–278.

Grant, M. E. and Jackson, D. S. (1976). The biosynthesis of procollagen. *Essays Biochem.* **12**, 77–113.

Jones, D. B. (1969). Mucosubstances of the glomerulus. *Lab. Invest.* **21**, 119–125.

Kefalides, N. A. (1977). Basement membranes. In *Mammalian Cell Membranes*, Vol. II (G. A. Jamieson and D. M. Robinson, eds), Butterworth, London and Boston, pp. 298–323.

Kefalides, N. A. (1978). Current status of chemistry and structure of basement membranes. In *Biology and Chemistry of Basement Membranes* (N. A. Kefalides, ed.), Academic Press, New York and London, pp. 215–229.

Latta, H., Johnston, W. H. and Stanley, T. M. (1975). Sialoglycoproteins and filtration barriers in the glomerular capillary wall. *J. Ultrastruct. Res.* **51**, 354–376.

Rennke, H. G. and Venkatachalam, M. A. (1977). Glomerular permeability: *in vivo* tracer studies with polyanionic and polycationic ferritins. *Kidney Int.* **11**, 44–53.

Rennke, H. G., Cotran, R. S. and Venkatachalam, M. A. (1975). Role of molecular charge in glomerular permeability: tracer studies with cationized ferritins. *J. Cell Biol.* **67**, 638–646.

Rennke, H. G., Patel, Y. and Venkatachalam, M. A. (1978). Glomerular filtration of proteins: clearance of anionic, neutral and cationic horseradish peroxidase in the rat. *Kidney Int.* **13**, 278–288.

Ryan, G. B. and Karnovsky, M. J. (1976). Distribution of endogenous albumin in the rat glomerulus: role of hemodynamic factors in glomerular barrier function. *Kidney Int.* **9**, 36–45.

Rodewald, R. and Karnovsky, M. J. (1974). Porous structure of the glomerular slit diaphragm in the rat and mouse. *J. Cell Biol.* **60**, 423–433.

Schurer, J. W., Hoedemaeker, Ph. J. and Molenaar, I. (1977). Polyethyleneimine as tracer particle for (immuno) electronmicroscopy. *J. Histochem. Cytochem.* **25**, 384–387.

Schurer, J. W., Kalicharan, D., Hoedemaeker, Ph. J. and Molenaar, I. (1978). Demonstration of anionic sites in basement membranes and in collagen fibrils. *J. Histochem. Cytochem.* **26**, 688–689.

Seiler, M. W., Rennke, H. G., Venkatachalam, M. A. and Cotran, R. S. (1977). Pathogenesis of polycation-induced alterations ("fusion") of glomerular epithelium. *Lab. Invest.* **36**, 48–61.

Venkatachalam, M. A., Karnovsky, M. J., Fahimi, H. D. and Cotran, R. S. (1970). An ultrastructural study of glomerular permeability using catalase and peroxidase as tracer proteins. *J. exp. Med.* **132**, 1153–1167.

8
Isolation and Characterization of Rat Glomerular Cells *in vitro*

Morris J. Karnovsky and Jeffrey I. Kreisberg

Introduction

The renal glomerulus contains at least three cell types: (1) endothelial cells; (2) glomerular epithelial cells (GEC); and (3) mesangial cells. The endothelial cell which lines the glomerular capillary wall is characterized by the presence of fenestrae approximately 1000 Å in diameter. Although the role these cells play in glomerular function is not clear, studies by Ryan and Karnovsky (1976) demonstrate that under good flow conditions in the rat, plasma albumin and immunoglobulin G molecules do not penetrate significantly beyond the fenestrae, suggesting that this layer may participate in the restriction of macromolecular passage across the glomerular capillary wall. GEC display multiple foot processes (podocytes) applied to the outside of the glomerular basement membrane (GBM). There is good evidence to suggest that GEC participate (1) in the synthesis of the GBM (Kurtz and Feldman, 1962; Walker, 1973); (2) in the filtration process through pinocytosis of filtered proteins that may have leaked through the GBM (Farquhar, 1975); and (3) in the filtration process by exerting an influence upon water flux during ultrafiltration (Ryan and Karnovsky, 1975). In addition, it has been demonstrated that intrinsic negatively charged glycoproteins in the filtration barrier restrict the passage of dextran sulfate (Chang *et al.*, 1975) and native ferritin (Rennke *et al.*, 1975), and the highly charged cell coat of the podocytes may participate in this effect. The mesangial cell may be phagocytic (Farquhar and Palade, 1961, 1962) and, hence, one of its proposed functions includes the clearing of debris from the mesangial region. Also, the mesangial cell contains myofibrillar bundles and may, therefore, regulate glomerular size and blood flow by appropriate contractile activity. Isolation and characterization of homogeneous populations of glomerular cells would aid in the study of their normal metabolism as well as their altered metabolism in disease states.

We have previously reported the isolation and characterization of a phagocytic cell from the mesangium of the rat glomerulus (Camazine *et al.*, 1976). These cells were also highly adherent to glass, developed C3 and Fc receptors after 24 h in culture, but could not be maintained *in vitro*.

In the present study, we have isolated and maintained in culture three additional and distinct cell types from rat glomeruli. One cell type has been characterized as the GEC (Kreisberg *et al.*, 1978*a*), the second cell type has not been completely characterized, although it contains many bundles of microfilaments, and the third cell type contains renin (Kreisberg *et al.*, 1978*b*). None of these cell types are phagocytic *in vitro*.

Materials and Methods

Culture of whole glomeruli and dissociated glomerular cells
Glomeruli were isolated using a graded sieving technique (Burlington and Cronkite, 1973) from male CD® (Charles River Breeding Laboratories, North Wilmington, Mass.) rat kidneys which were perfused *in situ* with Hanks Balanced Salt Solution (HSS) (Grand Island Biological Corporation, Grand Island, NY) to remove red blood cells. Aliquots of isolated glomeruli were examined by scanning electron microscopy (SEM). The procedure employed for isolating homogeneous populations of glomerular cells has been described in great detail in a previous report (Kreisberg *et al.*, 1978*a*). Briefly, glomeruli were either plated directly onto Falcon Tissue Culture Flasks (Falcon Plastics, Oxnard, Calif.) for outgrowths of cells, or dissociated in 0·2 per cent trypsin (12 700 BAEE units/mg; Sigma Chemical Co., St. Louis, Mo.), 0·1 per cent collagenase (190 units/mg; Sigma Chemical Co.) and 0·01 per cent de-oxyribonuclease (1115 Kientz units/mg protein, Sigma Chemical Co.) in HSS at 37 °C for 30 min. Before plating dissociated glomerular cells were filtered through 10 μm Nitex (TETKO, Inc., Elmsford, NY) to remove any intact glomeruli. Primary cultures from outgrowths of whole glomeruli (filtered through 10 μm Nitex (TETKO, Inc.) to remove glomeruli) and dissociated glomerular cells were plated for cloning at 4000 cells per 100 cm² Falcon Tissue Culture Dish (Falcon Plastics). The tissue culture media (RIC) used in this study was RPMI 1640 medium (Microbiological Associates, Bethesda, Md) buffered with 15 mM Hepes buffer (Sigma Chemical Co.), pH 7·4, supplemented with 20 per cent fetal calf serum (FCS), diluted in half with conditioned medium (CM) with 0·66 units/ml of insulin (Eli Lilly and Co., Indianapolis, Ind.). The RIC medium contained 100 units of

penicillin and 100 μg of streptomycin per millilitre. Conditioned medium was prepared from Swiss 3T3 cells in log phase growth maintained in Dulbecco's Modification of Minimum Essential Medium (DMEM) (Microbiological Associates) with 10 per cent FCS for 24 h. The conditioned medium was removed and filtered through 0·22 μm Millipore filters (Millipore Corp., Bedford, Mass.) before use. Clones were randomly isolated with penni-cylinders, and passaged with a 0·025 per cent trypsin–0·5 mM ethylenedia-minetetraacetic acid (EDTA) in Ca^{2+}–Mg^{2+}-free buffered salt solution (trypsin-versene) into Costar multiwell plates (Costar, Cambridge, Mass.) in RIC. All cells were tested for fibroblast contamination by their ability to grow in RPMI 1640 containing 20 per cent dialyzed FCS and D-valine substituted for L-valine (Gilbert and Migeon, 1975). Fibroblasts do not grow in D-valine-containing media.

Morphologic studies
Transmission electron microscopy was performed on all cloned cell types by usual techniques. Scanning electron microscopy (SEM) was performed on isolated glomerular preparations to determine the percentage of glomeruli with capsules intact and the degree of contamination with tubules. SEM was also performed on cloned cell types. Isolated glomeruli were fixed in suspension in 2 per cent glutaraldehyde in HSS, pH 7·2, washed twice in HSS and lightly suctioned onto silver membranes (Selas Flotronics, Spring House, Penn.) which had been coated with poly-L-lysine (1 mg/ml) (Sigma Chemical Co.). Cloned cell types were allowed to settle on coverslips which had been cleaned previously by boiling for 2 h in detergent solution (7X) (Linbro Scientific, Inc., Hamden, Conn.) and then washed thoroughly with distilled water. Coverslips with cells attached were fixed in 2 per cent glutaraldehyde in 0·1 M phosphate buffer, pH 7·2, for 1 h at room tempera-ture, and washed in buffer overnight. Both silver membranes with fixed glomeruli and coverslips with cells were postfixed in 1 per cent osmium tetroxide for 30 min at 4 °C, and prepared for SEM by routine methods.

Immunological studies
For immunocytochemical studies rabbit antisera to rat antihemophilic factor (Factor VIII) was kindly supplied by Drs Roger E. Benson and W. Jean Dodds (Benson and Dodds, 1976a,b). Reactivity of this antisera to rat glomerular and vascular endothelium was verified by indirect immuno-fluorescence on rat frozen sections. Coverslips of cell monolayers were washed and fixed in cold acetone for 3 min followed by a 10 min wash in phosphate-buffered saline. Coverslips were then stained for 30 min at 37 °C by the indirect method (Booyse et al., 1975). Dissociated cells were tested for the

presence of Factor VIII 6 days after plating, and cloned cell types were also tested.

Identifications of receptors for immunoglobulin and complement (rosette formation) were performed on rat glomerular cells maintained in tissue culture for 2 months. To identify Fc receptors, the glomerular cells were incubated at room temperature for 30 min with a suspension of sheep red blood cells (SRBC) (Colorado Serum Co., Denver, Colo.) which had been coated with a subagglutinating amount of rabbit IgM antibody to SRBC (1 : 200 dilution) (Becker and Benacerraf, 1966); negative controls were incubated with uncoated SRBC, positive controls were incubated with mouse peritoneal macrophages. To identify C3 receptors, glomerular cells were incubated at room temperature for 30 min with a suspension of SRBC which had been treated first with a subagglutinating amount of rabbit IgM antibody to SRBC (Cordis Laboratories, Miami, Fla) and second with C-5 deficient mouse serum (from A/St mice) (Lay and Nussenzweig, 1968). Negative controls were incubated with uncoated SRBC; positive controls included identifying C3 receptors on human GEC *in situ*. Preparations were examined for the presence of rosettes by phase microscopy and SEM.

Phagocytosis in vitro
Rat glomerular cells maintained in tissue culture were exposed to polystyrene spherules (1·1 μm diameter, Dow Chemical Co., Midland, Mich.), zymosan (Nutritional Biochemicals Corporation, Cleveland, Ohio), ferritin 2x crystalline, cadmium-free (Nutritional Biochemicals Corporation, Cleveland, Ohio), and carbon (Gunther Wagner, Hanover, Federal Republic of Germany) in RIC. Dissociated cells were tested for phagocytosis 6 days after plating, and cloned cell types were also tested. Phagocytosis was assessed by phase contrast and transmission electron microscopy.

Renin determinations
Angiotensin I generation from sonicated and unsonicated cell preparations was measured by a radioimmunoassay technique (Clinical Assays, Inc., Cambridge, Mass.) (Haber *et al.*, 1969). One millilitre of 10^6 unsonicated and sonicated cells was incubated with renin substrate in maleate buffer of pH 6·0 containing phenylmethylsulfonyl fluoride, to inhibit conversion and degradation of angiotensin I, at 37 °C for 90 min.

Studies with aminonucleoside of puromycin (AMNS)
Confluent monolayers of the different cloned cell types were treated with 0·1, 1·0, 10, and 100 μg/ml of AMNS in RIC for 24 h and the percentage of cells detaching from the monolayer was determined. Control monolayers were maintained in RIC alone.

Results

Isolation of glomeruli
SEM of glomerular preparations revealed that $85·0 \pm 6·0$ per cent were free of capsules, $15·0 \pm 5·0$ per cent contained capsules, and $3·0 \pm 2·1$ per cent contained vascular poles. SEM also revealed very little contamination of the preparations with tubules. Two hundred glomeruli were evaluated in each isolation.

Culture of cells from whole glomeruli and dissociated glomerular cells
In a previous report, we compared RIC to other growth media and determined that, with RIC as the tissue culture media, glomeruli attached and cells could be seen growing out from them after 1 day in culture (Kreisberg *et al.*, 1978a). In addition, although encapsulated glomeruli attached to the flask, cells did not grow from them. Also, attachment and growth of dissociated glomerular cells with RIC as the growth media was far superior to all the other media previously tested. Primary cell cultures from outgrowths of glomeruli and dissociated glomerular cells reached confluency after 1 week in culture, and clones established either from primary cultures of outgrowths of glomeruli or directly dissociated glomerular cells, became recognizable for cloning after 1–2 weeks in culture.

Characteristics of isolated cells
One cell type (cell type A) isolated by cloning was polygonal in shape by phase contrast microscopy and displayed a cobblestone appearance when confluency was reached. The doubling time was 15 h. This cell has been positively characterized as the GEC (Kreisberg *et al.*, 1978a) because it has receptors for C3, but not for Fc, bears cilia on its surface (Fig. 1) and forms junctions in culture. Also, the AMNS at low concentrations is cytotoxic towards this cell (Table I). Ultrastructurally, these cells bear a glycocalyx rich in sialic acid. Cell type B is a very large and flat cell by phase contrast microscopy. It has an average doubling time of 10 h. Ultrastructurally, it contains many bundles of microfilaments (Fig. 2). This cell did not possess receptors for C3 or Fc nor did the AMNS have any effect on it. The third cell type (cell type C) isolated in this study was spindle-shaped and criss-crossed and underlapped each other in culture. This cell had an average doubling time of 19 h. By transmission electron microscopy, it was found to contain numerous electron-dense granules in its cytoplasm when fixed in 2 per cent glutaraldehyde and stained with hafnium *en bloc* (J. I. Kreisberg and M. J. Karnovsky, unpublished data) or when fixed in a mixture of glutaraldehyde, osmium, and acrolein (Fig. 3). Cell type C did not possess

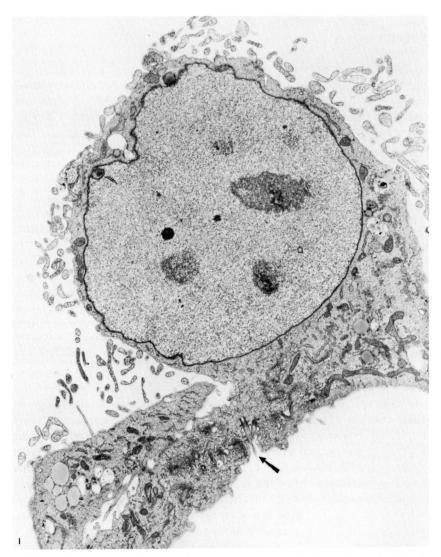

FIG. 1. *Transmission electron micrograph of a cultured glomerular epithelial cell. Note the two cilia on the cell surface (arrow). (From Kreisberg et al. (1978a).) × 9500.*

C3 or Fc receptors and was not affected by the AMNS in culture; however, extracts of this cell were able to convert angiotensinogen to angiotensin I, indicative of renin activity (Table I). As can also be seen in this table, the GEC had a small amount of renin activity. All three cell types isolated in this study grew in media containing D-valine and dialyzed FCS, indicating

TABLE I
Studies performed on purified rat glomerular cells in vitro

Cell type	AHF[a]	C3	Fc	Cilia	Growth in D-valine substituted medium	Phago-cytosis	Cyto-toxicity of low doses of AMNS[b]	Renin[c]
GEC	0	+	0	+	+	0	+	±
Cell with MF	0	0	0	0	+	0	0	0
Renin cell	0	0	0	0	+	0	0	+

[a] AHF, anti-hemophilic factor.
[b] AMNS, aminonucleoside of puromycin.
[c] Renin cell, $2·1 \pm 0·44$; GEC, $0·45 \pm 0·12$; cell with MF, $0·09 \pm 0·07$ ng per 10^6 cells $\pm$ s.d.
[d] GEC, glomerular epithelial cell.
[e] MF, microfilaments.

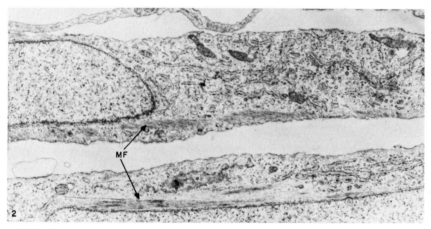

FIG. 2. *Transmission electron micrograph of a cultured cell that contains many bundles of microfilaments (MF).* × 9200.

that they were not fibroblasts (Gilbert and Migeon, 1975). Furthermore, none of the cell types were able to phagocytose any of the particles tested, nor did any of the cells contain Factor VIII (Table I). All three cell types have been maintained in culture for about 30 passages.

Discussion

In this study, we were able to isolate three cell types from rat glomeruli. One

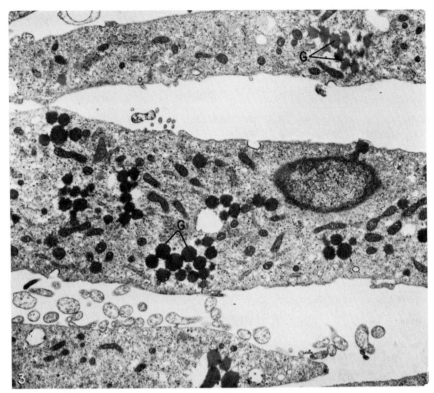

FIG. 3. *Transmission electron micrograph of a cultured renin cell. Note the presence of granules (G) in the cytoplasm.* × 9800.

of these cell types has been characterized as the GEC (Kreisberg *et al.*, 1978*a*). The presence of cilia on its surface, a characteristic of rat GEC *in situ* (Andrews and Porter, 1974; Andrews, 1975), and the cytotoxicity of the AMNS *in vitro* on GEC and not other glomerular cells helped us to identify it. The AMNS has been shown preferentially to injure GEC and not other kidney cells *in vivo* (Andrews, 1977; Glasser *et al.*, 1977; Velosa *et al.*, 1977). SEM of isolated glomeruli revealed that a great majority of the glomeruli did not have capsules, and there was little contamination of the preparations with tubular fragments. Furthermore, we observed, as did Bernik (1969), that cells did not grow from encapsulated glomeruli. These findings allowed us to eliminate the possibilities of our cells being parietal epithelial cells or proximal or distal tubule cells. Furthermore, we were able to isolate GEC from outgrowths of whole glomeruli which were easily distinguishable from tubules in culture by light microscopy.

None of the isolated cell types contained Factor VIII, a marker for endothelial cells (Hoyer *et al.*, 1973; Jaffe *et al.*, 1973). Since human endothelium (Jaffe *et al.*, 1973), calf endothelium (Booyse *et al.*, 1975), and rat aortic endothelium (R. L. Hoover, personal communication) retain Factor VIII in culture, we do not believe that one of our cell types merely lost its ability to synthesize Factor VIII *in vitro*. Since the fenestrated glomerular endothelium represents a highly differentiated type of cell, it probably requires particular conditions for growth which are not available in our growth medium. There have been numerous studies on the isolation and culture of human and animal glomerular cells *in vitro* (Bernik, 1969; Quadracci and Stricker, 1970; Dechenne *et al.*, 1975; Scheinman *et al.*, 1976; Burkholder *et al.*, 1977; Scheinman and Fish, 1978), and in none of these studies were glomerular endothelial cells isolated and grown in culture.

Since one of the proposed functions of mesangial cells is phagocytosis of debris from the mesangium (Farquhar and Palade, 1961, 1962), we tested our cell types for their ability to phagocytose particles *in vitro*. None of our cells were phagocytic. There are several explanations why we have not been able to isolate a phagocytic cell, which could possibly be a mesangial cell: (1) one or more of these cells may have been phagocytic *in vivo* and merely lost its ability to phagocytose in culture (Bernik, 1969); (2) there may be more than one type of mesangial cell, i.e. one phagocytic and one not phagocytic *in vivo*; and (3) that perhaps the function of the mesangial cell is controlling glomerular size and blood flow by contractility and not phagocytosis of debris from the mesangium. The third explanation is most intriguing. If the mesangial cell is not phagocytic, then perhaps phagocytic cells such as the blood monocytes percolate through the mesangium to clear debris. In a previous report from this laboratory, the isolation of a phagocytic cell from rat glomeruli was described (Camazine *et al.*, 1976). Briefly, glomeruli were isolated from animals that had been injected with ferritin. These glomeruli were subjected to prolonged enzymic digestions, and cells that had adhered to glass overnight were examined morphologically. Epithelial cells were rarely seen, indicating their susceptibility to the prolonged enzymic digestion. The cells adhering to glass were not only phagocytic but also had receptors for Fc and C3, and could be maintained in culture only for a short time which would be in line with the short survival time of macrophages in culture. These phagocytic cells were morphologically distinct from the cells we isolated and reported in this study. They had large, indented nuclei, large nucleus: cytoplasm ratios, and by SEM these cells showed extensive foldings of the cell surface. In time-lapse cinematographic studies by Thomson *et al.* (1978), they showed macrophages populating the normal glomerulus. Thomson observed macrophages migrating from isolated human glomeruli. In addition, Schneeberger *et al.* (1977), from electron micrographic studies, suggested that monocytes might be capable of invading the mesangium. We believe that the phagocytic cell previously isolated in our laboratory is a blood-derived monocyte that travels into and out from the mesangium to remove debris.

One of the cell types isolated in the present study contained many bundles of microfilaments but was not phagocytic. Scheinman *et al.* (1976) described a cell isolated from human glomeruli which had actomyosin and, based on the findings by Becker (1972), who described actomyosin by immunofluorescence in the mesangium and hilus of the human kidney, identified his isolated cell as "smooth muscle (mesangial)". Actin and myosin are now known to exist in a variety of non-muscle cells in culture (Lazarides and Weber, 1974; Pollack *et al.*, 1975; Fujiwara and Pollard, 1976) and, therefore, actomyosin does not appear to be a marker for a single mesangial cell type. Until specific markers for mesangial cells are found, the identity of the cell with microfilaments remains unknown.

Direct evidence that renin was concentrated in the vascular pole of the glomerulus was provided by the microdissection studies of Bing and Kazimierczak (1960) and the studies of Cook and Pickering (1959), who separated out glomeruli with magnetic iron. Nairn *et al.* (1959), using indirect immunofluorescence with rabbit anti-pig renin, found renin activity by immunofluorescence in the glomerular tuft, and there was no suggestion of specific staining of the juxtaglomerular apparatus (JGA). Edelman and Hartroft (1961), using fluorescein-labeled anti-hog renin, found a correlation between the degree of granulation of rabbit juxtaglomerular (JG) cells, immunofluorescence staining, and renin content; that is, the tissue giving greater granulation had the greatest fluorescent staining and highest renin content. In contrast to the results obtained by Nairn *et al.*, all the staining in this study was limited to the JGA.

It appears that granulated cells are not limited to the JGA. Barajas (1970), who examined serial sections of the JGA, found that granulated as well as agranulated cells entered the glomerulus and became continuous with the glomerular mesangial cell, confirming Goormaghtigh's (1944) suggestion that mesangial cells and granulated cells are closely related. In certain physiological conditions agranulated mesangial cells appear to develop granules. Dunihue and Boldosser (1963) observed in cats that underwent bilateral adrenalectomy that glomerular mesangial cells underwent hypertrophy and hyperplasia, and developed cytoplasmic granules similar to those of the JG cells. Since only 3 per cent of the glomeruli isolated in this study had vascular poles attached, we believe that the isolated renin cells described in this report were obtained from cells populating the glomerulus.

Isolation of pure renin-producing cells, when hemodynamic, tubular, and extrarenal influences are removed, could aid in an understanding of the action of various stimuli on renin release. For example, *in vivo* experiments have not established that renin is released by the direct action of cate-cholamines with β receptors on renin-producing cells (Reid *et al.*, 1972; Assaykeen *et al.*, 1974; Johnson *et al.*, 1974). There are also conflicting reports on the action of catecholamines on renal cortical slices *in vitro* (DeVito *et al.*, 1970; Aoi *et al.*, 1974). In isolated glomeruli, Morris *et al.* (1976) found that isoprenaline, adrenalin, and noradrenaline stimulated release of renin. Robertson *et al.* (1976) demonstrated in cultured human renal cortical cells the presence of a population of cells that contained granules that stained with Bowie's stain and anti-human renin antibody. In this study, we have obtained purified homogeneous renin-producing cell lines from isolated rat glomeruli.

Conclusions

Utilizing a tissue culture medium containing fetal calf serum (FCS), con-ditioned medium (from Swiss 3T3 cells in log phase growth) (CM), and insulin, we have been able to clone and maintain in culture three distinct cell types from isolated, dissociated glomeruli and explants of whole isolated glomeruli. Rat glomeruli were isolated by a graded sieving technique. Scanning electron microscopy (SEM) of glomerular preparations revealed that $85 \pm 6 \cdot 0$ per cent of the glomeruli were free of capsules, 15 ± 5 per cent contained capsules, and $3 \cdot 0 \pm 2 \cdot 1$ per cent of the glomeruli contained vascular poles. The problem with identifying glomerular cells *in vitro* is the current paucity of specific markers for these cell types. We have been able to characterize one of the three cells as the glomerular epithelial cell (GEC). It has cilia on its surface, receptors for complement (C3), and the aminonu-cleoside of puromycin (AMNS) is cytotoxic towards it. The second cell type has not been completely characterized. Ultrastructurally it contains many bundles of microfilaments, which have been used as a marker for mesangial cells by many investigators. This cell type, as well as the other two cell types, is not able to phagocytose, *in vitro*, particles such as polystyrene, zymosan, ferritin, or carbon. The third cell type has been characterized as a renin-producing cell because extracts of these cells are capable of generating angiotensin I as measured by a radioimmunoassay. Since only a small proportion of the isolated glomeruli contain vascular poles, we suggest that cells potentially capable of producing renin normally populate the glomeru-lus. In addition, a phagocytic cell type has previously been isolated, but not cultured, from the mesangium: this may represent a subset of mesangial cells, which are either resident, or are blood-derived.

Acknowledgements

This investigation was supported by Grant AM 13132 from the NIH, USPHS. We would like to thank Dr Roger E. Benson and Dr W. Jean Dodds for the preparation and gift of the anti-Factor VIII antibody. Their work was supported by Grant HL 09902 from the NIH, USPHS. We would also like to thank Dr Walter Flamenbaum for his assistance in performing the renin radioimmunoassays. The assistance of Denise Wayne, Robert Rubin, and Mary Mauri is greatly appreciated.

References

Andrews, P. M. (1975). Scanning electron microscopy of human and rhesus monkey kidneys. *Lab. Invest.* **32**, 610–618.

Andrews, P. M. (1977). A scanning and transmission electron microscopic comparison of puromycin aminonucleoside-induced nephrosis to hyperalbuminemia-induced proteinuria with emphasis on kidney podocyte pedical loss. *Lab. Invest.* **36**, 183–197.

Andrews, P. M. and Porter, R. (1974). A scanning electron microscopic study of the nephron. *Am. J. Anat.* **140**, 81–116.

Aoi, W., Wade, M. B., Rosner, D. R. and Weinberger, M. H. (1974). Reinin release by rat kidney slices *in vitro*: effects of cations and catecholamines. *Am. J. Physiol.* **227**, 630–634.

Assaykeen, T. A., Tanigawa, H. and Allison, D. J. (1974). Effect of adrenoceptor-blocking agents on the renin response to isoproterenol in dogs. *Eur. J. Pharmac.* **26**, 285–297.

Barajas, L. (1970). The ultrastructure of the juxtaglomerular apparatus as disclosed by three dimensional reconstructions from serial sections. The anatomical relationship between the tubular and vascular components. *J. Ultrastruct. Res.* **33**, 116–146.

Becker, C. G. (1972). Demonstration of actomyosin in mesangial cells of the renal glomerulus. *Am. J. Path.* **66**, 97–110.

Becker, A. and Benacerraf, B. (1966). Properties of antibodies cytophilic for macrophages. *J. exp. Med.* **123**, 119–144.

Benson, R. E. and Dodds, W. J. (1976a). Physical relationship between canine Factor VIII coagulant activity and Factor VIII related antigen. *Proc. Soc. exp. Biol. Med.* **153**, 339–343.

Benson, R. E. and Dodds, W. J. (1976b). Immunologic characterization of canine Factor VIII. *Blood* **48**, 521–529.

Bernik, M. B. (1969). Contractile activity of human glomeruli in culture. *Nephron* **6**, 1–10.

Bing, J. and Kazimierczak, J. (1960). Renin content of different parts of the periglomerular circumference. *Acta path. microbiol. scand.* **50**, 1–11.

Booyse, F. M., Sedlak, B. J. and Rafelson, M. E. (1975). Culture of arterial endothelial cells. Characterization and growth of bovine aortic cells. *Thrombos. diathes. haemorrh., Stuttgart* **35**, 825–839.

Burkholder, P. M., Oberly T. D., Barber, T. A., Beacom, A. and Koehler, C. (1977). Immune adherence in renal glomeruli. Complement receptor sites on glomerular capillary epithelial cells. *Am. J. Path.* **76**, 635–654.

Burlington, H. and Cronkite, E. P. (1973). Characteristics of cell cultures derived from renal glomeruli. *Proc. Soc. exp. Biol. Med.* **142**, 143–149.

Camazine, S. M., Ryan, G. B., Unanue, E. R. and Karnovsky, M. J. (1976). Isolation of phagocytic cells from the rat renal glomerulus. *Lab. Invest.* **35**, 315–326.

Chang, R. L. S., Robertson, C. R., Deen, W. M. and Brenner, B. M. (1975). Permselectivity of the glomerular capilllary wall. III. Restricted transport of polyanions. *Kidney Int.* **8**, 212–218.

Cook, W. F., Pickering, G. W. (1959). The localization of renin in the rabbit kidney. *J. Physiol., Lond.* **149**, 526–536.

Dechenne, C., Foidart-Willems, J. and Mahieu, P. M. (1975). Ultrastructural studies on dog renal glomerular and tubular cells in culture. *J. submicr. Cytol.* **7**, 165–184.

DeVito, E., Gordon, S. B., Cabrera, R. R. and Fasciolo, J. C. (1970). Release of renin by rat kidney slices. *Am. J. Physiol.* **219**, 1036–1041.

Dunihue, F. W., and Boldesser, W. G. (1963). Observations on the similarity of mesangial to juxtaglomerular cells. *Lab. Invest.* **12**, 1228–1240.

Edelman, R. and Hartroft, P. M. (1961). Localization of renin in juxtaglomerular cells of rabbit and dog through the use of the fluorescent antibody technique. *Circulation Res.* **9**, 1065–1077.

Farquhar, M. G. (1975). The primary glomerular filtration barrier—basement membrane or epithelial cells? *Kidney Int.* **8**, 197–211.

Farquhar, M. G. and Palade, G. E. (1961). Glomerular permeability. II. Ferritin transfer across the glomerular capillary wall in nephrotic rats. *J. exp. Med.* **114**, 699–716.

Farquhar, M. G. and Palade, G. E. (1962). Functional evidence for the existence of a third cell type in the renal glomerulus: phagocytosis of filtration residue by a "distinct" third cell. *J. Cell Biol.* **13**, 55–87.

Fujiwara, K. and Pollard, T. D. (1976). Fluorescent antibody localization of myosin in the cytoplasm, cleavage furrow, and mitotic spindle of human cells. *J. Cell Biol.* **71**, 848–875.

Gilbert, S. F. and Migeon, B. R. (1975). D-Valine as a selective agent for normal human and rodent epithelial cells in culture. *Cell* **5**, 11–17.

Glasser, R. S., Velosa, J. A. and Michael, A. F. (1977). Experimental model of focal sclerosis. I. Relationship to protein excretion in aminonucleoside nephrosis. *Lab. Invest.* **36**, 519–526.

Goormaghtigh, N. (1944). *Le fonction endocrinedes arterioles renales,* Libraire R. Fonteyn, Louvain.

Haber, E., Koerner, T., Page, L. B., Kliman, B. and Purnode, A. (1969). Application of a radioimmunoassay for angiotensin I to the physiological measurements of plasma renin activity in normal human subjects. *J. clin. Endocr. Metab.* **29**, 1349–1355.

Hoyer, L. W., De Los Santos, R. P. and Hoyer, J. R. (1973). Antihemophilic factor antigen. Localization in endothelial cells by immunofluorescent microscopy. *J. clin. Invest.* **52**, 2737–2744.

Jaffe, E. A., Hoyer, L. W. and Nachman, R. L. (1973). Synthesis of antihemophilic factor antigen by cultured human endothelial cells. *J. clin. Invest.* **52**, 2757–2764.

Johnson, L. A., Davis, J. O., Braverman, R., Gotshall, W., David, J. L., Lohmeier,

T. E. and Freeman, R. H. (1974). Inhibition of renin release in Na depleted dogs by intrarenal infusion of propanolol. *Fedn Proc. Fedn Am. Socs exp. Biol.* **33**, 339a.

Kreisberg, J. I., Hoover, R. L. and Karnovsky, M. J. (1978a). Isolation and characterization of rat glomerular epithelial cells *in vitro*. *Kidney Int.* **14**, 21–30.

Kreisberg, J. I., Karnovsky, M. J., Emmett, N. L. and Barger, A. C. (1978b). Isolation and culture of a "renin" containing cell from rat glomeruli. Abstracts, VIIth International Congress of Nephrology, Montreal.

Kurtz, S. M. and Feldman, I. D. (1962). Experimental studies on the formation of the glomerular basement membrane. *J. Ultrastruct. Res.* **6**, 19–27.

Lay, W. H. and Nussenzweig, V. (1968). Receptors for complement on leukocytes. *J. exp. Med.* **128**, 991–1009.

Lazarides, E. and Weber, K. (1974). Actin antibody: the specific visualization of actin filaments in non-muscle cells. *Proc. natn. Acad. Sci. U.S.A.* **71**, 2268–2272.

Morris, B. J., Nixon, R. L. and Johnston, C. I. (1976). Release of renin from glomeruli isolated from rat kidney. *Clin. exp. Pharmac. Physiol.* **3**, 37–47.

Nairn, R. C., Fraser, K. B. and Chadwick, C. S. (1959). The histological localization of renin with fluorescent antibody. *Br. J. exp. Path.* **40**, 155–163.

Pollack, R., Osborn, M. and Weber, K. (1975). Patterns of organization of actin and myosin in normal and transformed cultured cells. *Proc. natn. Acad. Sci. U.S.A.* **72**, 994–998.

Quadracci, L. J. and Stricker, G. F. (1970). Growth and maintenance of glomerular cells *in vitro*. *Proc. Soc. exp. Biol. Med.* **135**, 947–950.

Reid, I. A., Schrier, R. W. and Earley, L. E. (1972). An effect of extrarenal β-adrenergic stimulation of release of renin. *J. clin. Invest.* **51**, 1861–1869.

Rennke, H. G., Cotran, R. S. and Venkatachalam, M. A. (1975). Role of molecular charge in glomerular permeability. Tracer studies with cationized ferritins. *J. Cell Biol.* **67**, 638–646.

Robertson, A. L., Smeby, R. R., Bumpus, P. M. and Page, I. H. (1966). Production of renin by human juxtaglomerular cells *in vitro*. *Circulation Res.* **18**, I-131–142.

Ryan, G. B. and Karnovsky, M. J. (1975). An ultrastructural study of the mechanisms of proteinuria in aminonucleoside nephrosis. *Kidney Int.* **8**, 219–232.

Ryan, G. B. and Karnovsky, M. J. (1976). Distribution of endogenous albumin in the rat glomerulus: role of hemodynamic factors in glomerular barrier function. *Kidney Int.* **9**, 36–45.

Scheinman, J. I., and Fish, A. J. (1978). Human glomerular cells in culture. Three subcultured cell types bearing glomerular antigens. *Am. J. Path.* **92**, 125–145.

Scheinman, J. I., Fish, A. S., Brown, D. M. and Michael, A. J. (1976). Human glomerular smooth muscle (mesangial) cells in culture. *Lab. Invest.* **34**, 150–158.

Schneeberger, E. E., Collins, A. B. Latta, H. and McCluskey, R. T. (1977). Diminished glomerular accumulation of colloidal carbon in autologous immune complex nephritis. *Lab. Invest.* **37**, 9–19.

Thomson, N. M., Holdsworth, S. R., Glasgow, E. F., Atkins, R. C. (1978) The macrophage in crescentic glomerulonephritis. Abstracts, VIIth International Congress of Nephrology, Montreal.

Velosa, J. A., Glasser, R. J., Nevins, T. E. and Michael, A. F. (1977). Experimental model of focal sclerosis. II. Correlation with immunopathologic changes, macromolecular kinetics, and polyanion loss. *Lab. Invest.* **36**, 527–534.

Walker, F. (1973). The origin, turnover and removal of glomerular basement membrane. *J. Path.* **110**, 233–244.

9
Basement Membrane Biosynthesis by Rat Glomerular Cells in Culture

Jacqueline B. Foidart, Charles A. Dechenne
and Philippe R. Mahieu

Introduction

Knowledge of the nature of the glomerular cells which synthesize basement membrane polypeptides is gradually beginning to increase. It has been shown that, *in vivo*, normal glomerular epithelial cells are able to synthesize some basement membrane polypeptides (Walker, 1973). Furthermore, it has been demonstrated that, *in vitro*, normal glomerular epithelial cells retain their ability to synthesize some basement membrane collagenous polypeptides (Foidart *et al.*, 1975). However, since the glomerular basement membrane (GBM) contains dissimilar polypeptide subunits (Kefalides, 1972), the possibility that glomerular endothelial or mesangial cells also play a role in the biosynthesis of basement membrane glycoproteins cannot be excluded.

We have recently described a method allowing the propagation of homogeneous cell lines derived from normal rat glomeruli, showing that epithelial and mesangial cell lines can be cultivated and subcultivated up to five times without any appreciable morphological alterations (Foidart *et al.*, 1979). In the present work, the biosynthesis of GBM polypeptides by confluent cultures of normal epithelial or mesangial cells has been studied by immunofluorescence microscopy and radiolabelled amino acid analyses. Some biochemical and immunochemical characteristics of the GBM polypeptides synthesized by each type of glomerular cells have been determined and compared.

Materials and Methods

Materials
Insoluble GBM, GBM-soluble antigens and anti-GBM antibodies were prepared as previously described (Mahieu *et al.*, 1974). Procollagen and α chains of type I collagen were a gift from Prof. C. M. Lapière (Liège). Rabbit anti-type IV collagen antiserum was kindly provided by Dr N. A. Kefalides (Philadelphia, Penn.); type IV collagen and rabbit anti-type IV collagen antibodies were also prepared according to the method of Gunson and Kefalides (1976). Sheep anti-rabbit Ig antiserum was purchased from Organon (Oss, Netherlands), fluorescein-labelled goat anti-rabbit Ig antiserum from Nordic Laboratories (Tilburg, Netherlands), [^{14}C]proline (42 mCi/mmol) and [^{14}C]lysine (25 mCi/mmol) from the Radiochemical Centre (Amersham, Bucks, UK), RPMI medium and fetal bovine serum from Flow Laboratories (Irvine, Ayrshire, UK), cycloheximide from Sigma Chemical Co (London, UK), 2,2′-bipyridyl from Calbiochem (Los Angeles, Calif.), and highly purified collagenase from Worthington (Freehold, NJ).

Cell cultures
Cultures and subcultures of rat glomerular epithelial and mesangial cells were prepared as previously described (Foidart *et al.*, 1979). Immunofluorescence and biochemical studies were always performed at complete confluency. The density at cell saturation, evaluated by counting the cells with a haemocytometer, was about 1×10^4 cells/cm^2 for the epithelial cells and 0.5×10^4 cells/cm^2 for the mesangial cells.

Immunofluorescence studies
Glomerular cells were subcultivated using 0·05 per cent trypsin and 0·005 M ethylenediaminetetraacetate in phosphate-buffered saline (PBS) solution without Ca^{2+} and Mg^{2+}, pH 7·2, and were grown to confluency in RPMI medium containing 15 per cent fetal bovine serum on glass coverslips. The coverslips were washed twice in PBS and were then fixed for 8 min in absolute ether : ethanol (1 : 1) at room temperature. They were washed three times in PBS for 5 min each time and stained with the various antisera for 30 min using an indirect immunofluorescence method (Lambert and Dixon, 1968). Following staining, the coverslips were washed three times in PBS for 5 min each time and mounted in 50 per cent glycerin. The cells were then examined by phase contrast or fluorescence microscopy in a Leitz light microscope equipped with an HBO 50 mercury lamp. The specificity of rabbit anti-GBM or anti-type IV collagen antisera was demonstrated by immunofluorescence microscopy performed on normal rat kidney slices. Both antisera

stained the GBM, the tubular basement membranes and the Bowman's capsules linearly.

Biochemical studies
Incorporation experiments were performed at 2, 4, 6 and 8 h, when epithelial and mesangial cells reached confluency. At that time, the RPMI medium was supplemented with 10–50 μCi of the radioactive precursors and with freshly prepared ascorbate (50 μg/ml). The incubations were stopped by adding 2 μmol each of cycloheximide and 2,2'-bipyridyl, in a volume of 0·2 ml, to inhibit further protein synthesis and hydroxylation during the immediate post-incubational period. Collected media were chilled to 4 °C, exhaustively dialysed against distilled water and lyophilized. Lyophilized supernatants were chromatographed on Sephadex G-100 columns as previously described (Foidart *et al.*, 1975), and the presence of cross-reactive GBM or type IV collagen antigenic material in the chromatographic fractions was searched for by radioimmunoassay (Mahieu *et al.*, 1974; Gunson and Kefalides, 1976). The molecular size of GBM polypeptides was evaluated by gel filtration on columns of 6 per cent agarose (Bio-Gel, A-5 m, 200–400 mesh), equilibrated and eluted with 0·1 per cent dodecylsulphate in 0·1 M sodium phosphate buffer, pH 7·4 (Mahieu *et al.*, 1979). The production of hydroxy[^{14}C]proline *in vitro* was taken as an index of GBM collagenous polypeptide biosynthesis. The hydroxy[^{14}C]proline content was assayed by the method of Juva and Prockop (1966), after hydrolysis of the samples in 6 N HCl for 24 h at 100 °C. The degree of glycosylation of hydroxylysine was determined using GBM polypeptides obtained after incubation of the cultivated cells with [^{14}C]lysine. Peaks of radioactivity corresponding to the elution positions of standards of glucosylgalactosylhydroxylysine, galactosyl-hydroxylysine and hydroxylysine were obtained as previously described (Mahieu *et al.*, 1973).

Results and Discussion

Immunofluorescence studies
At confluency, the extracellular material of both epithelial and mesangial cells was strongly stained by the anti-GBM antiserum (Figs 1 and 2). In epithelial cell cultures, this material exhibited an amorphous linear appearance and generally surrounded the cell membranes. In mesangial cell cultures, the extracellular material also exhibited an irregular, linear appearance and was present in fine strands which were not in close connection with the cell membranes. The anti-type IV collagen antiserum stained, with a similar pattern, the extracellular material of epithelial cells, while this antiserum did

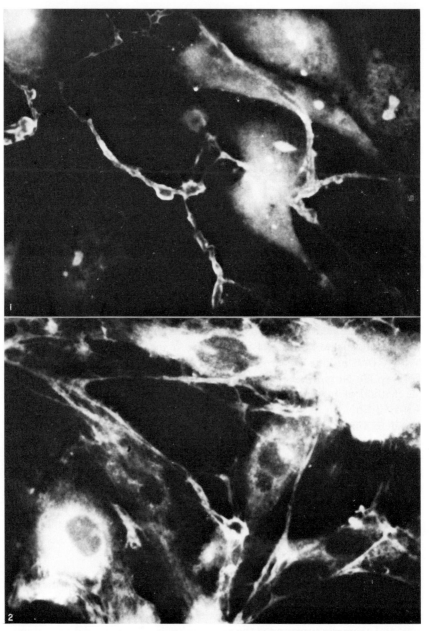

FIG. 1. *Confluent glomerular epithelial cells stained with the anti-GBM antiserum by indirect immunofluorescence. Extracellular material is strongly stained. ×500.*

FIG. 2. *Confluent glomerular mesangial cells stained with the anti-GBM antiserum by indirect immunofluorescence. Extracellular irregular strands of amorphous material are strongly stained. ×500.*

not stain the extracellular material of mesangial cells, after otherwise identical experimental conditions. The staining of the extracellular material of epithelial cells by both anti-GBM and anti-type IV collagen antisera suggests that, *in vitro*, these cells synthesize and secrete into the culture medium basement polypeptides sharing some antigenic determinants with type IV collagen. On the other hand, the staining of the extracellular material of mesangial cells by the anti-GBM antibodies only, suggests that these cells synthesize and secrete into the culture medium basement membrane polypeptides differing from type IV collagen polypeptides.

Biochemical studies

The incorporation rate of [^{14}C]proline into extracellular non-dialysable peptide material was found to be linear for up to 8 h, for both epithelial and mesangial cells. Moreover, the presence of 4-hydroxy[^{14}C]proline in this material demonstrated that some of the ^{14}C-labelled polypeptides synthesized by these cells were collagenous in nature. Glomerular cells were incubated with 50 μCi [^{14}C]lysine and the proportions of hydroxy[^{14}C]lysine, galactosyl-hydroxy[^{14}C]lysine, and glucosylgalactosylhydroxy[^{14}C]lysine were determined after a 6 h incubation (Table I). The results indicated that about

TABLE I

Percentage of glycosylated hydroxylysine in basement membrane polypeptides synthesized by epithelial and mesangial cells in culture[a]

	Percentage of total labelled hydroxylysine	
	Epithelial cells	Mesangial cells
Hydroxy[^{14}C]lysine	7·4	44·5
Galactosylhydroxy[^{14}C]lysine	9·2	5·7
Glucosylgalactosylhydroxy[^{14}C]lysine	83·4	49·8

[a] Confluent cultures were incubated for 6 h with [^{14}C]lysine and the extent of glycosylation of hydroxylysine determined as previously described (Foidart *et al.*, 1975).

90 per cent of the hydroxy[^{14}C]lysine synthesized by the epithelial cells were glycosylated and that about 80 per cent of glycosylated hydroxy[^{14}C]lysine was found as glucosylgalactosylhydroxy[^{14}C]lysine units. For the mesangial cells, the extent of glycosylation of hydroxy[^{14}C]lysine was only 55 per cent and about 50 per cent of glycosylated hydroxy[^{14}C]lysine was present as disaccharide units.

Confluent cultures of epithelial and mesangial cells were incubated for 6 h with 10 μCi [^{14}C]proline. At that time, the incubation media were ex-

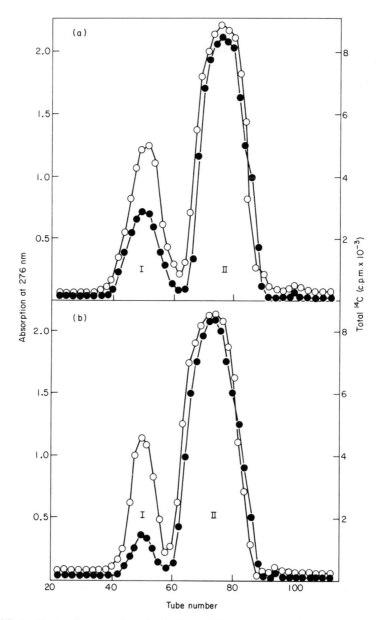

FIG. 3. *Elution diagrams from Sephadex G-100 columns of culture media of epithelial (a) or mesangial (b) cell lines incubated with [¹⁴C]proline. Columns were eluted, at room temperature, with 0·1 M phosphate buffer, pH 7·2 ; 2·4 ml per tube were collected and the samples were characterized by their absorption at 276 nm (●————●) or by their ¹⁴C (○————○) content. Tubes 40–57 (fraction I) and 64–85 (fraction II) were pooled, exhaustively dialysed against distilled water, and lyophilized. (From Foidart et al. (1978).)*

haustively dialysed against distilled water and lyophilized. Gel filtration of lyophilized supernatants on Sephadex G–100 columns is presented in Fig. 3. Two fractions (called I and II), characterized by their radioactivity and their absorption at 276 nm, were eluted using the incubation media of mesangial or epithelial cells. After dialysis and lyophilization, the presence of cross-reactive GBM or type IV collagen antigenic material in fractions I and II was searched for by radioimmunoassay, using specific anti-GBM and anti-type IV collagen antibodies. Increasing amounts (1–1000 μg) of fractions I and II were added to a solution of rabbit anti-GBM antibodies diluted 1000 times and binding specifically 60 per cent of labelled GBM antigens (Mahieu et al., 1974). One hundred micrograms of fractions I inhibited 80 per cent of the binding of labelled membrane antigens to antibodies, while 100 μg of fractions II reduced the specific precipitation by only 15 per cent. These results demonstrate the presence of an antigenic material immunologically related to GBM in both fractions I. In order to further characterize the GBM material of fractions I, similar experiments were realized using a specific anti-type IV collagen antiserum. The radioimmunoassay was performed according to the method of Gunson and Kefalides (1976). The results are given in Table II. It should be stressed that (a) in

TABLE II

Binding of fractions I, and of type IV collagen, to anti-type IV collagen antibodies[a]

Antigen	Amount[b] (μg)	Specific precipitation (per cent)
[14]C-labelled fraction I (epithelial cells)	10	12·4
[14]C-labelled fraction I (mesangial cells)	10	0·8
[125]I-labelled type IV collagen	0·1	69·4

[a] Anti-type IV collagen antiserum diluted 1000 times with 10 per cent normal rabbit serum in phosphate-buffered saline.
[b] The protein content was measured by the method of Lowry et al. (1951), using bovine serum albumin as a standard.

the presence of 10 μg of the fraction I obtained from epithelial cell culture media, the specific precipitation of ^{14}C-labelled polypeptides reached 12·4 per cent; (b) in the presence of similar amounts of the fraction I obtained from mesangial cell culture media, the specific precipitation was only 0·8 per cent; (c) in the presence of 100 ng of ^{125}I-labelled type IV collagen prepared according to the method of Gunson and Kefalides (1976), the specific precipitation was about 70 per cent. These results clearly show that cross-reactive type IV collagen antigenic material is present only in the

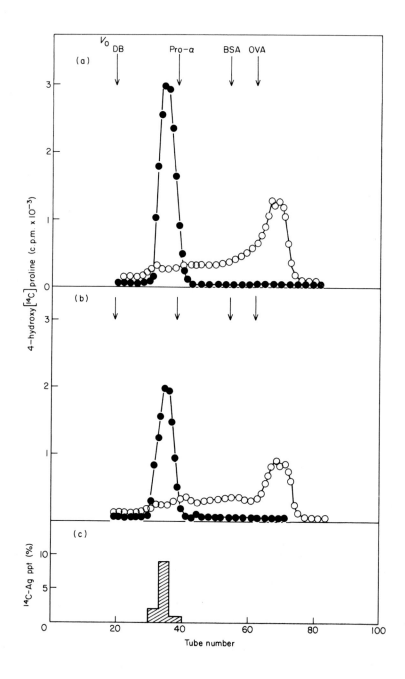

fraction I obtained from the culture medium of epithelial cells and therefore confirm the immunofluorescence microscopy data described above.

The ^{14}C-labelled polypeptides of fractions I were chromatographed on a dodecylsulphate–agarose column. The elution diagrams of labelled polypeptides are represented in Fig. 4. After reduction and denaturation with 2-mercaptoethanol and sodium dodecylsulphate, one major fraction, characterized by its 4-hydroxy[^{14}C]proline content, was eluted just ahead of the internal procollagen marker. Using various standard proteins, the molecular weight was evaluated at about 140 000 daltons. No major difference was observed in the molecular weight of 4-hydroxy[^{14}C]proline-containing polypeptides purified from the epithelial or mesangial cell culture media. After incubation of labelled GBM polypeptides with purified collagenase, most of the 4-hydroxy[^{14}C]proline was recovered into small peptide fragments (Fig. 4), thus confirming the collagenous nature of these polypeptides.

Samples (0·2 ml) from fractions 30–33, 34 and 37–40 (Fig. 4) were pooled, exhaustively dialysed against distilled water, and lyophilized. They were then tested by radioimmunoassay using anti-GBM antibodies. It was found that significant amounts of cross-reactive GBM antigenic material was present in fractions 34–36 from both epithelial or mesangial cell culture media.

Conclusions

Glomerular cells were isolated from rat kidneys using enzymic digestion, sieving and differential centrifugations. They were cultivated in RPMI medium containing 15 per cent fetal bovine serum. Two cell populations were

---

FIG. 4. *Gel filtration on dodecylsulphate–agarose of ^{14}C-labelled fractions I synthesized by epithelial (a) or mesangial (b) cells in culture. After reduction and denaturation with 2-mercaptoethanol and sodium dodecylsulphate (Foidart et al., 1975), labelled polypeptides were chromatographed on Biogel A-5 m columns equilibrated and eluted with 0·1 M sodium phosphate buffer, pH 7·4, containing 0·1 per cent sodium dodecylsulphate. The void volume (V_0) was in fraction 20 and the total volume was in fraction 82. Fractions of 2 ml were collected and aliquots were used for detection of 4-hydroxy[^{14}C]proline (●———●) by the method of Juva and Prockop (1966). The position of the markers used for calibrating the columns prior to the run are indicated (↓): DB, dextran blue 2000, excluded from the column (V_0); pro-α, pro-α chains of the type 1 procollagen; BSA, bovine serum albumin; OVA, ovalbumin. In control experiments, 4-hydroxy[^{14}C]proline (○———○) was measured after enzymic digestion of ^{14}C-labelled polypeptides by purified collagenase, prior to reduction, denaturation and gel filtration of the samples as described above. Samples (0·2 ml) of fractions 30–33, 34–36 and 37–40 were pooled, exhaustively dialysed against distilled water, and lyophilzed. The presence of cross-reactive GBM antigenic material in these samples was searched for by means of the radioimmunoassay (c).*

identified by phase contrast and immunofluorescence microscopy. Both cell lines synthesized and secreted a collagen differing from that of fibroblasts into the culture medium. Moreover, the basement membrane collagenous polypeptides synthesized by the epithelial or the mesangial cells were dissimilar with respect to some of their biochemical and antigenic properties.

Acknowledgements

This work was supported by a grant from the "Délégation Générale à la Recherche Scientifique et Technique Française". We are indebted to Mlle Y. Pirard and to Mme C. Flamand for their skillful technical assistance.

References

Foidart, J., Dechenne, C. and Mahieu, P. (1975). Biosynthesis of basement membrane collagen in cultures of renal glomerular and tubular epithelial cells. *Diabète Métabolisme* **1**, 227–234.

Foidart, J., Dechenne, C. and Mahieu, P. (1978). The biosynthesis of basement membrane collagen by mesangial cell lines derived from normal and diabetic (db/db) mouse glomeruli. In *Cellular and Biochemical Aspects in Diabetes Retinopathy* (F. Regnault and J. Dyhault, eds), INSERM Symposium 7, Elsevier North-Holland, Amsterdam, pp. 113–120.

Foidart, J., Dechenne, C. and Mahieu, P. (1979). Tissue culture of normal rat glomeruli. Isolation and morphological characterization of two homogeneous cell lines. *Invest. Cell Path.* **2**, 15–26.

Gunson, D. E. and Kefalides, N. A. (1976). The use of the radioimmunoassay in the characterization of antibodies to basement membrane collagen. *Immunology* **36**, 563–569.

Juva, K. and Prockop, D. J. (1966). Modified procedure for the assay of ^{3}H- or ^{14}C-labeled hydroxyproline. *Analyt. Biochem.* **15**, 77–83.

Kefalides, N. A. (1972). The chemistry of antigenic components isolated from glomerular basement membrane. *Connective Tissue Res.* **6**, 63–107.

Lambert, P. H. and Dixon, F. J. (1968). Pathogenesis of the glomerulonephritis of the NZB/W mice. *J. exp. Med.*, **127**, 507–516.

Lowry, O. H., Rosebrough, N. J., Farr, A. L. and Randall, R. J. (1951). Protein measurement with the folin phenol reagent. *J. biol. Chem.* **193**, 265–274.

Mahieu, P., Lambert, P. H. and Maghuin-Rogister, G. (1973). Primary structure of a small glycopeptide isolated from human glomerular basement and carrying a major antigenic site. *Eur. J. Biochem.* **40**, 599–606.

Mahieu, P., Lambert, P. H. and Miescher, P. A. (1974). Detection and antiglomerular basement membrane antibodies by a radioimmunological method. *J. clin. Invest.* **54**, 128–137.

Mahieu, P., Foidart, J. and Dechenne, C. (1979). Biosynthesis of basement membrane polypeptides by glomerular cells in culture. In *Frontier of the Biological Matrix* (L. Robert, ed.), Karger, Basel, pp. 60–71.

Walker, F. (1973). The origin, turnover and removal of glomerular basement membrane. *J. Path.* **110**, 233–244.

10
Enlargement of the Glomerular Capillary Surface and Increased Glomerular Function in Early Diabetes

R. Østerby, H. J. G. Gundersen, J. P. Kroustrup,
C. E. Mogensen and K. Seyer-Hansen

In patients with diabetes mellitus a remarkable pattern of development concerning kidney function is observed. During the first several years after the onset of diabetes, kidney function tests reveal an increased glomerular filtration rate (GFR) (Mogensen, 1972). The renal plasma flow at the same time is within the normal level, so that the filtration fraction is increased.

This phenomenon of hyperfunction is present at the time the diagnosis of diabetes is made and it may remain for many years. In contrast to this early renal hyperfunction are the later events. When diabetic patients are followed over the years, it is seen that eventually kidney function shows a gradual decrease so that the normal range is reached, and later still the continuous decline may end in kidney insufficiency. This is the well known clinical or symptomatic stage of diabetic kidney disease. The functional decrease in long-term diabetics is easily understood as a consequence of the glomerular basement membrane thickening which at this point of time has led to closure of many glomeruli (Gundersen and Østerby, 1977).

The early increase in GFR has been well known for many years, but the mechanism behind it has previously been unexplained. Various causes could be involved: an increased pressure gradient across the filtration barrier, an increased permeability of the filter, or an increased area available for filtration. The capillary pressure is not accessible for measurement in patients. As regards the permeability characteristics, it has been shown that the profile of graded dextran clearances is normal in diabetics with increased GFR (Mogensen, 1972). The last-mentioned possibility—a change in glomerular morphology—could be tested by measuring the area of the capillary wall.

The glomerular filtration surface was determined in kidney biopsy material from six young recently diagnosed diabetics and from eight comparable non-diabetic controls.

The first part of the study concerned determination of glomerular size. This was done by using a standard stereological technique (Saltikov, 1967), measuring the distribution of random glomerular cross-sectional areas. From each area distribution the glomerular size is derived. The results are shown in Table I. It was found that the glomerular volume in diabetic patients was nearly doubled (Østerby and Gundersen, 1975). The glomerular enlargement fits well with the demonstration of enlarged kidneys in such patients (Mogensen and Andersen, 1973). However, since the glomeruli occupy only about 5 per cent of the kidney volume, no conclusions about glomerular size can be immediately deduced from the renal enlargement.

TABLE I

Size of glomeruli and of filtration surface in recently diagnosed diabetic patients and in control subjects (geometric mean values)

	Glomerular volume ($\mu m^3 \times 10^6$)	Filtration surface area[a] ($\mu m^2 \times 10^6$)
Control subjects	0·83	0·136
Diabetics	1·41	0·244
2p	0·014	0·0096

[a] The filtration surface given here is that of the peripheral basement membrane (PBM) in an average-size glomerulus. PBM is the basement membrane in the capillary wall where the latter is a simple three-layered structure consisting of endothelium, basement membrane and epithelium, i.e. the capillary wall outside the mesangial regions.

One decisive morphological factor for the filtration rate is presumably the area of the peripheral capillary wall, and maybe also the surface of mesangial regions.

Estimation of the surface is based on the stereological formula

$$S_V = 2I/L,$$

where S_V is the surface density, i.e. the area of surface per unit containing volume. The estimator $2I/L$ is twice the number of intersections, I, between the surface and test lines of total length L (Weibel and Bolender, 1973).

The density of peripheral basement membrane within the glomeruli was determined on randomly cut and photographed cross-sections applying low magnification electron microscopy (Kroustrup *et al.*, 1977). From the relative surface area (surface area per unit volume) the absolute surface area per mean glomerulus was obtained, using the light microscopically determined glomerular size in the individual patients.

The result, shown in Table I, was that the capillary surface is increased by 80 per cent in the diabetic patients.

Under one simple and necessary assumption, that the filtration properties of the barrier are unchanged, this is a sufficient explanation of the increase in GFR. It makes the other two theoretically possible explanations unnecessary. Furthermore, it represents a nice structure–function relationship.

We have used an animal model to study further the development of morphological changes shortly after the onset of metabolic derangement. The injection of streptozotocin destroys the pancreatic β cells and thereby leads to an insulin-deficient, hyperglycaemic state. It has been known for some time that rats with experimentally induced diabetes develop kidney hypertrophy within a few days (Ross and Goldman, 1971; Seyer-Hansen, 1976). The increase in kidney weight is closely related to the degree of hyperglycaemia both in short-term (Seyer-Hansen, 1977) and in long-term experiments (Rasch, 1979).

In the animal with induced diabetes we have the possibility of mapping out in some detail the time course of the morphological changes, which might help us to answer some of the many questions that have arisen. For the quantitative morphological study, strictly randomized sections (Østerby and Gundersen, 1978) from perfusion-fixed kidneys were used at the light and electron microscopic level, applying standard stereological techniques. Female Wistar rats with a body weight of 250 g were used for the experiments. The duration of diabetes considered was between 4 and 47 days. Figure 1 shows kidney weight in groups of rats studied at the various points of time. A considerable increase is already seen after 4 days and the kidney continues to grow over the whole period (Seyer-Hansen et al., 1980).

In this very acute renal enlargement we have focused upon the glomeruli. Figure 2 shows the glomerular fractional volume which is about 5 per cent in the control rats. Rats which have been diabetic for 4 days show a strong tendency to an increase in glomerular volume fraction. At the later stages, on the other hand, it seems as if the non-glomerular renal structures are taking over the major part of the growth. The fact that there is no decrease in glomerular fractional volume initially shows that the glomeruli do participate in the growth from the very beginning. A triggering from a primary tubular hypertrophy is therefore not likely to occur.

From the glomerular fractional volume and the kidney weight the total glomerular volume is calculated, and it appears from Fig. 3 that this quantity is increased by about 30 per cent in a period of 4 days.

These dramatic changes in size lead us to the next questions. Referring to our knowledge of acute metabolic alterations in GFR in human diabetics,

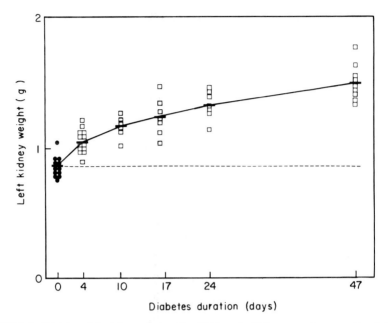

FIG. 1. *Weight of the left perfusion-fixed kidney in 250 g control rats and in diabetic rats after 4–47 days' duration of diabetes.*

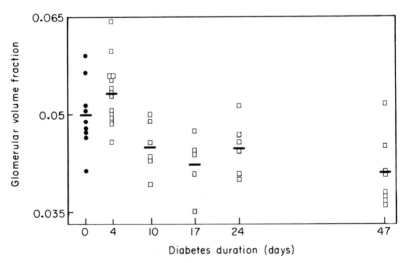

FIG. 2. *Glomerular volume expressed as fraction of the whole kidney, determined by point-counting on equidistantly spaced paraffin sections.*

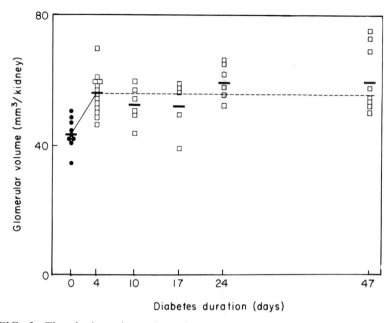

FIG. 3. *The absolute glomerular volume in cubic millimetres derived from the glomerular fraction and kidney weight.*

we are interested in the size of filtration surface; and with the alterations of basement membrane metabolism characterizing diabetic microangiopathy in mind we will focus on estimates of amounts of basement membrane in these glomeruli (Østerby and Gunderson, 1980).

It is generally accepted that the basement membrane turnover is a very slow process. In this particular situation we find that the basement membrane synthesis has accelerated considerably.

Table II shows the estimates of the filtration surface area and of the amount of peripheral basement membrane in control rats and rats which have had diabetes for 4 days. Both the surface of the peripheral capillary wall and that of the total tuft, i.e. including the surface of the mesangial regions, had increased. The enlargement of surface together with the unchanged thickness leads to a 40 per cent increase in total mass of peripheral basement membrane.

Two main points from the findings in this animal study should be emphasized.

The filtration surface was found to increase very rapidly in the acute metabolic derangement. This tells us that there could well be a close structure–function relationship in the diabetic patients concerning filtration surface and GFR. We know from many clinical studies that the changes

TABLE II

Peripheral basement membrane (PBM) in glomeruli from control rats and rats diabetic for 4 days (means ± s.d.)

	Number of animals	PBM thickness[a] (nm)	Surface area of PBM[b] (cm²/ kidney)	Amount of PBM[c] (mm³/ kidney)
Control rats	6	122 ± 9	84 ± 10	1·15 ± 0·14
Diabetic rats	5	119 ± 13	114 ± 14	1·56 ± 0·37
2p		0·75	0·00092	0·035

[a] PBM thickness is harmonic mean determined from orthogonal intercept distribution (Jensen et al., 1979).
[b] PBM surface area is (S_V of PBM in glomeruli) × (glomerular fraction of kidney) × (kidney weight).
[c] Amount of PBM is (total surface) × (thickness).

in the GFR depend on the metabolic state, and it is possible to normalize GFR by strict treatment (Mogensen, 1972).

So far we have only obtained data concerning the *onset* of structural changes in the animal model. The possible reversibility of the glomerular hypertrophy is presently under study.

The second main point concerns the basement membrane metabolism. One very serious aspect of the disease diabetes mellitus is the accumulation of capillary basement membrane over the years, showing up as basement membrane thickening. We do not yet know if this change in basement membrane metabolism is related to the very acute changes which occur within days after the onset of a hypoinsulinaemic and hyperglycaemic state. The two distinctly different basement membrane abnormalities might well have a common, metabolic cause which interferes with the normal control of basement membrane metabolism.

References

Gundersen, H. J. G. and Østerby, R. (1977). Glomerular size and structure in diabetes mellitus. II. Late abnormalities. *Diabetologia* **13**, 43–48.

Jensen, E. B., Gundersen, H. J. G. and Østerby, R. (1979). Determination of membrane thickness distribution from orthogonal intercepts. *J. Microscopie* **115**, 19–33.

Kroustrup, J. P., Gundersen, H. J. G. and Østerby, R. (1977). Glomerular size and structure in diabetes mellitus. III. Early enlargement of the capillary surface. *Diabetologia* **13**, 207–210.

Mogensen, C. E. (1972). Kidney function and glomerular permeability to macromolecules in juvenile diabetes. *Dan. med. Bull.* Suppl. 3.

Mogensen, C. E. and Andersen, M. J. F. (1973). Increased kidney size and glomerular filtration rate in early juvenile diabetes. *Diabetes* **22**, 706–712.

Rasch, R. (1979). Prevention of diabetic glomerulopathy in streptozotocin diabetic rats by insulin treatment. Kidney size and glomerular volume. *Diabetologia* **16**, 125–128.

Ross, J. and Goldman, J. K. (1971). Effect of streptozotocin-induced diabetes on kidney weight and compensatory hypertrophy in the rat. *Endocrinology* **88**, 1079–1082.

Saltikov, S. A. (1967). The determination of the size distribution of particles in an opaque material from a measurement of the size distribution of their sections. In *Stereology* (H. Elias, ed.), Springer, Berlin, pp. 163–173.

Seyer-Hansen, K. (1976). Renal hypertrophy in streptozotocin-diabetic rats. *Clin. Sci. molec. Med.* **51**, 551–555.

Seyer-Hansen, K. (1977). Renal hypertrophy in experimental diabetes: relation to severity of diabetes. *Diabetologia* **13**, 141–143.

Seyer-Hansen, K., Hansen, J. and Gundersen, H. J. G. (1980). Renal hypertrophy in experimental diabetes. A morphometric study. *Diabetologia* **18**, 501–505.

Weibel, E. R. and Bolender, R. P. (1973). Stereological techniques for electron microscopic morphometry. In *Principles and Techniques of Electron Microscopy*, Vol. 3 (M. A. Hayat, ed.), Van Nostrand Reinhold, New York, pp. 237–296.

Østerby, R. and Gundersen, H. J. G. (1975). Glomerular size and structure in diabetes mellitus. I. Early abnormalities. *Diabetologia* **11**, 225–229.

Østerby, R. and Gundersen, H. J. G. (1978). Sampling problems in the kidney. In *Lecture Notes in Biomathematics*, Vol. 23 (R. E. Miles and J. Serra, eds), Springer, Berlin, pp. 185–191.

Østerby, R. and Gundersen, H. J. G. (1980). Fast accumulation of basement membrane material and the rate of morphological changes in acute experimental diabetic glomerular hypertrophy. *Diabetologia* **18**, 493–500.

11
Correlation of Proteinuria and Ultrastructural Glomerular Changes in Toxaemia of Pregnancy

Pietro Zucchelli, Silvia Casanova, Mauro Sasdelli, Leonardo Cagnoli and Sonia Pasquali

Introduction

Epithelial cell changes consisting of a reduction in the number of foot processes, displacement of the filtration slits, formation of occluding junctions and appearance of ladder-like structures have been found in the course of puromycin aminonucleoside (PAN) nephrosis (Arakawa, 1970; Farquhar and Palade, 1961; Caulfield et al., 1976).

These changes seem to be associated with a decrease in glomerular polyanions and are thought to represent a secondary response to proteinuria (Caulfield et al., 1976). Attempts to induce foot process alterations by hyperalbuminaemia-induced proteinuria have yielded conflicting results (Andrews, 1977; Latta et al., 1975; Rodewald and Karnovsky, 1974; Seiler et al., 1977).

Studies on epithelial changes associated with human proteinuric disorders are uncommon. The aim of the present study was therefore to correlate permeability changes of the glomerulus for plasma protein with ultra-structural alterations of the capillary wall in some cases of toxaemia of pregnancy. In particular, the present study was undertaken in order to determine whether proteinuria *per se* may in some way damage epithelial cells. We therefore considered a proteinuric disorder, toxaemia of pregnancy, in which the earliest and most constant histological change is that of a thickening of the endothelial cell layer (endotheliosis) of the capillary wall, associated with deposits in the subendothelial layer of the glomerular basement membrane.

Patients and Methods

Patients
Following the definitions of the American Committee of Maternal Welfare, we selected for the study 13 patients suffering from hypertension, proteinuria and oedema occurring after the 24th week of pregnancy. To exclude the possibility that such a syndrome resulted from pre-existing renal diseases, hypertension or systemic disorders, we paid careful attention to the past obstetrical history of the patients and their clinical and laboratory findings. Renal biopsies were performed from 3 days to 1 month after delivery.

Proteinuria was determined in all cases after concentration of daily urine samples by dialysis, and protein concentration was estimated by the biuret technique. Selectivity was studied by direct observation of the electrophoretic cellulose acetate strips and by determination of the IgG/transferrin clearance ratio (Cameron and Blandford, 1966; Sasdelli *et al.*, 1974).

According to the amount of proteinuria at the time of the biopsy, the patients were divided into two groups. Group I consisted of six patients who had a proteinuria less than 200 mg/day (from 55 to 191 mg/day; mean value 105 ± 49 (s.d.) mg/day), with an age range of 18–43 years (mean 26·8 years). Group II consisted of seven patients who had minimal to moderate proteinuria (from 320 to 2550 mg/day, mean 1405 ± 729 (s.d.) mg/day), with an age range of 21–35 years (mean 27·8 years). Selectivity of proteinuria was high in one case and low in the others. All patients but one were primigravidae and became spontaneously normotensive at the time of biopsy.

Light microscopy
Renal biopsy specimens were obtained by percutaneous puncture using a Vim–Silverman needle modified by Franklin. For light microscopy, the tissue was immersed in Dubosq–Brazil fixative (80 per cent alcohol 150 ml, picric acid 1 g, 40 per cent formalin 60 ml, glacial acetic 15 ml), embedded in paraffin and cut at 2 µm. The following stains were used: haematoxylin and eosin, Masson trichome, periodic acid-Shiff and periodic acid silver methenamine. The degree of change in each histopathological feature was graded from 0 to 3+ according to Pirani *et al.* (1975). In evaluating the glomeruli, particular attention was paid to their cellularity, to the mesangial matrix, to the capillary basement membrane and to the capillary lumen. All specimens were examined by two observers.

Immunofluorescence microscopy was performed on biopsies from all patients with monospecific antisera for IgG, IgA, IgM, C3, Clq, C4, fibrinogen and albumin using the direct method reported by Zucchelli *et al.* (1976).

Electron microscopy
For electron microscopy renal biopsies were fixed by immersion in 2·5 per cent glutaraldehyde in 0·1 M cacodylate buffer, postfixed in 1 per cent OsO_4 in cacodylate buffer, dehydrated and embedded in an Epon–Araldite mixture. Sections 1 μm in thickness were stained with 1 per cent toluidine blue and periodic acid silver methenamine. Ultrathin sections were stained with uranyl acetate and lead citrate and examined in a Jeol T8 electron microscope.

At least four glomeruli were observed from each patient. The number of foot processes and the ultrastructure of the slit diaphragms and the innermost layer of glomerular basement membrane was investigated and the presence and degree of foot process fusion was assessed according to Powell (1976). Approximately 10 non-overlapping negatives (magnification × 2000) of glomerular peripheral capillary loops were taken of each glomerulus and care taken to avoid photographing the same structures in adjacent sections. The negatives were printed at a final magnification of × 7500 and slit pores were counted over a distance of 200 μm of basement membrane. The number of separate foot processes on a 10 μm long distance of the capillary basement membrane in 21 normal glomeruli was 18 with a range between 14 and 22. A similar number of slit pores has been reported in other studies (Powell, 1976).

Results

Light microscopy
Table I summarizes the mean scores of the semiquantitative histopathological

TABLE I
Histopathological changes by light microscopy in two groups of toxaemic patients[a]

	No proteinuria (Group I)	Moderate proteinuria (Group II)
Increased cellularity	0·66	1
Mesangial matrix increase	1	1·14
Mesangial interposition	0·5	1·14
Endotheliosis	1·8	2·85
Narrowing of capillary lumen	1·5	2·28

[a] Values represent average series on a scale from 0 to 3.

observations in the two groups. In Group I, patients without proteinuria, the increase of cellularity and mesangial matrix was doubtful to mild. Thickening of the capillary wall and narrowing of the capillary lumina was mild.

In Group II, patients with moderate proteinuria, the alterations were more prominent. Cellularity and mesangial matrix increase was slightly higher, splitting of the glomerular basement membrane was seldom observed, and the lumens of the capillary loops were narrowed by sheets of endothelial cytoplasm. There was a fairly good correlation between the degree of endotheliosis and the amount of proteinuria. In Table I the scores are average values on a scale 0–3. Only the mean value of endotheliosis showed a significant difference between the two groups (Wilcoxon's test).

Immunofluorescence microscopy
Material immunoreactive with antifibrinogen serum was found in all of the 13 biopsies examined; a positive immunofluorescence with IgM serum was present in three out of six cases of Group I and in six out of seven cases of Group II. The deposits were predominantly localized in subendothelial areas, but positive fluorescence was also present inside the endothelial cells and in the mesangium. The tubules, interstitial tissue or the wall of the small vessels contained very little reactive material.

Electron microscopy
Electron microscopy of glomeruli from patients in Group I confirmed the light microscopic findings: the glomeruli were slightly enlarged with a normal frequency of nuclei and showed an inconspicuous widening of the mesangial areas and occasional incomplete mesangial interpositions. Many capillary loops were patent, whilst others were still occupied by enlarged endothelial cells (Fig. 1). Endothelial oedema was occasionally observed, but this finding was considered an unspecific reaction, possibly representing a preparation artefact, as it is seldom observed in otherwise normal biopsies.

The epithelial cells were moderately swollen in a few areas, but the foot processes were generally unchanged, except for focal areas which showed loss of foot process. Similar limited zones of flattening can also be observed in normal glomeruli (Andrews, 1977). The glomerular basement membrane had a normal thickness, except in localized areas where fine fibrillar and slightly electron-dense material was present on the endothelial side of the capillary basement membrane.

In Group II alterations involving the endothelial cells were more prominent. Many capillary loops were bloodless and occupied by endothelial cells with an increased number of organelles, enlarged cytoplasm and arcade formation (endotheliosis) (Fig. 3). Some cells contained lipid vacuoles.

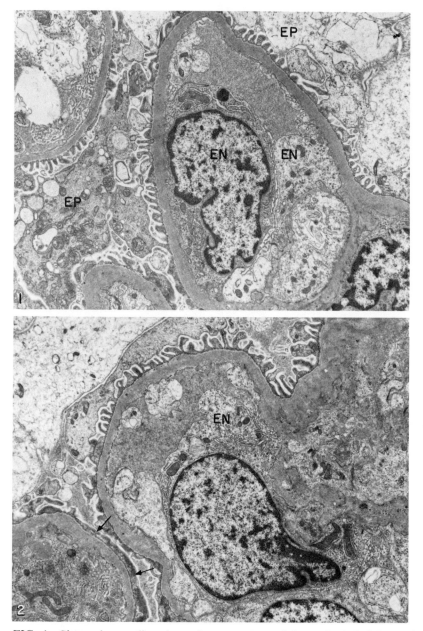

FIG. 1. *Glomerular capillary loops from a patient of Group I. Endothelial cells (EN) show increase in organelles and protrude into the capillary lumina. The epithelial cells (EO) to the right show pronounced cytoplasmic swelling, while the cell to the left contains large vacuoles.* × 6400.

FIG. 2. *Glomerular capillary from a patient of group I. The endothelial (EN) cells are activated and a podocyte (EP) shows fused foot processes.* × 5400.

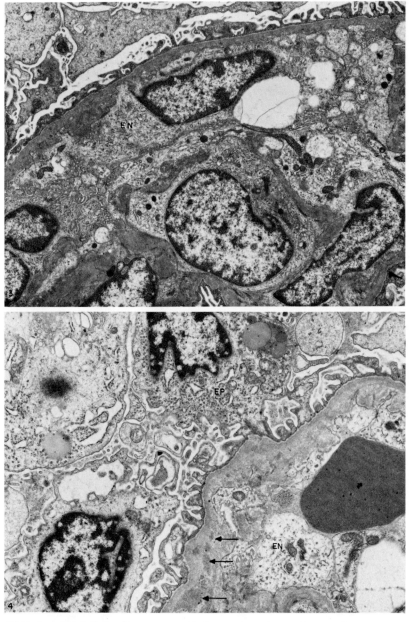

FIG. 3. *Endothelial cells in Group II show enlarged cytoplasm with an increased number of organelles, nuclear notching and arcade formation. A swollen mesangial cell is also present.* × 6000.

FIG. 4. *Epithelial cells (EP) in a biopsy from a patient of Group II. The main cell body contains rough-surfaced hypertrophic and dilated endoplasmic reticulum and a few lipid droplets; foot processes are preserved. Irregularly osmiophilic deposits (arrows) are present on the endothelial layer of the basement membrane and endothelial cells (EN) are swollen.* × 8400.

Mesangial cells were also more prominent and on occasion were displaced between the endothelium and the glomerular basement membrane.

Widening of the lamina rara interna caused by the presence of varying amounts of irregularly osmiophilic material was observed (Figs 4 and 5). Epithelial cells were generally enlarged and the cell body of some podocytes showed increased amounts of dilated, rough-surfaced endoplasmic reticulum and ribosomes, dilated vacuoles and few lipid droplets (Fig. 4). Some cells exhibited pronounced swelling of the cell body (Fig. 5) and a few contained protein inclusions. Major foot processes and pedicels were discrete and well preserved (Figs 4 and 5). The epithelial slits, measuring 300–500 Å across, were spanned by thin diaphragms which sometimes showed a central dot (Fig. 6).

No quantitative correlation was found between the width of the foot processes and proteinuria in our toxaemic patients (Fig. 7). The mean value in Group 1 (17 ± 2 (s.d.) foot processes per 10 μm of basement membrane) was not significantly different from the value in Group II ($16\cdot2 \pm 0\cdot9$ (s.d.) foot processes per 10 μm of basement membrane).

Discussion

The aim of the present study was to correlate permeability changes of the glomerulus for plasma protein with ultrastructural alterations of the capillary wall during toxaemia of pregnancy. The results indicate the following:

(1) Only minor changes in the epithelial cell covering of the glomerular basement membrane were present in all cases and no significant displacement or distortion of slit diaphragms was observed.

(2) The quantitative assessment of foot process fusion did not show a significant difference between groups with and without proteinuria. Furthermore, no correlation was found between the degree of proteinuria and the number of podocyte pedicels.

(3) The strongest correlation was found between endotheliosis and degree of proteinuria.

The results seem thus to indicate that in toxaemia of pregnancy, proteinuria is not associated with extensive epithelial cell spreading.

Our data differ from previous studies which indicate that generalized changes in the shape and organization of glomerular podocytes in the course of nephropathies occur following protein leakage through the glomerular capillary wall (Caulfield et al., 1976).

However, in keeping with our findings, Andrews (1977) recently observed, using a scanning electron microscope, that hyperalbuminaemia-induced

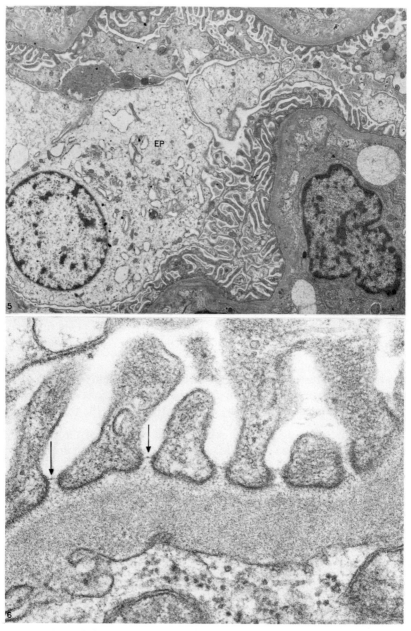

FIG. 5. *Epithelial cell (EP) from a patient in Group II showing cytoplasmic swelling and slender interdigitating foot process.* × 5200.

FIG. 6. *Higher magnification electron micrograph from a biopsy of a patient in Group II. The foot processes are regularly arranged with wide intervening slit pores (arrows).* × 78 000.

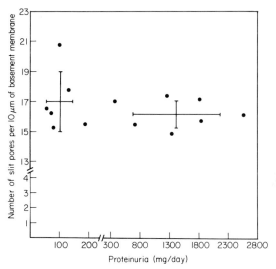

FIG. 7. *Correlation between number of slit pores and proteinuria in 13 patients with toxaemia of pregnancy. The point of intersection of each of the two lines indicates the mean value and the crossed lines show ± S.D. of the proteinuria and the number of slit pores for each of the two groups. There is no significant correlation between the number of slit pores and the amount of proteinuria (r = −0·216). Mean value (± S.D.) of number of foot processes does not appear significantly reduced in Group II patients compared with Group I patients.*

proteinuria failed to cause significant loss of pedicels. Similar results have been reported by others (Seiler *et al.*, 1977).

It should be stressed that the amount of proteinuria in our patients was not of a very high level, and it may be hypothesized that, at higher levels of proteinuria, extensive spreading of podocyte pedicels might become evident. In fact Andrews (1977) reports that pedicel distortion in rats became apparent when proteinuria greater than 1000 mg per 100 ml of urine was induced by injection of a very large amount of albumin. Nevertheless, in pre-eclampsia with massive proteinuria and nephrotic syndrome, First *et al.* (1978) noted the presence of fusion in only 5–10 per cent of the foot processes examined.

Comparing our present data on toxaemic patients with our unpublished observations of some patients with minimal change nephropathy (MCN) and the same levels of proteinuria, we found a far more evident fusion in MCN patients (10·2 ± 3 foot processes per 10 μm of basement membrane) in comparison with toxaemic patients (16·2 ± 0·9 foot processes per 10 μm of basement membrane; $p < 0·01$).

From our data it seems possible to postulate that, in the histogenesis of foot process changes, factors other than proteinuria may play an important role: in MCN it has been hypothesized by Eyres *et al.* (1976) that direct cytotoxic damage to the epithelial cells may occur, whilst in membranous glomerulonephritis others have suggested that local disturbances of the electrical environment in the subepithelial layer caused by large immune-complexes could play a role in the pathogenesis of foot process changes (Seiler *et al.*, 1977).

Haemodynamic changes may be responsible for the proteinuria during toxaemia when a hypertensive state is present. A marked increase in glomerular permeability was induced in rats (Hulme and Pessina, 1976) during renin or angiotensin infusion and ascribed to altered intrarenal haemodynamics resulting in an increased filtration fraction. All our patients, however, had returned to a normotensive state by the time of biopsy and plasma renin activity was normal in all cases. According to Hulme and Pessina (1976) induced proteinuria disappeared rapidly on termination of renin infusion.

In our experience, in agreement with the findings of Pollak and Nettles (1960), Mautner *et al.* (1962) and First *et al.* (1978), the histopathological data which showed the strongest correlation with proteinuria consisted of alterations of the lamina rara interna and the endothelial cells, and were presumably caused by intravascular coagulation in toxaemia.

Recent studies have suggested that the glomerular charge barrier may be created in part by anionic sites localized in the lamina rara interna (Brenner *et al.*, 1978). Damage of the innermost layer of the capillary wall could perhaps modify the electrical properties of this layer and alter its function as a barrier to proteins. At this stage, however, this possibility is merely put forward as a hypothesis and requires experimental verification.

References

Andrews, P. M. (1977). A scanning and transmission electron microscopic comparison of puromycin aminonucleoside-induced nephrosis to hyperalbuminemia-induced proteinuria with emphasis on kidney podocyte pedicel loss. *Lab. Invest.* **36**, 183–196.

Arakawa, M. (1970). A scanning electron microscopy of the glomerulus of normal and nephrotic rats. *Lab. Invest.* **23**, 489–496.

Brenner, B. M., Hostetter, T. H. and Humes, H. D. (1978). Molecular basis of proteinuria of glomerular origin. *New Engl. J. Med.* **298**, 826–833.

Cameron, J. S. and Blandford, G. (1966). Simple assessment of selectivity in heavy proteinuria. *Lancet ii*, 242–244.

Caulfield, J. P., Reid, J. J. and Farquhar, M. G. (1976). Alterations of the glomerular epithelium in acute aminonucleoside nephrosis. Evidence for formation of occluding junctions and epithelial cell detachment. *Lab. Invest.* **34**, 43–59.

Eyres, K., Mallick, N. P. and Taylor, G. (1976). Evidence for cell-mediated immunity to renal antigens in minimal-change nephrotic syndrome. *Lancet i*, 1158–1159.

Farquhar, M. G. and Palade, G. E. (1961). Glomerular permeability. II. Ferritin transfer across the glomerular capillary wall in nephrotic rats. *J. exp. Med.* **114**, 699–716.

First, M. R., Ooi, B. S., Jao, W. and Pollak, V. E. (1978). Pre-eclampsia with the nephrotic syndrome. *Kidney Int.* **13**, 166–177.

Hulme, B. and Pessina, A. (1976). Influence of renin and angiotensin II on macromolecular glomerular permeability. In *Proceedings of the VIth International Congress of nephrology, Florence 1975* (S. Giovannetti, V. Bonomini and G. D'Amico, eds), Karger, Basel, pp. 361–368.

Latta, H., Johnston, W. H. and Stanley, T. M. (1975). Sialoglycoproteins and filtration barriers in the glomerular capillary wall. *J. Ultrastruct. Res.* **51**, 354–376.

Mautner, W., Churg, J., Grishman, E. and Dachs, S. (1962). Pre-eclamptic nephropathy. An electron microscopic study. *Lab. Invest.* **11**, 518–530.

Pirani, C. L., Salinas-Madrigal, L. and Koss, M. (1975). Evaluation of percutaneous renal biopsies. In *Kidney Pathology Decennial, 1966–1975* (S. C. Sommers, ed.) Appleton-Century-Crofts, New York, pp. 108–163.

Pollak, V. E. and Nettles, J. B. (1960). The kidney in toxaemia of pregnancy: a clinical and pathologic study based on renal biopsies. *Medicine, Baltimore* **39**, 469–526.

Powell, H. R. (1976). Relationship between proteinuria and epithelial cell changes in minimal lesion glomerulopathy, *Nephron* **16**, 310–317.

Rodewald, R. and Karnovsky, M. J. (1974). Porous structure of the glomerular slit diaphragm in the rat and mouse. *J. Cell Biol.* **63**, 423–433.

Sasdelli, M., Rovinetti, C., Zuccalà, A., Toschi, P. and Fabbri, L. (1974). Lo studio delle proteine urinarie nella pratica nefrologica. *Terapia* **59**, 200–216.

Seiler, M. W., Rennke, H. G., Venkatachalam, M. A. and Cotran, R. S. (1977). Pathogenesis of polycation-induced alterations ("fusion") of glomerular epithelium. *Lab. Invest.* **36**, 48–61.

Zucchelli, P., Sasdelli, M., Cagnoli, L., Donini, U., Casanova, S. and Rovinetti, C. (1976). Membranoproliferative glomerulonephritis: correlations between immunological and histological findings. *Nephron* **17**, 449–460.

Part II

Tubules: Ion and Fluid Pathways

12
The Na$^+$, K$^+$-ATPase as a Regulator of the Intracellular Concentration of Na$^+$, K$^+$ and Cl$^-$. Its Function in Transcellular Transport of NaCl

Jens Chr. Skou

Introduction

An important part of the kidney's function is related to the regulation of the salt and the water content in the body. This is accomplished by a regulated reabsorption of the filtered NaCl. It leads to an excretion of the surplus NaCl, to an isosmotic reabsorption of water in the proximal tubule and to formation of an osmotic gradient in the interstitium which acts as a driving force for the hormone-regulated reabsorption of water from the collecting ducts.

Injection of ouabain into the renal artery decreases the reabsorption of NaCl and decreases the kidney metabolism (Sejersted *et al.*, 1971; Lie *et al.*, 1974). There is thus a chemical energy-dependent reabsorption of NaCl which is inhibited by ouabain. The effect of ouabain is most pronounced in the diluting segments of the kidney, i.e. the thick ascending limb of Henle's loop.

Studies on isolated segments of this part of the tubule show a net transfer of Na$^+$ as well as Cl$^-$ from lumen to bath against a transtubular potential gradient of about 6 mV, lumen positive; ouabain reduces the potential gradient (Burg and Green, 1973; Rocha and Kokko, 1973). From this it was proposed that the transcellular transport of NaCl consists of an active Cl$^-$ transport driven by an electrogenic Cl$^-$ pump and with a passive Na$^+$ transport along the resulting electrochemical gradient.

However, the diluting segment of the kidney is one of the tissues with the highest content of the transport system, the Na$^+$, K$^+$-ATPase (see Jørgensen, 1975), which is known to be responsible for active transport of Na$^+$ and

K^+ in other cells, and which is known specifically to be inhibited by ouabain (Skou, 1965). This makes it likely, as has been proposed (Jørgensen, 1976), that it is this system which is responsible for the active energy-dependent Na^+ reabsorption. The net Cl^- : Na^+ transport ratio in the above-mentioned experiments on the isolated segments of the ascending limb of Henle's loop was lower than 1. This would be compatible with a Cl^- transport driven by the Na^+ transport, and not the reverse.

But how can the Na^+, K^+ transport system which exchanges Na^+ for K^+ across the cell membrane give a net transepithelial transport of Na, and how can this be coupled to a Cl^- transport?

Regulation of the Na^+, K^+-ATPase Activity

The Na^+, K^+-ATPase is located in the cell membrane. It couples the passive flux of Na^+ out of and K^+ into the cell to a flux of the same cations in the opposite direction against their electrochemical gradient—the active transport (see Skou, 1975). The coupling is tight enough to give a steady state concentration of Na^+ and of K^+ in the cell which is away from thermodynamic equilibrium of the two cations.

The passive flux of Na^+ into the cell is coupled to the passive flux of K^+ out by the membrane potential, which again is set by the higher permeability of the membrane for K^+ than for Na^+, and by the concentration gradients.

But how is the passive flux coupled to the active transport, i.e. how is the information about a change in the intracellular concentrations of the cations transferred to the coupling system—the Na^+, K^+-ATPase?

It is characteristic of the Na^+, K^+-ATPase that it requires a combined effect of Na^+ and of K^+ for hydrolysis of ATP. Na^+ acts on a site in the system which is facing the internal solution in the intact membrane, the i-site in the following, and K^+ on a site facing the external solution, the o-site, i.e. a $^oK_m/^iNa_n$ form of the system (i for inside, o for outside, m and n are integers); each of the sites accepts a number of cations, probably three Na^+ or two K^+ ions, and on each site there is competition between Na^+ and K^+ (see Skou, 1975). It means that saturation of each of the sites with one or the other of the cations is a function of the absolute concentrations of Na^+ and K^+ and of the ratio between the concentrations of the two cations in the internal, and external, solutions respectively.

In vitro it is not possible to have the i- and the o-site in contact with different Na^+–K^+ concentrations. But the apparent affinity for Na^+ relative to K^+ on the i-site differs so much from that on the o-site that it is possible with a certain Na^+ : K^+ concentration ratio to have the main part of the system of the active $^oK_m/^iNa_n$ form (Fig. 1). The asymmetry of the curve reflects the difference in affinities at the two sites.

As seen from the left part of the curve in Fig. 1, the Na⁺ : K⁺ concentration ratio necessary to give the half-maximum Na⁺ activation (effect on i-site) is about 1 : 3, suggesting that the apparent affinity for Na⁺ on the i-site is about three times higher than for K⁺. From the right part of the curve it can be seen that the K⁺ : Na⁺ concentration ratio necessary for half-maximum K⁺ activation (effect on o-site) is about 1 : 60, suggesting that the apparent affinity for K⁺ on the o-site is about 60 times higher than for Na⁺. This is with saturating concentrations of ATP and at optimum pH 7·2–7·4.

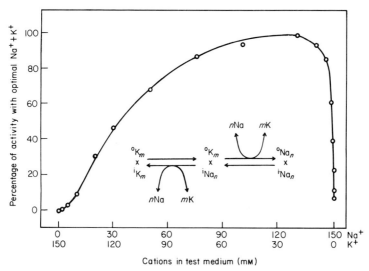

FIG. 1. *Activity of Na⁺, K⁺-ATPase as a function of the Na⁺ + K⁺ concentration. The activity was measured with 3 mM ATP, 3 mM magnesium, pH 7·4, 37 °C, and with the concentrations of Na⁺ + K⁺ shown.*

If it is correct that the i-site and the o-site on the system exist simultaneously (see Skou, 1975), and assuming that each site does not exist in a hybrid form, the enzyme molecules will be divided between four different forms which are in equilibrium.

And with the above-mentioned affinities and with the normal extra- and intracellular concentrations of Na⁺ and K⁺ in contact with the o- and the i-site respectively, the fractions of the enzyme molecules having the four different forms will be approximately as shown in Fig. 2; the Na⁺–K⁺-dependent rate of hydrolysis of ATP (the $^oK_m/^iNa_n$ form) will then be about 35 per cent of maximum (see Skou, 1975).

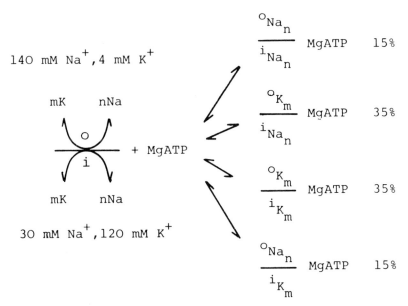

FIG. 2. *Fraction of enzyme molecules in the four different forms at the extra- and intracellular concentrations of Na⁺ and K⁺ shown. For further explanation, see text.*

The rate of the chemical reaction, the hydrolysis of ATP, will, as in any enzymic reaction, be dependent on the concentration of the substrate, ATP (and magnesium); for the Na^+ plus K^+-activated reaction the apparent K_m for MgATP is about 0·3 mM (Post *et al.*, 1965), and saturation is obtained with 3 mM.

However, ATP also influences the apparent affinity for Na^+ relative to K^+ both on the i- and on the o-site. On the i-site, where Na^+ activates, ATP increases the apparent affinity for Na^+ relative to K^+ from about 0·4:1 without ATP to about 3:1 with saturating concentrations of ATP (Skou, 1974*a,b*).

This means that with a given $Na^+:K^+$ ratio in the medium the number of enzyme molecules with a Na^+-saturated i-site increases with the ATP concentration, and thereby the number of enzyme molecules on the active $^oK_m/^iNa_n$ form. The effect is due to ATP as such, before ATP is hydrolysed (Skou, 1974*a*).

ATP also has, however, an effect on the apparent affinity for K^+ relative to Na^+ on the o-site. This seems to be an effect of MgATP (Robinson, 1967) and may be related to the rate of hydrolysis of ATP. MgATP decreases the apparent affinity for K^+ relative to Na^+, and with saturating concentrations of MgATP it is about 60:1.

At a given Na$^+$: K$^+$ concentration ratio, a decrease in the ATP concentration thus tends to decrease the saturation of the i-site with Na$^+$, and thereby decreases the fraction of the enzyme molecules on the ^{o}K$_m$/^{i}Na$_n$ form. On the other hand, a decrease in the MgATP concentration increases the apparent affinity for K$^+$ on the o-site, and because of this tends to increase the fraction of the molecules on the ^{o}K$_m$/^{i}Na$_n$ form.

The optimum pH for the reaction is dependent on the ATP concentration. With saturating concentrations of ATP it is 7·2–7·4. With a decrease in the ATP concentration the pH optimum is shifted to a higher pH value, and with a very low ATP concentration, 1 μM, it is about 8·0–8·2. Furthermore, pH has an effect on the apparent affinity for Na$^+$ relative to K$^+$ on the i-site, the effect depending on the ATP concentration. With saturating concentrations of ATP, an increase in pH leads to a decrease in apparent affinity for Na$^+$ relative to K$^+$. At low ATP concentrations the effect of an increase in pH is the opposite: it increases the apparent affinity for Na$^+$ relative to K$^+$. These effects seem to be related to pK changes in the system when it reacts with the different ligands. The functional significance of these changes is not known (J. C. Skou, unpublished).

The activity as a function of the Na$^+$: K$^+$ concentration ratio, shown in Fig. 1, is with saturating concentrations of ATP and at optimum pH. The left part of the curve, which shows the activating effect of Na$^+$, is S-shaped; it has its steepest part around the normal intracellular Na$^+$: K$^+$ concentration ratio, 30 : 120 mM, i.e. variations in the internal Na$^+$: K$^+$ concentration ratio around this value will give the largest change in activity. The activity is around 40 per cent of maximum. *In vitro* this Na$^+$: K$^+$ concentration ratio will give K$^+$ saturation of the o-site.

From the right-hand part of the bell-shaped curve in Fig. 1 it can be seen that, with the normal extracellular K$^+$: Na$^+$ concentration ratio of 4 : 145 mM, the K$^+$ activation is about 70–80 per cent of maximum; this is with a Na$^+$ concentration which gives Na$^+$ saturation of the i-site *in vitro*.

With the normal intracellular Na$^+$: K$^+$ concentrations in contact with the i-site and the normal extracellular concentrations in contact with the o-site, the activity will then be about 30–35 per cent of maximum (cf. Fig. 2).

The information about a change in the passive flux across the cell membrane which gives a change in the intra- and extracellular concentrations of Na$^+$ and K$^+$ is thus transferred to the transport system via a direct activating effect of the cations on the catalytic activity of the transport system. The activating effect of a given Na$^+$: K$^+$ concentration ratio depends on the apparent Na$^+$ relative to K$^+$ affinity of the sites on the system, and as seen from the effects of ATP and pH this is variable.

Due to the higher permeability of the cell membrane for K$^+$ than for Na$^+$, the gradient for the cations created by the Na$^+$, K$^+$ transport system leads to a membrane potential positive to the outside. This will influence the distribution of anions which can permeate the membrane, Cl^- and HCO_3^-; their electrochemical gradient across the membrane will be zero, i.e. the intracellular concentration will be lower than the extracellular.

The Na^+, K^+ transport system thus not only regulates the intracellular concentration of Na^+ and K^+ but also indirectly the concentrations of Cl^- and HCO_3^-, and thereby also the intracellular osmotic concentration—the water content, i.e. the cell volume.

The Na⁺, K⁺-ATPase as a Transcellular Na⁺–K⁺ Transport System

The active Na^+–K^+ transport system can accomplish two types of transport (Glynn and Karlish, 1974): one in which there is a net transport of the cations involved, and another in which there is no net transport but an exchange of similar cations.

The net transport can either be an exchange of Na^+ from inside for K^+ from outside, the $^oK_m/^iNa_n$ form, which requires ATP in the internal medium and is coupled to the exergonic chemical reaction, the hydrolysis of ATP; alternatively it can be a low net efflux of Na^+ to an external medium which contains choline but no Na^+ or K^+ (Lew et al., 1973; Garrahan and Glynn, 1967a; Karlish and Glynn, 1974), which requires ATP in the internal medium (Lew et al., 1973).

Finally, the net transport can be an exchange of Na^+ from outside for K^+ from inside, the $^oNa_n/^iK_m$ form: this requires ADP and P_i in the internal medium and is coupled to the endergonic reaction, the synthesis of ATP, a reversal of the pump (Garrahan and Glynn, 1967c; Glynn et al., 1970; Lant et al., 1970).

The exchange reaction with no net transport is either an exchange of Na^+ from inside for Na^+ from outside, the $^oNa_n/^iNa_n$ form, or an exchange of K^+ for K^+, the $^oK_m/^iK_m$ form (Glynn and Karlish, 1974).

The $Na^+ : Na^+$ exchange requires ATP (Garrahan and Glynn, 1967b) and ADP (Glynn and Hoffman, 1971; Baker et al., 1971) in the internal medium. There is no (or a very low) net hydrolysis of ATP, but probably a phosphorylation of the system from ATP followed by a reversal of the reaction, with formation of ATP by a reaction of the phosphoenzyme with ADP—an ADP–ATP exchange reaction.

The $K^+ : K^+$ exchange requires ATP (Glynn et al., 1971) and P_i (Glynn et al., 1970) in the internal medium, but the chemical reaction underlying the exchange is not known.

The nature and the direction of the transport is thus set by the nature of the cations on the o- and the i-sites, respectively, which again is determined by the ratio of the cations in the external and the internal medium and of the affinities of the sites for the cations. It is, however, the chemical potential for the ATP–ADP–P$_i$ system which determines whether the reaction with a given combination of cations on the two sites will proceed or not, and the rate of the reaction.

The tight coupling between the chemical reaction and the flow of the cations suggests that the cations cannot flow across the membrane through the system unless there is a reaction with the chemical substrate ATP–ADP–P$_i$.

With the normal intra- and extracellular Na$^+$ and K$^+$ concentrations and the normal high intracellular [ATP]/[ADP] × [P$_i$] concentration ratio, it is the exergonic reaction which proceeds, leading to a transport of Na$^+$ out and K$^+$ into the cell. There will probably be no net non-coupled Na$^+$ efflux and a low Na : Na and K : K exchange.

In the exergonic reaction three Na$^+$ ions are transported out and two K$^+$ ions in for each ATP molecule hydrolysed (see Glynn, 1968). The 3 : 2 ratio is not compensated for by a flow of an anion together with Na$^+$ or of another cation, a proton, with K$^+$; the transport is electrogenic (Thomas, 1972). It suggests that anions and protons cannot pass the membrane along the same route along which Na$^+$ and K$^+$ are transported.

A system which can exchange Na$^+$ from inside for K$^+$ from outside against an electrochemical gradient can, as proposed by Kofoed-Johnsen and Ussing (1958), give a net transepithelial flux of Na$^+$. It requires that a certain part of the membrane is permeable to Na$^+$ but not to K$^+$ and has no Na$^+$–K$^+$ pumps, while the other part of the membrane has the pumps, has a low or no Na$^+$ permeability, but has a high permeability for K$^+$. According to this the Na$^+$, K$^+$ exchange system should be located in the abluminal but not in the luminal part of the tubule cell in the thick ascending limb of Henle's loop in order to give a net transtubular reabsorption of Na$^+$. And the luminal membrane should be permeable to Na$^+$ but not to K$^+$, while the abluminal membrane should be permeable to K$^+$ but not to Na$^+$. Na$^+$ will flow passively into the cell across the luminal membrane and be transported actively out across the abluminal membrane in exchange for K$^+$, and K$^+$ will then flow out passively across the abluminal membrane. There will be a steady recirculation of K$^+$ across the abluminal membrane without any net movement.

The membrane potential set up by the K$^+$ gradient may be used as a driving force for Cl$^-$ transfer from intracellular to extracellular across the abluminal membrane. But to do this and to get a transepithelial net transfer of Cl$^-$ requires an uphill movement of Cl$^-$ from the lumen to the tubule cell. The reabsorption of Cl$^-$ is inhibited by ouabain (Burg and Green, 1973; Rocha and Kokko, 1973) and the reabsorption of Na$^+$ is inhibited by replacing Cl$^-$

in the tubule lumen with unreabsorbable anions (Kahn *et al.*, 1975). This seems to suggest that there is a coupling between the transport of Na^+ and Cl^-.

From what has been discussed, a coupling cannot occur on the transport ATPase. The information suggests that the energy for the uphill movement of the Cl^- from lumen to cell comes from the downhill movement of Na^+ from lumen to cell.

A coupling between the two fluxes could be accomplished by a carrier-mediated Cl^- transfer which is coupled to the transfer of Na^+ from lumen to cell, and where the influx of Cl^- is driven by the Na^+ gradient. The luminal membrane must be tight for passive Na^+ and Cl^- diffusion.

A coupling could either be via a Cl^- carrier, which would require the binding of Na^+ for Cl^- transfer, or it could utilize two carriers—a Cl^-–HCO_3^- exchange carrier and a Na^+–H^+ exchange carrier with a coupling via the intracellular $H_2CO_3 \rightleftharpoons H^+ + HCO_3^-$ reaction. The gradient for Na^+ will drive the intracellular $H_2CO_3 \rightleftharpoons H^+ + HCO_3^-$ reaction towards the right, the HCO_3^- will exchange for Cl^- from outside and extracellular $H^+ + HCO_3^-$ will form $CO_2 + H_2O$.

Cl^- flows out across the Cl^--permeable abluminal membrane, driven by the membrane potential set up by the K^+ gradient created by the Na^+–K^+ pump.

A Na^+–Cl^- coupled transfer across the luminal membrane with an active transfer of Na^+ across the abluminal membrane in exchange for K^+ and with a back-diffusion of K^+ could give a net transfer of Na^+ as well as of Cl^- against an electrochemical gradient. And for Cl^- this occurs without involving an active transfer, in the sense that the Cl^- transport is directly linked to a chemical reaction. Such a Cl^- transport will be inhibited by ouabain and an inhibition of the Cl^- transfer across the luminal membrane will give a decrease in Na^+ transport.

But what is the explanation of the ouabain-sensitive transtubular potential difference in the thick ascending limb of Henle's loop with the lumen positive? The Na^+, K^+-(ATPase) is not only located in the peritubular part of the abluminal membrane but also in that part of the membrane which faces the interstitium between the tubule cells (Maunsbach *et al.*, 1978). Na^+ flowing through the luminal membrane is then pumped out in the interstitium. And a back-diffusion of Na^+ through the tight junction could be responsible for the potential difference. Another possibility is that it is a transepithelial potential difference. The pumping activity is, according to what was discussed above, dependent on the intracellular $Na^+ : K^+$ concentration ratio. Na^+ flowing in through the luminal membrane and pumped out across the lateral membrane may lead to a gradient of Na^+ from luminal to peritubular end of the tubule cell, i.e. the pumping activity may decrease along the interstitium from the tight junctions towards the peritubular lumen. A higher rate of Na$^+$ pumping means a higher rate of K$^+$ uptake. With a limited amount of K$^+$ in the interstitium, and if the resistance for flow of K$^+$ along the interstitium is low, this may give a higher concentration gradient for K$^+$ and thereby a higher membrane potential in the luminal part of the cell than in the peritubular part of the cell.

Conclusions

The Na, K transport system, the Na$^+$, K$^+$-ATPase, is activated by a combined effect of intracellular Na$^+$ and extracellular K$^+$. Intracellular K$^+$ inhibits by competing with Na$^+$ for the Na$^+$ site, and extracellular Na$^+$ inhibits by competing with K$^+$ for the K$^+$ site. It is thus the intracellular and the extracellular Na$^+$:K$^+$ concentration ratios and the affinity for Na$^+$ relative to K$^+$ on the two activator sites which regulate the rate of active transport of the cations. The apparent Na$^+$ relative to K$^+$ affinity is variable, and is dependent on ATP concentration and pH.

The transport system exchanges Na$^+$ for K$^+$. Located in the abluminal part of a tubule cell membrane which is permeable to K$^+$ but not to Na$^+$, and with a luminal membrane which allows a flux of Na$^+$ but not of K$^+$ from lumen to cell, the Na–K exchange system can give a net active, transcellular transport of Na$^+$ from lumen to peritubular space. K$^+$ is transported into the cell across the abluminal membrane, but diffuses out across the same membrane (Kofoed-Johnsen and Ussing, 1958).

The lumen-to-cell gradient for Na$^+$ created by the Na–K transport abluminal may be used for an uphill transport of Cl$^-$ from lumen to cell, either on a Cl$^-$ carrier which is driven by the Na$^+$ gradient, or on a Cl$^-$–HCO$_3^-$ exchange carrier coupled to a Na$^+$–H$^+$ carrier via the intracellular H$_2$CO$_3 \rightleftharpoons$ H$^+$ + HCO$_3^-$ reaction. With a luminal membrane which only allows carrier-mediated coupled Na$^+$–Cl$^-$ transfer, and with an abluminal membrane which is permeable to Cl$^-$, Cl$^-$ transported into the cell from lumrn by the Na$^+$ gradient will flow passively out through the abluminal membrane, driven by its electrochemical gradient.

References

Baker, P. F., Foster, R. F., Gilbert, D. S. and Shaw, T. I. (1971). Sodium transport by perfused giant axons of Loligo. *J. Physiol., Lond.* **219**, 487–506.
Burg, M. B. and Green, N. (1973). Function of the thick ascending limb of Henle's loop. *Am. J. Physiol.* **224**, 659–668.

Garrahan, P. J. and Glynn, I. M. (1967a). The sensitivity of the sodium pump to external sodium. *J. Physiol., Lond.* **192**, 175–188.

Garrahan, P. J. and Glynn, I. M. (1967b). Factors affecting the relative magnitudes of the sodium : potassium and sodium : sodium exchanges catalysed by the sodium pump. *J. Physiol., Lond.* **192**, 189–216.

Garrahan, P. J. and Glynn, I. M. (1967c). The incorporation of inorganic phosphate into adenosine triphosphate by reversal of the sodium pump. *J. Physiol., Lond.* **192**, 237–256.

Glynn, I. M. (1968). Membrane ATPase and cation transport. *Br. med. Bull.* **24**, 165.

Glynn, I. M. and Hoffman, J. F. (1971). Nucleotide requirements for sodium–sodium exchange catalysed by the sodium pump in human red cells. *J. Physiol., Lond.* **218**, 239–256.

Glynn, I. M. and Karlish, S. J. D. (1974). The association of biochemical events and cation movements in (Na : K) dependent adenosine triphosphatase activity. In *Membrane Adenosine Triphosphatase and Transport Processes* (R. Bronk, ed.), Biochemical Society Special Publication 4, The Biochemical Society, London, pp. 145–158.

Glynn, I. M., Hoffman, J. F. and Lew, V. L. (1971). Some "partial reactions" of the sodium pump. *Phil. Trans. R. Soc. B* **262**, 91–102.

Glynn, I. M., Lew, V. L. and Lüthi, U. (1970). Reversal of the potassium entry mechanism in red cells, with and without reversal of the entire pump cycle. *J. Physiol., Lond.* **207**, 371–391.

Jørgensen, P. L. (1975). Isolation and characterization of the components of the sodium pump. *Q. Rev. Biophys.* **7**, 239–274.

Jørgensen, P. L. (1976). The function of Na, K-ATPase in the thick ascending limb of Henle's loop. In *Current Problems in Clinical Biochemistry*, Vol. 6, *Renal Metabolism in Relation to Renal Function* (U. Schmidt and C. Dubach, eds), Hans Huber Publishers, Bern, pp. 190–199.

Karlish, S. J. D. and Glynn, I. M. (1974). An uncoupled efflux of Na from human red cells probably associated with Na dependent ATPase activity. *Ann. N.Y. Acad. Sci.* **242**, 461–470.

Kahn, T., Bosch, J., Levitt, M. F. and Goldstein, M. H. (1975). Effect of sodium nitrate loading on electrolyte transport by the renal tubule. *Am. J. Physiol.* **229**, 746–753.

Kofoed-Johnsen, V. and Ussing, H. H. (1958). The nature of the frog skin potential. *Acta physiol. scand.* **42**, 298–308.

Lant, A. F., Priestland, R. N. and Whittam, R. (1970). The coupling of downhill ion movements associated with reversal of the sodium pump in human red cells. *J. Physiol., Lond.* **207**, 291–301.

Lew, V. L., Hardy, M. A. and Ellory, J. C. (1973). The uncoupled extrusion of Na^+ through the Na^+ pump. *Biochim. biophys. Acta* **323**, 251–266.

Lie, M., Sejersted, O. M., Raeder, M. and Kiil, F. (1974). Comparison of renal responses to ouabain and ethacrynic acid. *Am. J. Physiol.* **226**, 1221–1226.

Maunsbach, A. B., Deguchi, N. and Jørgensen, P. L. (1978). Ultrastructure of purified Na, K ATPase. In *Membrane Proteins, 11th FEBS Meeting, Copenhagen 1977* (P. Nicholls, J. V. Møller, P. L. Jørgensen and A. J. Moody, eds), Pergamon Press, Oxford, pp. 173–181.

Post, R. L., Sen, A. K. and Rosenthal, A. S. (1965). A phosphorylated intermediate in adenosine triphosphate dependent sodium and potassium transport across kidney membranes. *J. biol. Chem.* **240**, 1437–1445.

Robinson, J. D. (1967). Kinetic studies on a brain microsomal adenosine triphosphatase. Evidence suggesting conformational changes. *Biochemistry* **6**, 3250–3258.

Rocha, A. S. and Kokko, J. P. (1973). Sodium chloride and water transport in the medullary thick ascending limb of Henle: evidence for active chloride transport. *J. clin. Invest.* **52**, 612–623.

Sejersted, O. M., Lie, M. and Kiil, F. (1971). Effect of ouabain on metabolic rate in renal cortex and medulla. *Am. J. Physiol.* **220**, 1488–1493.

Skou, J. C. (1965). Enzymatic basis for active transport of Na$^+$ and K$^+$ across cell membrane. *Physiol. Rev.* **45**, 596–617.

Skou, J. C. (1974a). Effect of ATP on the intermediary steps of the reaction of the (Na$^+$ + K$^+$)-dependent enzyme system. I. Studied by the use of *N*-ethylmaleimide inhibition as a tool. *Biochim. biophys. Acta* **339**, 234–245.

Skou, J. C. (1974b). Effect of ATP on the intermediary steps of the reaction of the (Na$^+$ + K$^+$)-dependent enzyme system. II. Effect of a variation in the ATP/Mg^{2+} ratio. *Biochim. biophys. Acta* **339**, 246–257.

Skou, J. C. (1975). The (Na$^+$ + K$^+$) activated enzyme system and its relationship to transport of sodium and potassium. *Q. Rev. Biophys.* **7**, 401–434.

Thomas, R. C. (1972). Electrogenic sodium pump in nerve and muscle cells. *Physiol. Rev.* **52**, 563–594.

13
Quantification of Intracellular Elements in Frog Skin and Tubular Cells under Different Functional Conditions by Means of Electron Microprobe Analysis

Klaus Thurau, Adolf Dörge, Roger Rick, Richard Bauer, Franz Beck, June Mason and Christiane Roloff

Introduction

The understanding of transepithelial movements of elements presumes the knowledge of the cellular concentrations. Since most epithelia are composed of different cell types, with possibly different transport properties, the analysis of intracellular element concentrations has to be performed on a cellular scale. The present paper deals with the analysis of electrolyte concentrations in individual epithelial cells of frog skin and rat kidney cortex using the technique of electron microprobe analysis.

Methods

Energy dispersive X-ray microanalysis (EDAX, Link, FDR) was performed on freeze-dried cryosections in a scanning electron microscope (Cambridge S 4). The acceleration voltage used was 17 kV, and the probe current selected was 0·5 nA. Areas of 0·3–1 μm^2 were scanned for 200 s and the emitted X-rays were analysed in the energy range between 0·6 and 4 keV, including the K-lines of the elements Na to Ca. The discrimination between characteristic and uncharacteristic radiations (*Bremsstrahlung*) was performed using a computer program.

In order to avoid dislocation of electrolytes the biological tissue was shock-frozen in propane at −180 °C, cut into sections of about 1 μm thickness at −80 °C (Reichert OMU 2) and freeze-dried at −80 °C and 10⁻⁶ torr. Immediately prior to shock-freezing, the tissue was covered with a thin layer of 20 g per cent albumin Ringer's solution, thus providing an internal standard for quantification. The cellular electrolyte concentrations were evaluated by comparing the intensities of the characteristic radiations obtained in the cells with those in the albumin standard layer. Further details of the preparation procedure are published elsewhere (Dörge *et al.*, 1978).

Localization of the Na Transport Compartment in Frog Skin Epithelium

Since the fundamental work of Koefoed-Johnson and Ussing (1958) it is generally accepted that transepithelial Na transport in frog skin is achieved

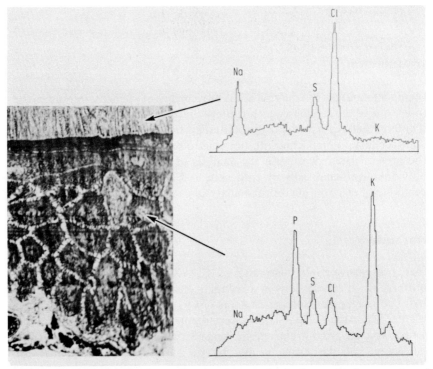

FIG. 1. *Scanning transmission electron micrograph of a freeze-dried cryosection of frog skin epithelium (about 1 μm thick) and two X-ray spectra obtained in the albumin standard layer (upper spectrum) and in a spiny cell (lower spectrum).*

by a passive entrance of Na into the cellular transport compartment at the apical side and an active extrusion at the basal side. In order to clarify the localization of this transport compartment, the influx or efflux of Na into or out of the transport compartment was altered and the electrolyte concentrations were measured in the different cell layers of the epithelium. The experiments were performed on isolated abdominal skins of *Rana temporaria* and *Rana esculenta* in Ussing-type chambers under short-circuited conditions.

Figure 1 shows a scanning electron micrograph of a freeze-dried frog skin section together with two energy-dispersive X-ray spectra. The different epithelial layers (stratum corneum, granulosum, spinosum and germinativum) are easily discernible. The slightly lighter pear-shaped cell corresponds to a mitochondria-rich cell. The upper spectrum was obtained in the albumin standard layer adherent to the epithelial surface, the lower spectrum in a cell in the stratum spinosum. Compared to the extracellular standard

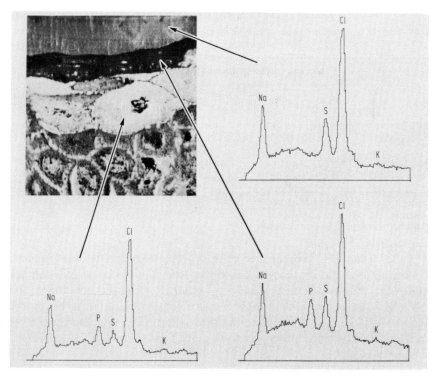

FIG. 2. *Scanning transmission electron micrograph of a freeze-dried cryosection of from skin epithelium (about 1 μm thick) and three X-ray spectra obtained in the albumin standard layer (upper spectrum), in the stratum corneum (lower spectrum, right) and in a light cell of the first living cell layer (lower spectrum, left).*

spectrum, the cellular spectrum shows lower peaks for Na and Cl and higher peaks for P and K.

Similar X-ray spectra as in the stratum spinosum cell were observed in almost all cell types, except in the cells of the stratum corneum and in a special cell type which was light and swollen and occasionally appeared as the first layer underneath the stratum corneum. Figure 2 shows that the characteristic peaks of Na, Cl and K of both these structures are very similar to those of the albumin standard layer. Since the intensities of these electrolytes in the stratum corneum and the light and swollen cells were reduced to almost zero when the outside bathing solution was replaced by Na-free Ringer's solution, and were not influenced by the action of substances like amiloride or ouabain, it has to be concluded that these cells represent extracellular compartments and are not at all involved in transepithelial Na transport.

TABLE I

Cytoplasmic and nuclear concentrations of elements in frog skin epithelium obtained by electron microprobe anlalysis[a]

	Concentration (mmol/kg wet weight)					
	Na	K	P	Cl	Ca	Dry weight (g%)
Cytoplasm	7·4	111·8	98·8	36·5	1·1	25·4
	± 4·5	± 12·1	± 19·2	± 5·0	± 1·2	± 2·3
Nucleus	5·1	115·0	144·4	32·9	0·3	21·8
	± 3·9	± 11·4	± 19·1[b]	± 3·7[b]	± 0·6[bc]	± 1·9[b]

[a] Mean values ± standard deviation, $n = 19$.
[b] Significantly different from the cytoplasmic value, $2p < 0.05$.
[c] Not significantly different from zero.

Table I shows a comparison of the cytoplasmic and nuclear element concentrations and dry weight content in frog skin epithelial cells. Under control conditions, as well as under all other experimental conditions, the Na and K concentrations in both compartments were found to be almost identical. In contrast, the P concentration of the cytoplasm was lower than in the nucleus, whereas the concentration of Cl and Ca and of the dry weight content was higher.

To get some more information about the localization of the Na transport compartment, the cellular electrolyte concentrations were measured after blocking the active transport step with ouabain (Zerahn, 1969; Nagel and Dörge, 1971) and the passive transport step with amiloride (Eigler *et al.*,

1967; Dörge and Nagel, 1970; Moreno *et al.*, 1973; Rick *et al.*, 1975) or Na-free Ringer's solution in the outside bathing medium.

As demonstrated by the two spectra in Fig. 3, which were obtained from spiny cells, the application of ouabain (10^{-4} M, 90 min) to the corial side caused an increase in Na and a decrease in K concentration. As can be seen from Fig. 4 these alterations in Na and K concentrations after ouabain treatment could be observed in all epithelial cell layers. The average Na concentration increased after ouabain treatment from 10 to 110, and the K concentration decreased by almost the same amount from 120 to 18 mmol/kg wet weight. However, the effect of ouabain upon cellular Na and K

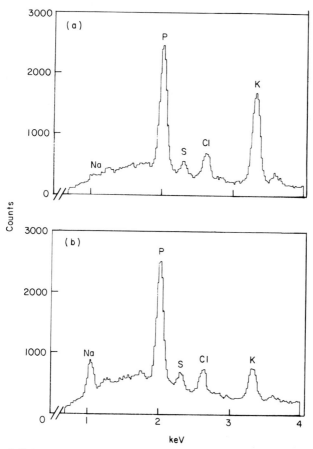

FIG. 3. *Cellular X-ray spectra obtained in the stratum spinosum under control conditions (a) and after ouabain treatment (b) (10^{-4}M, 90 min).*

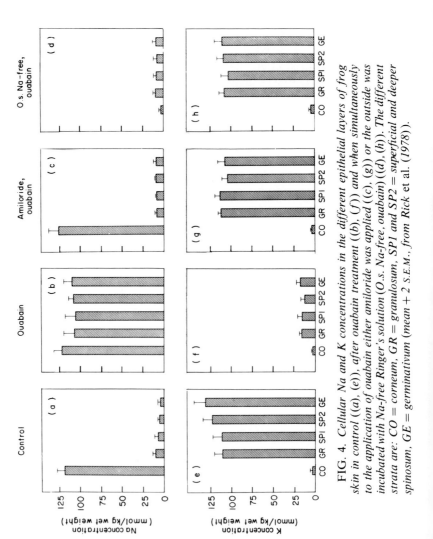

FIG. 4. *Cellular Na and K concentrations in the different epithelial layers of frog skin in control ((a), (e)), after ouabain treatment ((b), (f)) and when simultaneously to the application of ouabain either amiloride was applied ((c), (g)) or the outside was incubated with Na-free Ringer's solution (O.s. Na-free, ouabain) ((d), (h)). The different strata are: CO = corneum, GR = granulosum, SP1 and SP2 = superficial and deeper spinosum, GE = germinativum (mean + 2 s.e.m., from Rick et al. (1978)).*

concentrations was completely abolished, when, in addition to ouabain, either amiloride (10^{-4} M) was applied to the epithelial side, or the Ringer's solution of the epithelial side was Na-free. Under both experimental conditions the Na concentration remained as low and the K concentration as high as in the control.

The results demonstrate that the cellular accumulation of Na after oubain is caused by an influx of Na from the outside bathing medium. Therefore, all epithelial layers (aside from the stratum corneum) show the characteristic features of a Na transport compartment as suggested by Ussing and Windhager (1964).

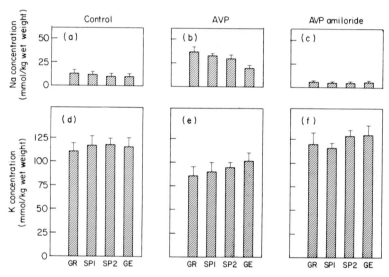

FIG. 5. *Cellular Na and K concentrations in the different epithelial layers of frog skin in control ((a), (d)), after arginine vasopressin (AVP) ((b), (e)) and when after 90 min incubation with arginine vasopressin amiloride was applied ((c), (f)). The abbreviations used for the different strata are the same as in Fig. 4 (mean $\pm$ 2 S.E.M.).*

Similar conclusions can be drawn from experiments performed under the action of antidiuretic hormone, which is thought to increase the transepithelial Na transport by increasing the Na permeability of the apical membrane (Cereijido and Rotunno, 1971; Biber and Cruz, 1973). Figure 5 shows that after application of arginine vasopressin (0·2 U/ml) to the corial side the Na concentration is increased, whereas that of K is decreased in all epithelial cell layers, and that this effect could be abolished by the additional application of amiloride. However, since the increase in Na concentration after arginine vasopressin was also abolished when the corial bathing medium was Na-free Ringer's solution, it is possible that the increased Na concentration is due to an enhanced cellular Na influx from the epithelial and from the corial side.

However, it appears that the syncytial Na transport compartment comprises only the cells of the various living epithelial layers, and does not include the gland cells and mitochondria-rich cells of the epithelium. Varying from the other epithelial cells, the gland cells showed only a small increase in their Na concentration after ouabain. In the mitochondria-rich cells, the increase in the cellular Na concentration after ouabain could not be abolished by amiloride. The most striking difference between gland cells and those of the different epithelial layers lay in the fact that their cellular electrolyte concentrations were almost unaffected by ouabain. Compared to the cells of the epithelial cell layers, the mitochondria-rich cells showed a much less pronounced K/Na exchange, which, however, could not be abolished by the action of amiloride. Also, the electrolyte concentrations of the mitochondria-rich cells were not affected by arginine vasopressin, providing an additional argument against the involvement of mitochondria-rich cells in the functional syncitium.

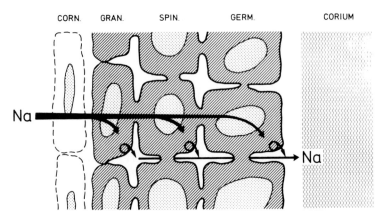

FIG. 6. *Diagrammatic representation of Na movement through the frog skin.*

Figure 6 shows schematically the transepithelial Na transport pathway in frog skin as derived from the present results. Na enters the cellular compartment across the outer cell membrane of the outermost living cell layer by a passive step, which can be blocked by amiloride. Compared to the inner facing cell membranes, this membrane is highly permeable to Na. Na passes via intercellular connections from the outer into the deeper cell layers and is extruded actively across the inner facing cell membranes into the intercellular spaces, from which it diffuses toward the corium.

The question, however, whether all cells of the different layers are involved to the same extent in the transepithelial Na transport can not be answered by the present data. In principle, the transepithelial Na transport could be accomplished by only a single cell type, to which the other cells of the epithelium are coupled. Since, however, recent distribution studies of ouabain binding sites (Mills *et al.*, 1977) have demonstrated that all the inner facing membranes of the epithelium are potential sites of active Na transport, it seems more probable that each cell layer contributes significantly to transepithelial Na transport.

Influence of Renal Ischaemia upon Tubular Electrolyte Concentrations

Temporary renal ischaemia, which has often been used as a model of acute renal failure, is known to result in a reduction of tubular salt and water reabsorption (Tanner *et al.*, 1973, 1976). In order to determine whether the impairment of tubular reabsorption is accompanied by alterations in cellular electrolyte concentrations, measurements were performed at different stages of renal ischaemia and after reflow of renal blood.

The experiments were conducted on male Sprague-Dawley rats, which were anaesthetized by intraperitoneal injection of 100 mg/kg body weight inactin. The left kidney was exposed by a flank incision, freed from adhering connective tissue and placed in a lucite cup. Rectal temperature was maintained at 37–38 °C by means of a heated operation table. A weakly sprung clip was used to clamp the renal artery. The sections were obtained from superficial regions of the renal cortex.

Since measurements in the region of the basolateral infoldings and the brush borders provided clear evidence that extracellular spaces are also excited during analysis, all the measurements were performed in the nuclei of the cells. However, the results obtained in the cytoplasm near the nuclei for Na, Cl and K were very similar to those of the nuclei themselves. It therefore seems justified to consider these measurements as representative for the entire cell.

Intracellular electrolyte concentrations in normal tubules
Figure 7 shows a scanning electron micrograph of a freeze-dried cryosection of rat kidney cortex under control conditions together with two X-ray spectra. The nuclei can easily be distinguished from the slightly darker surrounding cytoplasm. The characteristic feature which differentiates distal from

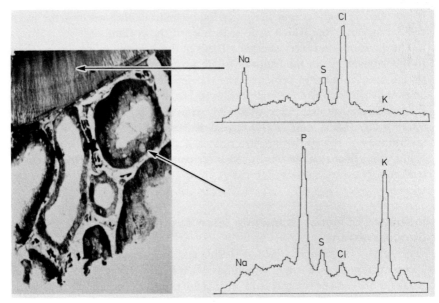

FIG. 7. *Scanning transmission electron micrograph of a freeze-dried section of rat kidney and X-ray spectra obtained in the albumin standard layer (upper spectrum) and in the nucleus of a proximal tubule (lower spectrum).*

proximal tubules is the pronounced appearance of microvilli in the latter. Compared to the upper X-ray spectrum obtained in the extracellular albumin standard layer, the lower spectrum obtained in the nucleus of a proximal tubular cell shows smaller peaks for Na and Cl and higher peaks for P and K.

Table II shows the mean intracellular concentrations in normal kidneys for the proximal and distal tubules. The Na and Cl concentrations of the proximal tubule (19 mmol/kg wet weight for Na and 25 for Cl) were significantly higher than those of the distal tubule (11 mmol/kg wet weight

TABLE II

Intracellular concentrations in proximal and distal tubules of normal kidneys[a]

	Concentrations (mmol/kg wet weight)			
	Na	K	Cl	P
Proximal tubules	19 ± 1	131 ± 3	25 ± 1	159 ± 3
Distal tubules	11 ± 1^{b}	131 ± 4	16 ± 1^{b}	187 ± 4^{b}

[a] Values are means $\pm$ S.E.M.;
[b] Significantly different from the cytoplasmic value, $2p < 0.05$.

for Na and 16 for Cl). In contrast, the P concentration of the proximal tubule
of 159 was somewhat lower than that of the distal tubule with 187 mmol/kg
wet weight. For K very similar values of about 131 mmol/kg wet weight
were found in both nephron segments.

Intracellular electrolyte concentrations during ischaemia
During ischaemia the kidney surface was either exposed to normal air or
to 100 per cent nitrogen gas. For ischaemic periods up to 60 min no
significant alteration of the cellular electrolyte concentrations in superficial
tubules were detected when the kidney was kept in air.

Figure 8 shows the Na, Cl and K concentrations after 20 min of ischaemia
in a nitrogen atmosphere. In the proximal tubules the Na and Cl concentrations increased to 76 and 36 mmol/kg wet weight, whereas K concentration
decreased to 89 mmol/kg wet weight. In contrast, in the distal tubule almost
no effect upon the cellular electrolyte concentrations was observed after 20
min ischaemia. At present three possible explanations for the different

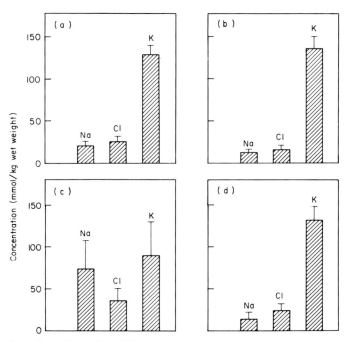

FIG. 8. *Cellular Na, Cl and K concentrations of the proximal and distal tubules
of rat kidney under control conditions and after 20 min of ischaemia (mean + S.D.).
(a) Proximal tubule, control conditions; (b) distal tubule, control conditions; (c)
proximal tubule after ischaemia; (d) distal tubule after ischaemia.*

behaviour of the two tubular segments after short-term ischaemia can be given. Firstly, because of larger energy stores the distal tubular cells may tolerate longer periods of ischaemia; secondly, the basolateral membranes of distal tubule may be less permeable to Na; and thirdly, the access of Na from the interstitium to the luminal membrane is hindered to a greater extent by the tight junctions of the distal than by those of the proximal tubules.

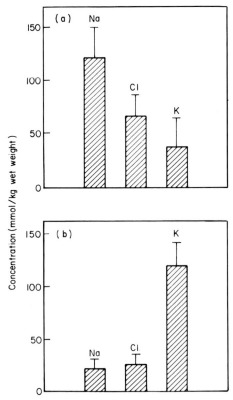

Fig. 9. *Cellular Na, Cl and K concentrations of rat kidney (a) after 60 min of ischaemia and (b) after 60 min of ischaemia and 60 min of renal blood reflow (mean + S.D.).*

Figure 9 shows the cellular electrolyte concentrations after 60 min of ischaemia in a nitrogen atmosphere and after 60 min of renal blood reflow. Since, under this condition, the electrolyte concentrations of the proximal and distal tubules showed no systematic differences, the data in Fig. 9 were pooled. After ischaemia the Na concentration increased to 121 mmol/kg wet weight while the K concentration decreased by almost the same amount of about 100 to 37 mmol/kg wet weight. At the same time the Cl concentration increased to 66 mmol/kg wet weight.

The cell swelling during ischaemia known from morphological studies (Flores *et al.*, 1972; Frega *et al.*, 1976; Glaumann *et al.*, 1977) is reflected in the present investigation by a decrease in the P concentration of about 25 per cent. In addition, the observed increase in the cellular Cl concentration agrees well with the view of cellular uptake of extracellular fluid.

In order to determine whether the changes in cellular electrolyte concentrations resulting from ischaemia were reversible, reflow was permitted for 60 min after the ischaemic period. As can be seen from Fig. 9(b), 60 min after opening the arterial clamp, the Na, K and Cl values had almost returned to their control levels.

The observed differences in the electrolyte concentrations in the proximal and distal tubule in the control and after short-term ischaemia may result from functional differences between the two nephron segments. On the other hand, the impairment of renal functions following ischaemia is apparently not reflected in a disturbance of the cellular electrolyte distribution since electrolyte concentrations were found to be almost completely restored after 60 min of blood reflow.

Acknowledgement

Supported by the Deutsche Forschungsgemeinschaft.

References

Biber, T. U. L. and Cruz, L. J. (1973). Effect of antidiuretic hormone on sodium uptake across the outer surface of frog skin. *Am. J. Physiol.* **225**, 912–917.

Cereijido, M. and Rotunno, C. A. (1971). The effect of antidiuretic hormone on Na movement across frog skin. *J. Physiol., Lond.* **213**, 119–133.

Dörge, A. and Nagel, W. (1970). Effect of amiloride on sodium transport in the frog skin. II. Sodium transport pool and unidirectional fluxes. *Pflügers Arch. ges. Physiol.* **321**, 91–101.

Dörge, A., Rick, R., Gehring, K. and Thurau, K. (1978). Preparation of freeze-dried cryosections for quantitative X-ray microanalysis of electrolytes in biological soft tissues. *Pflügers Arch. ges. Physiol.* **373**, 85–97.

Eigler, J., Kelter, J. and Renner, E. (1967). Wirkungscharakteristika eines neuen Acylguanidins—Amiloride-HCl (MK 870)—an der isolierten Haut von Amphibien. *Klin. Wschr.* **14**, 737–738.

Flores, J., DiBona, D. R., Frega, N. and Leaf, A. (1972). Cell volume regulation and ischemic tissue damage. *J. Membrane Biol.* **10**, 331–343.

Frega, N. S., DiBona. D. R., Guertler, B. and Leaf, A. (1976). Ischemic renal injury. *Kidney Int.* **10**, S17–S25.

Glaumann, B., Glaumann, H., Berezesky, I. K. and Trump, B. F. (1977). Studies on cellular recovery from injury. II. Ultrastructural studies on the recovery of the pars convoluta of the proximal tubule of the rat kidney from temporary ischaemia. *Virchows Arch. B. Cell Path.* **24**, 1–18.

Koefoed-Johnson, V. and Ussing, H. H. (1958). The nature of the frog skin potential. *Acta physiol. scand.* **42**, 298–308.

Mills, J. W., Ernst, S. A. and DiBona, D. R. (1977). Localization of Na^+-pump sites in frog skin. *J. Cell Biol.* **73**, 88–110.

Moreno, J. H., Reisin, I. L., Rodriguez Boulan, E., Rotunno, C. A. and Cereijido, M. (1973). Barriers to sodium movement across frog skin. *J. Membrane Biol.* **11**, 99–115.

Nagel, W. and Dörge, A. (1971). A study of the different sodium compartments and the transepithelial sodium fluxes of the frog skin with the use of ouabain. *Pflügers Arch. ges. Physiol.* **324**, 267–278.

Rick, R., Dörge, A. and Nagel, W. (1975). Influx and efflux of sodium at the outer surface of frog skin. *J. Membrane Biol.* **22**, 183–196.

Rick, R., Dörge, A., v. Arnim, E. and Thurau, K. (1978). Electron microprobe analysis of frog skin epithelium: evidence for a syncytial sodium transport compartment. *J. Membrane Biol.* **39**, 313–331.

Tanner, G. A., Sloan, K. L. and Sophasan, S. (1973). Effects of renal artery occlusion on kidney function in the rat. *Kidney Int.* **4**, 377–389.

Tanner, G. A. and Sophasan, S. (1976). Kidney pressures after temporary renal artery occlusion in the rat. *Am. J. Physiol.* **230**, 1173–1181.

Ussing, H. H. and Windhager, E. (1964). Nature of shunt path and active sodium transport path through frog skin epithelium. *Acta physiol. scand.* **61**, 484–504.

Zerahn, K. (1969). Nature and localization of the sodium pool during active transport in the isolated frog skin. *Acta physiol. scand.* **77**, 272–281.

14
Morphologic Evaluation of Paracellular Pathways in the Mammalian Nephron

C. Craig Tisher

Introduction

There is mounting evidence derived from various physiologic and electro-physiologic studies that many epithelia possess a low resistance paracellular shunt pathway in parallel with a high resistance pathway, the latter located across the apical and basolateral plasmalemma of the cell (Boulpaep and Seely, 1971; Frömter, 1972; Frömter and Diamond, 1972; Frizzell and Schultz, 1972; Grandchamp and Boulpaep, 1974; Berry and Boulpaep, 1975; Schafer *et al.*, 1975). These so-called "leaky" epithelia are characterized by a relatively low transepithelial potential difference when bathed in solutions having identical ionic composition and offer limited resistance to trans-epithelial ionic diffusion (Schultz, 1977). Most investigators believe that the shunt pathway is composed of a non-occluding tight junction (*zonula occludens*) and the basolateral intercellular space. While there appears to be little doubt that paracellular pathways afford the opportunity for trans-epithelial ionic diffusion, in some epithelia there is evidence that this shunt pathway may also provide a major route for transepithelial water flow in response to an osmotic pressure difference. The data supporting this hypothesis have been summarized recently by Schultz (1977).

The morphologic technique of freeze-fracture electron microscopy and the use of certain ultrastructural tracers combined with improved methods of tissue preservation have proven useful in the delineation of both transcellular and extracellular routes of solute and fluid movement in several trans-porting epithelia, including the various segments of the mammalian renal tubule. In general an excellent correlation has been found in the renal tubule between the electrophysiologic evidence and the ultrastructural tracer data that support the presence of paracellular shunt pathways (Tisher and Yarger, 1973, 1975; Martinez-Palomo and Erlij, 1973). With certain possible exceptions, a similar positive correlation has been appreciated with freeze-fracture electron microscopy (Claude and Goodenough, 1973). These structural–functional relationships will be explored in subsequent sections of this presentation. The ultrastructural tracer studies to be described were performed with lanthanum hydroxide and lanthanum chloride using standard micropuncture techniques as previously described (Tisher and Yarger, 1973, 1975). The freeze-fracture studies were performed on kidneys derived from non-diseased Sprague-Dawley rats and from Long Evans hooded rats with hereditary hypothalamic diabetes insipidus (M. Dratwa and C. C. Tisher, unpublished observations).

Proximal Tubule

In the mammalian kidney observations derived from ultrastructural tracer studies employing lanthanum have been limited to the proximal convoluted tubule (PCT). No attempt has been made to evaluate either the pars recta (PR) or the individual segments (S_1–S_3) that are known to characterize the rat proximal tubule (Maunsbach, 1966c). The tight junction of the PCT is a belt-like structure that surrounds the entire cell and is quite shallow, ranging in depth from 200 to 400 Å in the rat as viewed with thin section electron microscopy (Farquhar and Palade, 1963). The tight junction of the PCT is freely permeable to lanthanum (Fig. 1). In studies from our laboratory (Tisher and Yarger, 1973) the tracer was found to be capable of penetrating the tight junction when introduced from either the luminal or antiluminal side. The intermediate junction or *zonula adherens* offered no resistance to lanthanum penetration. Similar observations have been reported by Martinez-Palomo and Erlij (1973), also in rat proximal tubules. Larsson (1975) observed that the tight junctions of proximal tubules of immature non-filtering nephrons were completely permeable to colloidal lanthanum and horse-radish peroxidase, while complete penetration by colloidal lanthanum was not found in proximal tubules of mature nephrons. Lanthanum permeability of the tight junction has also been demonstrated in the proximal tubule of the toad kidney (Wittembury and Rawlins, 1971).

Freeze-fracture electron microscopy of the rat PCT (Fig. 2) reveals a tight junction that is usually composed of one or two strands (equivalent to ridges on the P face and grooves on the E face[a]) (Pricam et al., 1974; Roesinger

---

[a] According to the freeze-etching nomenclature recently proposed by Branton et al. (1975), the membrane fracture face closest to the protoplasm is designated the P face, the E face corresponding to the face closest to the extracellular space.

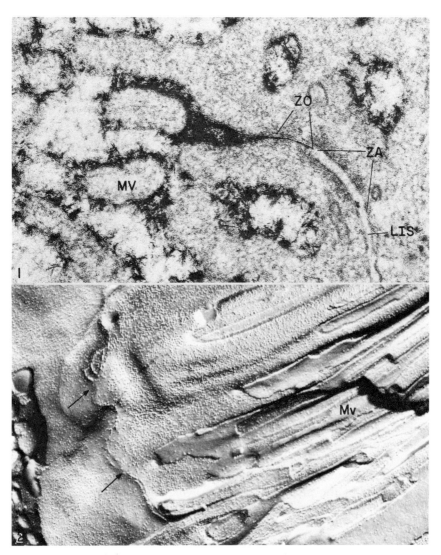

FIG. 1. *Oblique section through apical region of epithelium of a PCT from a normovolemic rat. Individual microvilli (MV) in oblique and cross section on the left are surrounded by lanthanum. The tracer has penetrated the entire* zonula occludens *(ZO) from the luminal surface to the region of the* zonula adherens *(ZA). LIS, lateral intercellular space. (From Tisher and Yarger (1973).)* × 90 000.

FIG. 2. *Freeze-fracture replica through the apical region of rat PCT. In this region the tight junction is composed of two strands that are often discontinuous (arrows). Mv, microvilli.* × 30 000.

et al., 1978). Kühn and Reale (1975) have reported similar findings in the human kidney. Up to 10 per cent of the strands are discontinuous in the rat PCT (Roesinger *et al.*, 1978). It appears quite possible that lanthanum may penetrate some of the tight junctions of the rat PCT by infiltrating through the gaps of these discontinuous strands. Although there is little interspecies variation in junctional morphology in the PCT, it has been observed that the rat and the tree shrew (*Tupaia belangeri*) have discontinuous strands, while the PCT of cat, dog, rabbit and golden hamsters lack such gaps (Roesinger *et al.*, 1978). With the exception of the rabbit the tight junction of the PR has been found to be considerably more elaborate in those animals in which it has been examined (Roesinger *et al.*, 1978).

The demonstration that the tight junction of the rat PCT is permeable to lanthanum and is formed by just one or two strands, many of which are discontinuous, provides strong morphologic evidence that this particular segment of the renal tubule is "leaky" in character due to the presence of a paracellular shunt pathway. The morphologic findings correlate nicely with published electrophysiologic data derived from the rat that also indicate the existence of the shunt pathway. For instance, Hegel *et al.* (1967) recorded a transepithelial electrical resistance of only 5–7 Ω cm^2.

Several studies have provided evidence that alterations in the structure of the tight junction can be seen in physiologic conditions in which enhanced movement of solutes and water, presumably via the paracellular pathway, has been demonstrated. Bentzel (1972), studying *Necturus* kidney during volume expansion, noted that the mean length of the tight junction of proximal tubules decreased and the juxtaluminal portion of the tight junction widened during volume expansion. Bulger *et al.* (1974) demonstrated non-fusion of many of the adjacent cell membranes in the region of the tight junction of proximal tubules in which the intraluminal pressure was elevated via partial renal vein occlusion or an increase in ureteral pressure. Both conditions are known to be associated with an increase in the permeability of the proximal tubule (Lorentz *et al.*, 1972). Elevation of intraluminal pressure in flounder proximal tubules results in the passage of ferritin and thorotrast from lumen to intercellular space, probably via reversible opening of the tight junctions (Ottosen, 1976). The passage of the tracer, microperoxidase (molecular weight 1800 daltons), through the tight junctions of isolated proximal tubules of neonatal rabbits under conditions

FIG. 3. *Electron micrograph illustrating lanthanum penetration of the tight junction (arrow) in a TALH from a rat with hypothalamic diabetes insipidus.* × 56 000.

FIG. 4. *Freeze-fracture replica through the apical region of a TALH from a rat. The tight junction is formed by four to six anastomosing strands that are closely packed (arrow).* × 81 000.

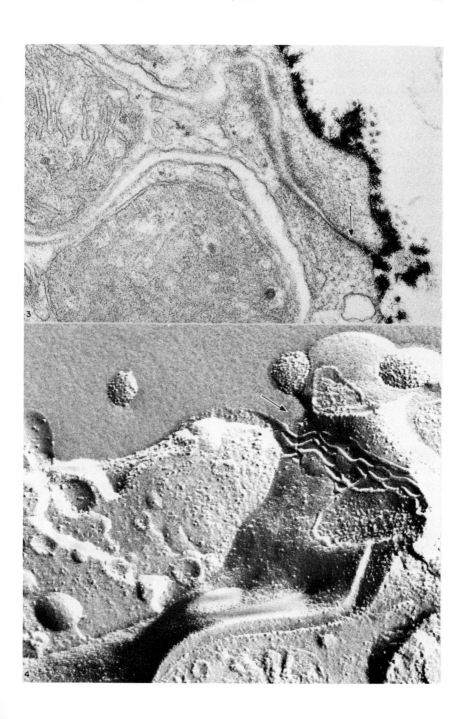

of increased intraluminal pressure has also been described (Horster and Larsson, 1976). However, in contradistinction to the earlier findings of Bulger *et al.* (1974) derived from the rat, intraluminal pressure elevations of 20 cm H_2O failed to cause similar alterations in the tight junctions of proximal tubules dissected from mature rabbits.

Recently, Humbert *et al.* (1976), employing freeze-fracture techniques, found that tight junctions of proximal tubules of *Necturus maculosus* were markedly altered during saline diuresis. When compared with control tubules, there was a reduction in the number of individual strands or fibrils forming the tight junction and those that were present had more frequent and extensive gaps or interruptions. Enhanced back-leak of sodium, presumably via a paracellular pathway, has been demonstrated under similar physiologic conditions (Boulpaep, 1972).

The establishment of a transtubular osmotic gradient by making the tubule lumen hypertonic with urea or mannitol has also been demonstrated to widen the tight junction reversibly and, in the case of urea, to increase the magnitude of lanthanum crossing the tight junction from the antiluminal surface (Rawlins *et al.*, 1975). Earlier studies conducted under similar physiologic conditions demonstrated enhanced movement of several non-electrolyte extracellular marker molecules into the tubule lumen from the portal circulation, presumably via a functional paracellular pathway (Pérez-Gonzalez and Whittembury, 1974). Thus, there is considerable structural–functional evidence pointing toward the existence of a functional paracellular shunt pathway for ion and fluid movement in the renal proximal tubule of several animals.

Distal Tubule[a]

Standard thin section electron microscopy of the thick ascending limb of Henle (TALH) reveals a tight junction that is quite deep and has an appearance similar to "occluding" types of tight junctions usually found in epithelia that possess a relatively large transepithelial electrical resistance. However, studies with lanthanum (C. C. Tisher and W. E. Yarger, unpublished observations) reveal penetration of the extracellular tracer into the tight junction (Fig. 3). Preliminary data (M. Dratwa and C. C. Tisher, unpublished observations) derived from freeze-fracture studies in the rat reveal tight junctions in the TALH formed by four to six strands that are closely

[a] The distal tubule of the rat kidney, as defined by the morphologist, is composed of three segments or specialized regions that are histologically distinct. These include the thick ascending limb of Henle (*pars recta*), the macula densa (*pars maculata*) and the distal convoluted tuble (*pars convoluta*).

packed and exhibit occasional anastomoses with one another (Fig. 4). The appearance resembles that of the tight junction in the distal convoluted tubule. Kühn and Reale (1975) reported that tight junctions of the pars recta of the distal tubule in the human kidney generally had five or more strands arranged linearly that ran parallel to one another with only partial anastomoses. In a few cases only one strand was observed. If the ability of lanthanum to penetrate a tight junction is sufficient to establish the presence of a potential paracellular shunt pathway, the presence of such a pathway in the TALH would not appear to be of major importance for transepithelial water flow in light of the fact that this region of the nephron is relatively impermeable to water (Rocha and Kokko, 1973; Burg and Green, 1973). *In vivo* measurements of transepithelial resistance in this region of the renal tubule have not been performed because of a lack of accessibility to standard micropuncture and electrophysiologic techniques.

In the distal convoluted tubule (DCT) of the rat, early studies using thin section electron microscopy (Farquhar and Palade, 1963) revealed a tight junction with a depth of approximately 0·3 μm. Despite this configuration, however, lanthanum was found to penetrate freely the tight junction between individual cells of the DCT (Fig. 5) (Tisher and Yarger, 1973), findings that have been confirmed by other investigators (Martinez-Palomo and Erlij, 1973).

Freeze-fracture electron microscopic studies of rat (Pricam *et al.*, 1974), mouse (Claude and Goodenough, 1973), and human (Kühn and Reale, 1975) kidney have demonstrated the presence of five or six ridges or strands that usually run parallel to one another and are relatively closely packed in the DCT (Fig. 6). While the strands exhibit relatively few branchings, abrupt transitions in the number of strands and their overall appearance are common. Discontinuities are frequently visible and, as in the PCT, may account for the ability of lanthanum to enter the tight junction. Thus, both the tracer and the freeze-fracture data are consistent with the presence of a potential paracellular shunt pathway. These morphologic findings correlate quite well with the electrophysiologic data of Malnic and Giebisch (1972) that also support the existence of a paracellular shunt pathway in the DCT. These investigators reported a transepithelial electrical resistance of approximately 350 Ω cm² in the distal tubule[a] of the rat.

---

[a] The distal tubule as defined at the micropuncture table, that is, that segment of the nephron beginning at the *macula densa* and extending to the first junction with another renal tubule, is composed of at least two morphologically distinct types of epithelium all of which are accessible to micropuncture. It was not stated explicitly by the authors (Malnic and Giebisch, 1972) whether the values for transepithelial electrical resistance were obtained from that region of the distal tubule that morphologically is composed of epithelium that is typical of the DCT (early "distal" tubule) or the initial collecting tubule (late "distal" tubule).

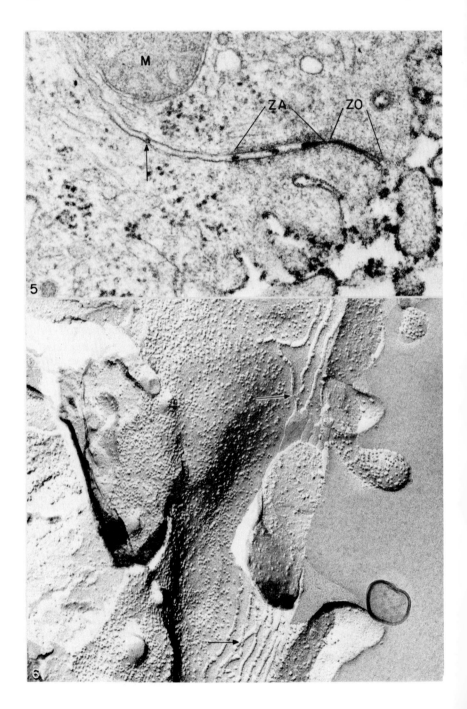

Collecting Duct

For the purposes of this discussion the collecting duct is divided into three major regions, including the cortical segment, the outer medullary segment, and the inner medullary segment. The cortical segment includes the initial collecting tubule, which begins after the transition with the DCT and extends to the first junction with another renal tubule, an arched portion and a medullary ray portion. The inner medullary segment also includes the papillary ducts or ducts of Bellini. As depicted in Fig. 7, ultrastructural tracer studies have demonstrated that the tight junctions of the cortical and outer medullary segments of the collecting duct resist lanthanum penetration (Tisher and Yarger, 1973, 1975). In contrast, those of the inner medullary collecting duct, including the papillary collecting ducts, are freely permeable to lanthanum (Fig. 8) (Tisher and Yarger, 1975). The observations in the cortical collecting duct have been confirmed by others (Martinez-Palomo and Erlij, 1973). These results were not influenced by the presence of vasopressin in any region of the collecting duct that was examined (Tisher and Yarger, 1975), nor were the results in the cortical collecting duct altered by isotonic volume expansion (Tisher and Yarger, 1973).

Freeze-fracture examination of the cortical and outer medullary collecting duct reveals the presence of eight or nine individual strands that form a rather complex anastomosing network (Figs 9 and 10) with an average overall apico-basal depth of 0·3–0·4 μm. Examination of collecting ducts from the inner medulla, including the papilla, reveals a similar configuration of the tight junctions (Fig. 11) despite the fact that these junctional complexes do not resist lanthanum penetration. Thus, in the inner medulla of the rat, a discrepancy does appear to exist in the permeability characteristics of the tight junction when comparing the results of lanthanum tracer data with those derived from freeze-fracture electron microscopy.

The morphologic data derived from the cortical collecting duct correlate well with measurements of transepithelial electrical resistance that have been reported previously (Helman et al., 1971). Working with isolated segments

---

FIG. 5. *Electron micrograph from the apical region of a DCT from a normovolemic rat. Lanthanum is present in the* zonula occludens (ZO) *and has entered the* zonula adherens (ZA) *and the lateral intercellular space (arrow).* M. *mitochondrion. (From Tisher and Yarger (1973).)* ×66 000.

FIG. 6. *Freeze-fracture replica through the apical region of a rat DCT. The tight junction is formed by five or six parallel strands that are relatively closely packed and demonstrate both branching and discontinuities (arrows). (Courtesy of Dr Max Dratwa.)* ×72 000.

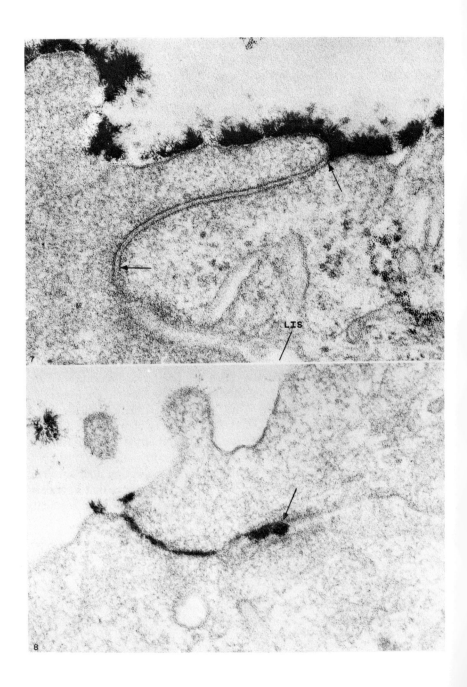

of rabbit cortical collecting tubules these workers recorded a relatively high transepithelial electrical resistance of 867 Ω cm² that was not affected appreciably by the addition of vasopressin to the antiluminal surface of the tubule. Thus, in the cortical collecting duct, and probably throughout the outer medullary collecting duct, the available morphologic and electrophysiologic data are in agreement and fail to provide evidence for the presence of a paracellular shunt pathway for ion and water movement.

In contrast, ultrastructural tracer data support the existence of such a shunt pathway in the inner medullary and papillary segments of the collecting duct. Unfortunately measurements of transepithelial electrical resistance are not currently available in these regions of the collecting duct of the rat or rabbit. However, Rau and Frömter (1974), using indirect techniques, reported an estimated transepithelial electrical resistance value of approximately 1000 Ω cm² in what appears to be the inner medullary collecting duct of the golden hamster. In the absence of lanthanum tracer studies performed in the inner medullary collecting duct of the golden hamster, it is difficult to relate the electrophysiologic data to the morphologic data derived from the rat.

The second major component of the paracellular shunt pathway is the lateral or basolateral intercellular space. Despite general agreement that this compartment is a part of the shunt pathway, attempts to demonstrate changes in its configuration during manipulation of transepithelial ionic diffusion or osmotically driven transepithelial water flow in the kidney have met with varied success. This variation in results can be ascribed, in part, to difficulties in obtaining adequate preservation of the kidney for morphologic investigation. Maunsbach (1966a,b) has clearly established that the size and configuration of the lateral intercellular space can be greatly influenced by the method of fixation that is employed.

In our own laboratory we have utilized the isolated perfused tubule model to evaluate the potential role of the lateral intercellular space in the paracellular shunt pathway (Tisher and Kokko, 1974). Isolated segments of rabbit PCT were subjected to oncotic pressure gradients of varying magnitude known to enhance net transepithelial solute and water flux from lumen to

---

FIG. 7. *Section through apical region of cortical collecting tubule from a normovolemic rat. Lanthanum on the luminal surface of two adjacent cells does not penetrate the tight junction (arrows). LIS, lateral intercellular space. (From Tisher and Yarger (1973).) × 96 000.*

FIG. 8. *Electron micrograph illustrating lanthanum penetration of the tight junction in the papillary segment of a collecting duct from an untreated rat with hypothalamic diabetes insipidus. The lanthanum has extended beyond the tight junction to the level of the intermediate junction (arrow). (From Tisher and Yarger (1975).) × 100 000.*

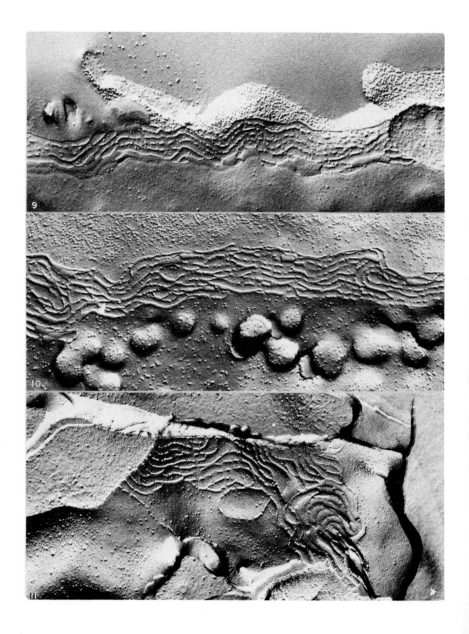

bath. A statistically significant difference in the width of the lateral intercellular space was observed in those tubules subjected to iso-oncotic
(333 ± 36 s.d. Å) and hyperoncotic (367 ± 15 s.d. Å) baths in comparison
with tubules exposed to a protein-free bath of identical osmolality (260 ± 38
s.d. Å; $p < 0.001$). Autoradiographic studies employing ^{125}I-labeled albumin
revealed that the intercellular spaces of those tubules bathed in protein contained albumin which presumably crossed the basement membrane from the
bath. Since albumin is capable of crossing the basement membrane of the
tubule, the oncotic effect of protein in this model is probably not mediated
solely across the basement membrane, but may also affect an osmotic driving
force across the tight junction. If a major component of the increased sodium
and water reabsorption in response to the increase in ambient protein concentration occurs via the paracellular pathway, possibly by decreasing back-
leak, then the studies provide an excellent positive correlation between net
fluid reabsorption and the size of the intercellular space in this particular
model. The studies of Imai and Kokko (1972) also provide additional indirect evidence that the paracellular pathway is involved in the increase in
net sodium and water reabsorption in this model. They found that the
transepithelial potential difference was not affected by altering the concentration of the bath protein, while ^{14}C-labelled sucrose permeability from bath
to lumen, thought to reflect paracellular ion movement, was increased when
the protein concentration was decreased.

In other studies the response of the lateral intercellular space of proximal
tubules to a variety of manipulations that alter the permeability of the renal
tubule and enhance solute and water movement through the paracellular pathway has been varied. Bulger et al. (1974), working with the rat kidney, were
unable to demonstrate consistent widening of the lateral intercellular spaces
of the proximal tubule during elevation of ureteral pressure, a condition that
is known to be associated with an increase in both the intraluminal pressure

---

FIG. 9. *Freeze-fracture replica of a tight junction at the transition from the E to the P face from the cortical collecting duct of a rat. Usually eight or nine strands form a closely packed network. Anatomoses are frequent. The tubule lumen is above. (Courtesy of Dr Max Dratwa.) × 48 000.*

FIG. 10 *Freeze-fracture replica of a tight junction at the transition from the E to the P face from a segment of rat outer medullary collecting duct. The structural organization closely resembles that of the cortical collecting duct (Fig. 9). (Courtesy of Dr Max Dratwa.) × 48 000.*

FIG. 11. *Freeze-fracture replica of a tight junction from a segment of rat papillary collecting duct. The junction is composed of eight to ten closely packed branched strands that have frequent gaps or discontinuities. The tubule lumen is at the extreme right. (Courtesy of Dr Max Dratwa.) × 60 000.*

and the permeability of the proximal tubule (Lorentz *et al.*, 1972). However, in the same study certain tubules exhibited an increased frequency of enlargement of the lateral intercellular space that was said to be especially prominent in the apical region of the cell in animals with partial renal venous constriction, a condition also believed to effect the paracellular shunt pathway. Evan *et al.* (1976) reported that dilatation of lateral intercellular spaces of proximal tubules occurred following volume expansion amounting to 7 per cent of body weight with Ringer–Locke solution. However, these investigators were unable to detect any structural differences in the tight junctions of the proximal tubules in comparison with those of control animals. Thus, while conceptually the role of the lateral intercellular space in the paracellular pathway seems obvious, the actual demonstration of its involvement has met with limited success.

Acknowledgments

Segments of the work from the laboratory of the author were supported by Public Health Service grant AM 13845. The author gratefully acknowledges the technical assistance of Mrs Helen Parks, Mrs Kathy Blake, and Mrs Betty Waller. Mrs Jessie Calder prepared the illustrative material and Miss Fran Wilson provided secretarial support.

References

Bentzel, C. J. (1972). Proximal tubule structure–function relationships during volume expansion in *Necturus*. *Kidney Int.* **2**, 324–335.

Berry, C. A. and Boulpaep, E. L. (1975). Nonelectrolyte permeability of the paracellular pathway in *Necturus* proximal tubule. *Am. J. Physiol.* **228**, 581–595.

Boulpaep, E. L. (1972). Permeability changes of the proximal tubule of *Necturus* during saline loading. *Am. J. Physiol.* **222**, 517–531.

Boulpaep, E. L. and Seely, J. F. (1971). Electrophysiology of proximal and distal tubules in the autoperfused dog kidney. *Am. J. Physiol.* **221**, 1084–1096.

Branton, D., Bullivant, S., Gilula, N. B., Karnovsky, M. J., Moor, H., Mühletaler, K., Northcote, D. N., Packer, L., Satir, B., Satir, P., Speth, V., Staehelin, L. A., Steere, R. L., and Weinstein, R. S. (1975). Freeze-etching nomenclature. *Science, N.Y.* **190**, 54–56.

Bulger, R. E., Lorentz, W. B., Jr, Colindres, R. E., and Gottschalk, C. W. (1974). Morphologic changes in rat renal proximal tubules and their tight junctions with increased intraluminal pressure. *Lab. Invest.* **30**, 136–144.

Burg, M. B. and Green, N. (1973). Function of the thick ascending limb of Henle's loop. *Am. J. Physiol.* **224**, 659–668.

Claude, P. and Goodenough, D. A. (1973). Fracture faces of zonulae occludentes from "tight" and "leaky" epithelia. *J. Cell Biol.* **58**, 390–400.

Evan, A. P., Baker, J. T. and Bengele, H. H. (1976). Zonulae occludentes of the rat nephron under conditions of experimental expansion of blood and/or fluid volume. *Anat. Rec.* **186**, 139–150.

Farquhar, M. G. and Palade, G. E. (1963). Junctional complexes in various epithelia. *J. Cell Biol.* **17**, 375–412.

Frizzell, R. A. and Schultz, S. G. (1972). Ionic conductances of extracellular shunt pathway in rabbit ileum: influence of shunt on transmural sodium transport and electrical potential differences. *J. gen. Physiol.* **59**, 318–346.

Frömter, E. (1972). The route of passive ion movement through the epithelium of *Necturus* gallbladder. *J. Membrane Biol.* **8**, 259–301.

Frömter, E. and Diamond, J. (1972). Route of passive ion permeation in epithelia. *Nature new Biol.* **235**, 9–13.

Grandchamp, A. and Boulpaep, E. L. (1974). Pressure control of sodium reabsorption and intercellular backflux across proximal kidney tubule. *J. clin. Invest.* **54**, 69–82.

Hegel, U., Frömter, E., and Wick, T. (1967). Der elektrische Wandwiderstand des proximalen Konvolutes der Rattenniere. *Pflügers Arch. ges. Physiol.* **292**, 274–290.

Helman, S. I., Grantham, J. J. and Burg, M. B. (1971). Effect of vasopressin on electrical resistance of renal cortical collecting tubules. *Am. J. Physiol.* **220**, 1825–1832.

Horster, M. and Larsson, L. (1976). Mechanisms of fluid absorption during proximal tubule development. *Kidney Int.* **10**, 348–363.

Humbert, F., Grandchamp, A., Pricam, C., Perrelet, A., and Orci, L. (1976). Morphological changes in tight junctions of *Necturus maculosus* proximal tubules undergoing saline diuresis. *J. Cell Biol.* **69**, 90–96.

Imai, M. and Kokko, J. P. (1972). Effect of peritubular protein concentration on reabsorption of sodium and water in isolated perfused proximal tubules. *J. clin. Invest.* **51**, 314–325.

Kühn, K. and Reale, E. (1975). Junctional complexes of the tubular cells in the human kidney as revealed with freeze-fracture. *Cell Tissue Res.* **160**, 193–205.

Larsson, L. (1975). Ultrastructure and permeability of intercellular contacts of developing proximal tubule in the rat kidney. *J. Ultrastruct. Res.* **52**, 100–113.

Lorentz, W. B., Jr, Lassiter, W. E. and Gottschalk, C. W. (1972). Renal tubular permeability during increased intrarenal pressure. *J. clin. Invest.* **51**, 484–492.

Malnic, G. and Giebisch, G. (1972). Some electrical properties of distal tubular epithelium in the rat. *Am. J. Physiol.* **223**, 797–808.

Martinez-Palomo, A. and Erlij, D. (1973). The distribution of lanthanum in tight junctions of the kidney tubule. *Pflügers Arch. ges. Physiol.* **343**, 267–272.

Maunsbach, A. B. (1966a). The influence of different fixatives and fixation methods on the ultrastructure of rat kidney proximal tubule cells. I. Comparison of different perfusion fixation methods, and of glutaraldehyde, formaldehyde and osmium tetroxide fixatives. *J. Ultrastruct. Res.* **15**, 242–282.

Maunsbach, A. B. (1966b). The influence of different fixatives and fixation methods on the ultrastructure of rat kidney proximal tubule cells. II. Effects of varying osmolality, ionic strength, buffer system and fixative concentration of glutaraldehyde solutions. *J. Ultrastruct. Res.* **15**, 283–309.

Maunsbach, A. B. (1966c). Observations on the segmentation of the proximal tubule in the rat kidney. Comparison of results from phase contrast, fluorescence and electron microscopy. *J. Ultrastruct. Res.* **16**, 239–258.

Ottosen, P. D. (1976). Effect of intraluminal pressure on the ultrastructure and protein transport in the proximal tubule. *Kidney Int.* **9**, 252–263.

Pérez-Gonzalez, M. and Whittembury, G. (1974). Widening of the paracellular pathway in the kidney tubule by a transtubular osmotic gradient. Passage of graded size non-electrolytes. *Pflügers Arch. ges. Physiol.* **351**, 1–12.

Pricam, C., Humbert F., Perrelet, A., and Orci, L. (1974). A freeze-etch study of the tight junctions of the rat kidney tubules. *Lab Invest.* **30**, 286–291.

Rau, W. S. and Frömter, E. (1974). Electrical properties of the medullary collecting ducts of the Golden hamster kidney. II. The transepithelial resistance. *Pflügers Arch. ges. Physiol.* **351**, 113–131.

Rawlins, F. A., González, E., Pérez-González, M. and Whittembury, G. (1975). Effect of transtubular osmotic gradients on the paracellular pathway in toad kidney proximal tubule. Electron microscopic observations. *Pflügers Arch. ges. Physiol.* **353**, 287–302.

Rocha, A. S. and Kokko, J. P. (1973). Sodium chloride and water transport in the medullary thick ascending limb of Henle. *J. clin. Invest.* **52**, 612–623.

Roesinger, B., Schiller, A., and Taugner, R. (1978). A freeze-fracture study of tight junctions in the pars convoluta and pars recta of the renal proximal tubule. *Cell Tissue Res.* **186**, 121–133.

Schafer, J. A., Patlak, C. S., and Andreoli, T. E. (1975). A component of fluid absorption linked to passive ion flows in the superficial pars recta. *J. gen. Physiol.* **66**, 445–471.

Schultz, S. G. (1977). The role of paracellular pathways in isotonic fluid transport. *Yale J. Biol. Med.* **50**, 99–113.

Tisher, C. C. and Kokko, J. P. (1974). Relationship between peritubular oncotic pressure gradients and morphology in isolated proximal tubules. *Kidney Int.* **6**, 146–156.

Tisher, C. C. and Yarger, W. E. (1973). Lanthanum permeability of the tight junction (zonula occludens) in the renal tubule of the rat. *Kidney Int.* **3**, 238–250.

Tisher, C. C. and Yarger, W. E. (1975). Lanthanum permeability of tight junctions along the collecting duct of the rat. *Kidney Int.* **7**, 35–43.

Whittembury, G. and Rawlins, F. A. (1971). Evidence of a paracellular pathway for ion flow in the kidney proximal tubule: electronmicroscopic demonstration of lanthanum precipitate in the tight junction. *Pflügers Arch. ges. Physiol.* **330**, 302–309.

15
Influence of Hydrostatic Pressure Changes on Paracellular Shunt Ultrastructure in Proximal Tubule

Arvid B. Maunsbach and Emile L. Boulpaep

Introduction

Ultrastructural and physiological studies have demonstrated that the lateral intercellular spaces participate in the transport of salt and water across epithelial barriers in different tissues (Tormey and Diamond, 1967; Voûte and Ussing, 1970; Boulpaep, 1971; Grantham, 1971; Spring and Hope, 1978). In the renal proximal tubule a number of different experimental conditions have been observed to change the ultrastructure of the paracellular pathway, but it has often been difficult to relate the ultrastructural alterations to specific functional changes.

The aim of this investigation was to evaluate the effects of changes in hydrostatic pressure gradients on the ultrastructure of the paracellular pathway in the *Necturus* proximal tubule during normal conditions and during reduced fluid reabsorption in volume-expanded animals. Particular care was taken to control the hydrostatic and osmotic pressure in the kidney before and during fixation of the tissue since the ultrastructure of renal tubules may be greatly influenced by the preparatory procedure for electron microscopy (Maunsbach *et al.*, 1962; Maunsbach, 1966).

Experimental Model

The kidneys of *Necturus maculosus* were prepared for micropuncture as described by Grandchamp and Boulpaep (1972). Control animals were

infused with Ringer's solution at a rate of 0.1 μl min^{-1} g^{-1} body weight
for 2 h and volume-expanded animals with 1 μl min^{-1} g^{-1} body weight.
The caudal portion of the abdominal vein was cannulated for rapid infusion
of fixative in the renal portal vein at the end of the experiment. The
hydrostatic pressure was determined in proximal tubules and peritubular
capillaries by means of the Wiederhielm technique (Wiederhielm, 1966).

Proximal tubules from five experimental conditions were analysed, and
each condition in at least five animals:

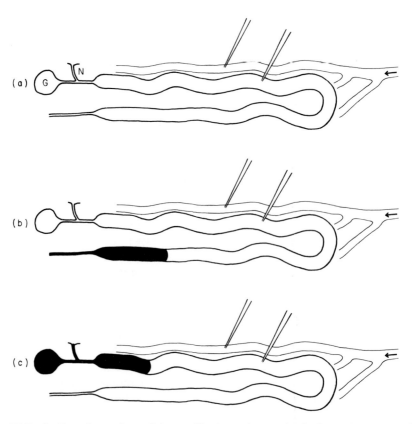

FIG. 1. *Experimental conditions utilized to change the hydrostatic pressure in
proximal tubules of* Necturus *kidney. Free-flow tubules have a normal pressure (a) while
tubules with a distal oil block have a high pressure (b) and tubules with a proximal oil
block a low luminal hydrostatic pressure (c). Micropipettes used to measure the
hydrostatic pressures are shown in the proximal tubule and a peritubular capillary. The
arrow indicates the direction of the blood flow in the peritubular capillaries which
originate from the renal portal vein. G, glomerulus; N, nephrostome.*

(1) Control animals, free-flow proximal tubules (Fig. 1(a)).

(2) Control animals, stop-flow tubules with increased luminal hydrostatic pressure caused by an end-proximal block with silicone oil (Grandchamp and Boulpaep, 1972) (Fig. 1(b)).

(3) Control animals, stop-flow tubules with decreased luminal pressure. Glomeruli, neck segments and early proximal tubules were filled with silicone oil which interrupted tubular flow and caused the luminal hydrostatic pressure to decrease or even reverse as compared to the peritubular capillary hydrostatic pressure (Fig. 1(c)).

(4) Volume-expanded animals, free-flow proximal tubules.

(5) Volume-expanded animals, stop-flow tubules with increased luminal pressure caused by end-proximal oil block.

Fixation of the kidneys were carried out by perfusion of osmium tetroxide in Veronal buffer (osmolality 215–220 mosmol/kg H_2O), through the renal portal veins which branch into the capillary network around the proximal tubules. The hydrostatic pressure in a peritubular capillary was recorded before and during the fixation through a pressure-measuring micropipette to ensure that the hydrostatic pressure in the capillaries was kept constant. After fixation experimental tubules as well as adjacent free-flow tubules were dehydrated and embedded in Vestopal. Semithin sections were cut for light microscopy and ultrathin sections were placed on one-hole grids to enable the observation of entire tubular cross-sections in the electron microscope.

All tubules were analysed in cross-sections oriented at right angles to the axis of the tubule. Overlapping electron micrographs were obtained from the whole tubule wall and assembled in montages. The luminal and peritubular diameter of the tubules and the cell height were measured on the montages. Stereological methods, described in detail elsewhere (Maunsbach and Boulpaep, 1980) were used to determine (per millimetre length of tubule) the tubular wall volume, the cell volume, the lateral intercellular space (LIS) volume, the LIS volume density, the total length of the tight junctions and

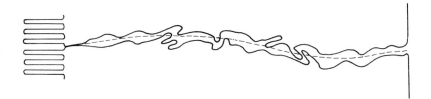

FIG. 2. *Schematic drawing of the lateral intercellular space between two proximal tubule cells. The dashed line indicates the location of the surface at half-width of LIS which was determined in the stereological analysis.*

the length of the peritubular opening of the LIS. In addition we defined and measured an (imaginary) surface (surface at half-width of LIS) which followed the general course of the lateral intercellular space except for the small irregularities and folds of the lateral cell membranes (Fig. 2). We then determined the true area of the lateral cell membranes as the product of the surface at half-width of LIS and a stereologically determined convolution factor of the lateral cell membranes. These stereological determinations were used to calculate the average minimum and average maximum path depth of LIS as well as the average minimum and average maximum width of LIS (Fig. 3).

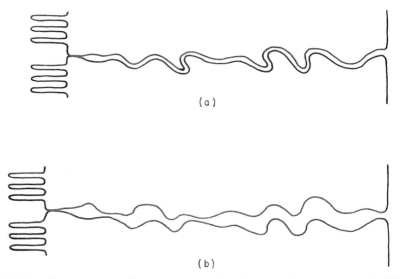

FIG. 3. *When adjacent cell membranes are placed in apposition the path depth of the lateral intercellular space shows its maximum value (a) and when the lateral intercellular space is dilated the path depth shows its minimum value (b).*

Ultrastructure of the Paracellular Pathway in *Necturus*

The paracellular pathway in *Necturus* tubules consists of the tight junction and the lateral intercellular space (Fig. 4). Within the tight junctions the two cell membranes showed at least one, but usually a few, touching points (Fig. 5). An open space through the junction was never observed in any of the present experimental conditions. The reported presence of an open space through the tight junctions (Bentzel, 1972) was probably caused by incomplete staining of the outermost layers of the plasma membranes.

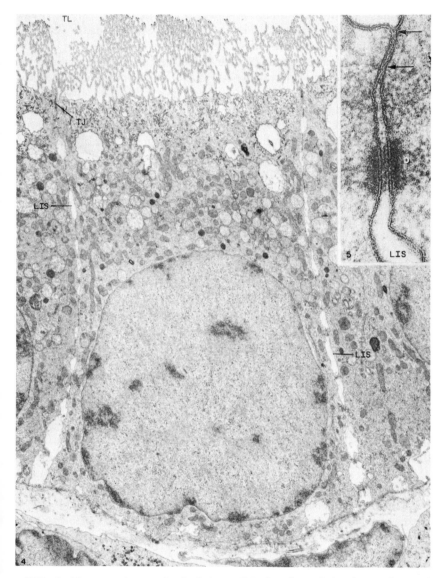

FIG. 4. *Electron micrograph of tubular wall in free-flow tubule of control animal.*
LIS, lateral intercellular space; TJ, tight junction; TL, tubule lumen. × 4500.

FIG. 5. *Higher magnification of tight junction between proximal tubule cells. The cell*
membranes show touching points within the junction (arrows). LIS, lateral intercellular
space; D, desmosome.

The proximal tubule cells in *Necturus* are cuboidal and less complex in shape than the interdigitating cells of the mammalian proximal tubule (Himmelhoch and Karnovsky, 1961; Claude, 1968; Maunsbach, 1973). While the lateral intercellular spaces in mammalian tubules approximate regular slits of constant width, the lateral cell membranes that formed the walls of the interspace in *Necturus* were only in part parallel and the interspaces therefore not geometrically simple slits (Fig. 4). In many regions there were interdigitations between folds from the cell membranes lining the lateral intercellular space. Analysis of serial sections demonstrated that the interdigitations occurred between true folds of the lateral cell membrane and not between fingerlike projections (Fig. 6). Due to the cell interdigitations the path depth of the lateral intercellular space is greater than the shortest distance between the tight junction and the peritubular opening of the lateral intercellular space (compare depths of interspace in Fig. 3). Only if the interspace is dilated to such an extent that the membrane folds do not interdigitate is the path depth approximately similar to the distance between the tight junction and the peritubular opening of LIS. The lateral cell membranes were also in close contact at gap junctions and desmosomes, but these cell contacts covered only small areas of the lateral cell membranes and presumably offered little hindrance for fluid transport in the lateral intercellular spaces.

Effects of Hydrostatic Pressure on the Lateral Intercellular Space

The ultrastructure of the proximal tubule epithelium was greatly influenced by the hydrostatic pressure gradients over the epithelium. In control animals an increase in luminal hydrostatic pressure from 25 to 57 mm H_2O increased the diameter of the tubule lumen from an average of 55 μm in free-flow tubules to 87 μm in high pressure tubules and decreased the cell height and the width of the lateral intercellular space (Fig. 7). On the other hand, a decrease of the luminal hydrostatic pressure to 10 mm H_2O, which corresponded to a negative transepithelial hydrostatic pressure gradient of 13 mm H_2O, caused a decrease of the diameter of the tubule lumen to 23 μm. Furthermore, it increased the cell height from 20 to 27 μm and increased the volume of

---

FIG. 6. *Serial sections of basal part of lateral intercellular space (LIS) between proximal tubule cells in free-flow tubules of control* Necturus *kidney. The drawings and the electron micrograph ((a)–(i)) show the course of adjacent cell membranes in every second section in a series of 18 sections with an average thickness of 340 Å. Notice that the projections of the lateral cell membranes, such as those indicated by arrows in (e), do not represent single finger-like projections, but true folds, since they appear in several consecutive sections.* × 46 000.

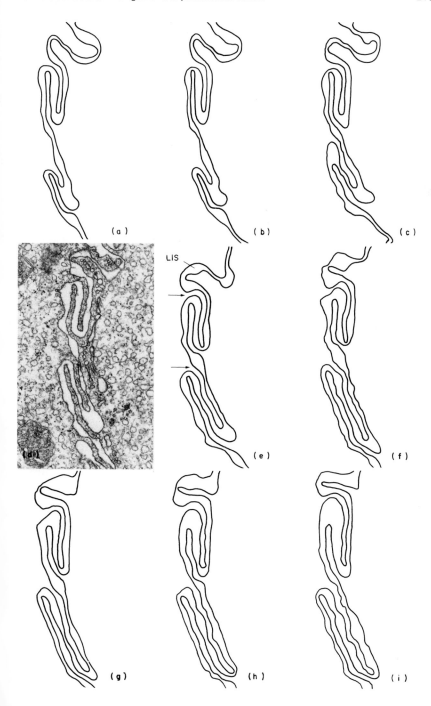

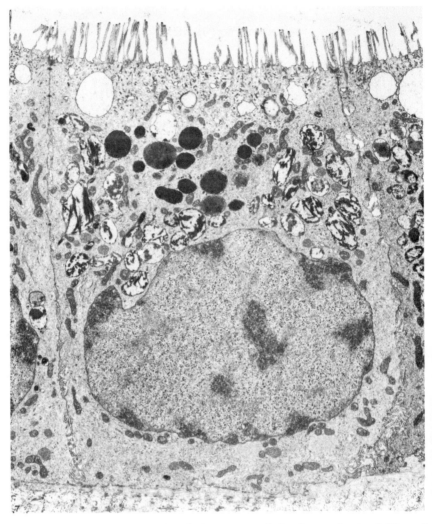

FIG. 7. *Part of tubular wall in high pressure tubule of control animal. The cell height is lower and the lateral intercellular spaces less wide than in free-flow tubules.* × 4500.

the lateral intercellular space by a factor of three (Fig. 8). The three-dimensional lengths of the tight junctions and the peritubular openings of the lateral intercellular space averaged 19 and 34 mm per millimetre of tubule length, respectively, in free-flow tubules of control animals and were not statistically different in high pressure and low pressure tubules. When the

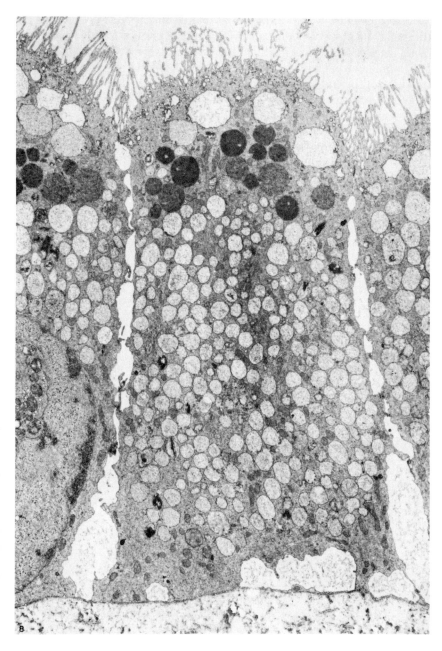

FIG. 8. *Tubule wall from low pressure tubule in control animal. The cells are taller than in control animals and the lateral intercellular spaces widened.* × *4500.*

average maximum width of the lateral intercellular space was calculated as the intercellular space volume divided by the surface area at half-width of the lateral intercellular space there was a significant narrowing of the average maximum intercellular space width in high pressure tubules and a significant widening of the width in low pressure tubules (Fig. 9). The same differences were obtained when the average minimum width of the lateral intercellular space was calculated for a situation when the path depth was a maximum, i.e. when the paracellular path was assumed to follow all convolutions of the lateral cell membrane. Also in volume-expanded animals there was a decrease of the average maximum width of the lateral intercellular spaces in tubules with increased luminal hydrostatic pressure (Fig. 9).

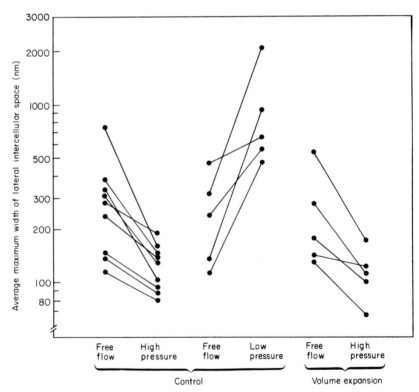

FIG. 9. *Average maximum width of lateral intercellular space in control and volume-expanded animals. Each pair of measurements is derived from one animal. The values were obtained through stereological analysis of complete tubular cross-sections. The width of the lateral intercellular space decreased in high pressure tubules both in control and volume-expanded animals and increased in low pressure tubules.*

In electrophysiological studies it has been demonstrated that the electrical resistance per unit tubule length increases significantly both in control and volume-expanded animals in tubules with a high hydrostatic pressure as compared to free-flow tubules in the same experimental conditions (Grand-champ and Boulpaep, 1974). Since the change in hydrostatic pressure, in control or volume-expanded animals, caused no difference in the reabsorptive capacity of the tubules, and no indication of a modification of the permeability of the junctional complex, the increase in resistance in both groups is interpreted as an effect of decreased width of the lateral intercellular spaces even if the path depths are assumed to be the same. However, it is likely that the effective diffusion path in high pressure tubules is longer than in free-flow tubules since the folds of the lateral membranes show a maximum of interdigitation (Figs 3 and 7). In low pressure tubules, on the other hand, the lateral intercellular space is dilated and adjacent folds of the lateral cell membranes separated to the extent that they do not interdigitate. These alterations in the effective path lengths of the lateral intercellular space work contradictory to the alterations in path depth caused by the changes in cell height at high or low luminal hydrostatic pressures and may also be important in the regulation of the transepithelial electrical resistance.

Effects of Volume Expansion on the Lateral Intercellular Space

Volume expansion caused a significant increase in the luminal diameter of free-flow tubules and a small decrease in the cell height. There was also a small decrease in the volume in the lateral intercellular space and the calculated average maximum and average minimum width of the lateral intercellular space. However, the average maximum and average minimum path depth of the lateral intercellular space was unchanged. Also the lengths of the tight junctions and the peritubular openings of the lateral intercellular space per millimetre of tubule length were similar in control and volume-expanded animals.

The transepithelial electrical resistance of the *Necturus* proximal tubule is approximately three times smaller in free-flow tubules of volume-expanded animals than in free-flow tubules of controls (Boulpaep, 1972). A similar difference exists between high pressure tubules of volume-expanded animals and high pressure tubules of controls. However, the transepithelial resistance as predicted from the width and path depth of the lateral intercellular space, both using the average maximum and the average minimum width or path depth, predicts an unaltered or slightly increased transepithelial resistance if the resistance per millimetre tubule is calculated as $r = \rho d/wL$, where ρ is the volume resistivity of *Necturus* Ringer's solution, d the path depth, w the

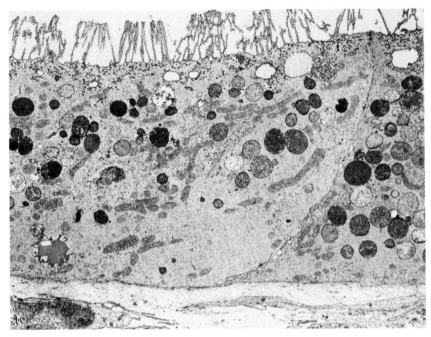

FIG. 10. *Tubule wall from free-flow tubule in volume-expanded animal. The cells are flattened and the lateral intercellular spaces decreased in width as compared to free-flow tubules in control animals.*

width of the lateral intercellular space and L the length of the interspace. The difference between the observed and the predicted transepithelial resistance is probably due to a decrease in the resistance of the junctional complex in volume-expanded animals. This interpretation is supported by the increase in the apparent permeability for NaCl and raffinose in volume expansion despite the fact that the intercellular space did not widen. However, the sucrose permeability coefficient, measured in the absence of solute and solvent flow (Berry and Boulpaep, 1975), decreased during volume expansion in parallel with the observed decrease in the width of the lateral intercellular space.

Fluid Transport and Geometry of Paracellular Pathway

The importance of the size of the lateral intercellular space was first emphasized in studies of gallbladder epithelium (Tormey and Diamond, 1967) and subsequently of other epithelia, and it was suggested that dilatation of the lateral intercellular spaces was associated with maximum salt and water transport and that the interspaces were collapsed when transport was decreased or inhibited. During isotonic extracellular volume expansion or changed hydrostatic pressure gradients there are no changes in active transport in a proximal tubule. Nevertheless, the present study demonstrated pronounced alterations in the geometry of the lateral intercellular space. We therefore conclude that dilated lateral intercellular spaces are not necessarily caused by active transport, but that hydrostatic pressure gradients have an overriding influence on the geometry of the paracellular pathway. Furthermore, it is apparent that the distended lateral intercellular spaces previously recorded in volume-expanded kidneys (Caulfield and Trump, 1961; Bentzel, 1972; Bengele and Evan, 1975) may be more related to alterations in hydrostatic pressure gradients than to volume expansion.

Different models have been proposed for isotonic or near isotonic water transport (Diamond and Bossert, 1967; Sackin and Boulpaep, 1975; Schafer et al., 1977; Welling et al., 1978). Among these models the standing gradient model (Diamond and Bossert, 1967) requires a long path depth and a small width of the lateral intercellular space. The geometrical parameter that influences the concentration of the absorbate at the peritubular opening of the pathway is $d^2/(w/2)$, where d is the depth of the channel and w the width (Segel, 1970).

The present morphometric analysis of the *Necturus* proximal tubule predicts values for $d^2/(w/2)$ ranging from 1·4 mm to 61·9 mm (Maunsbach and Boulpaep, 1980). The maximum value was calculated for high pressure control tubules assuming that the flow of water in the interspaces has to follow all convolutions of the lateral cell membranes and the minimum value was computed for low pressure control tubules assuming negligible interdigitations of the lateral cell membranes. Both values are considerably smaller than the value of 500 mm which was calculated to be necessary for isotonic transport in models of constant geometry (Hill, 1975).

However, it is questionable if $d^2/(w/2)$ can be used to predict the osmolality of the reabsorbate emerging from the interspace since the osmotic permeability coefficient is controversial (Diamond, 1977). Moreover, it is evident from the electron micrographs that the degree of interdigitation of the lateral cell membranes is variable along the depths of the lateral intercellular space and that some localized segments would predict a very high and some a very low value for $d^2/(w/2)$. In addition, stereological information from single sections is insufficient to evaluate the relative contributions of narrow and wide portions of the lateral intercellular space since it does not take into account the three-dimensional variability in pathway geometry. There are no relevant weighing techniques which can be proposed as a valid solution to this problem unless specifically applied to a simple physical process such as convection or diffusion, and no existing model for epithelial transport has considered such complex boundary conditions as those that are observed in the lateral intercellular spaces of the *Necturus* proximal tubule. However, since fluid transport is probably iso-osmotic in *Necturus* proximal tubule despite the variations in intercellular space geometry, the present observations favour models of near isotonic transport which do not require long and narrow interspaces.

Conclusions

(1) The width of the lateral intercellular space in the *Necturus* proximal tubule is dependent upon the hydrostatic pressure gradient over the epithelium and is not primarily correlated to the rate of fluid reabsorption.

(2) Pressure-induced changes in the transepithelial resistance and in the permeability coefficient for water correlated with the geometry of the lateral intercellular space.

(3) The changes in electrical resistance or the permeability coefficients for solutes which are induced by volume expansion appear not to be dependent on the geometry of the lateral intercellular space.

(4) The lateral intercellular space of the *Necturus* proximal tubule does not have the long diffusion path required for isotonic transport in the standing gradient model for fluid transport.

Acknowledgement

The authors are indebted to Mrs Marianne Ellegaard for excellent technical assistance. This work was supported by the Danish Medical Research Council and by USPHS Grants AM–13844 and AM–17433 from the National Institutes of Arthritis, Metabolic and Digestive Diseases.

References

Bengele, H. H. and Evan, A. P. (1975). The effects of Ringer–Locke or blood infusions on the lateral intercellular spaces of the rat proximal tubule. *Anat. Rec.* **182**, 201–214.

Bentzel, C. J. (1972). Proximal tubule structure–function relationships during volume expansion in *Necturus*. *Kidney Int.* **2**, 324–335.

Berry, C. A. and Boulpaep, E. L. (1975). Nonelectrolyte permeability of the paracellular pathway in *Necturus* proximal tubule. *Am. J. Physiol.* **228**, 581–595.

Boulpaep, E. L. (1971). Electrophysiological properties of the proximal tubule: importance of cellular and intercellular transport pathway. In *Electrophysiology of Epithelial Cells* (G. Giebisch, ed.), F. K. Schattauer Verlag, Stuttgart and New York, pp. 91–112.

Boulpaep, E. L. (1972). Permeability changes of the proximal tubule of *Necturus* during saline loading. *Am. J. Physiol.* **222**, 517–531.

Caulfield, J. B. and Trump, B. F. (1962). Correlation of ultrastructure with function in the rat kidney. *Am. J. Path.* **40**, 199–218.

Claude, P. (1968). An electron microscopic study of the urinary tubules of *Necturus maculosus*. PhD dissertation, University of Pennsylvania, Philadelphia.

Diamond, J. M. (1977). The epithelial junction : bridge, gate, and fence. *Physiologist* **20**, 10–18.

Diamond, J. M. and Bossert, W. H. (1967). Standing-gradient osmotic flow. A mechanism for coupling of water and solute transport in epithelia. *J. gen. Physiol.* **50**, 2061–2083.

Grandchamp, A. and Boulpaep, E. L. (1972). Effect of intraluminal pressure on proximal tubular sodium reabsorption. A shrinking drop micropuncture study. *Yale J. Biol. Med.* **45**, 275–288.

Grandchamp, A. and Boulpaep, E. L. (1974). Pressure control of sodium reabsorption and intercellular backflux across proximal kidney tubule. *J. clin. Invest.* **54**, 69–82.

Grantham, J. J. (1971). Mode of water transport in mammalian renal collecting tubules. *Fedn Proc. Fedn Am. Socs exp. Biol.* **30**, 14–21.

Hill, A. E. (1975). Solute–solvent coupling in epithelia: a critical examination of the standing-gradient osmotic flow theory. *Proc. R. Soc. B* **190**, 99–114.

Himmelhoch, S. R. and Karnovsky, M. J. (1961). Oxidative and hydrolytic enzymes in the nephron of *Necturus maculosus*. *J. biophys. biochem. Cytol.* **9**, 893–908.

Maunsbach, A. B. (1966). The influence of different fixatives and fixation methods on the ultrastructure of rat kidney proximal tubule cells. I. Comparison of different perfusion fixation methods and of glutaraldehyde, formaldehyde and osmium tetroxide fixatives. *J. Ultrastruct. Res.* **15**, 242–282.

Maunsbach, A. B. (1973). Ultrastructure of the proximal tubule. In *Handbook of Physiology*, Sect. 8, *Renal Physiology* (J. Orloff and R. W. Berliner, eds) American Physiological Society, Washington, DC, pp. 31–79.

Maunsbach, A. B. and Boulpaep, E. L. (1980). Hydrostatic pressure changes related to paracellular shunt ultrastructure in proximal tubule. *Kidney Int.*, **17**, 732–748.

Maunsbach, A. B., Madden, S. C. and Latta, H. (1962). Variations in fine structure of renal tubular epithelium under different conditions of fixation. *J. Ultrastruct. Res.* **6**, 511–530.

Sackin, H. and Boulpaep, E. L. (1975). Models for coupling of salt and water transport. Proximal tubular reabsorption in *Necturus* kidney. *J. gen. Physiol.* **66**, 671–733.

Schafer, J. A., Patlak, C. S. and Andreoli, T. E. (1977). Fluid absorption and active and passive ion flows in the rabbit superficial pars recta. *Am. J. Physiol.* **233**, F154–F167.

Segel, L. A. (1970). Standing-gradient flows driven by active solute transport. *J. theor. Biol.* **29**, 233–250.

Spring, K. R. and Hope, A. (1978). Size and shape of the lateral intercellular spaces in a living epithelium. *Science, N. Y.* **200**, 54–57.

Tormey, J. M. and Diamond, J. M. (1967). The ultrastructural route of fluid transport in rabbit gall bladder. *J. gen. Physiol.* **50**, 2031–2060.

Voûte, C. L. and Ussing, H. H. (1970). Quantitative relation between hydrostatic pressure gradient, extracellular volume and active sodium transport in the epithelium of the frog skin. *Exptl Cell Res.* **62**, 375–383.

Welling, D. J., Welling, L. W. and Hill, J. J. (1978). Phenomenological model relating cell shape to water reabsorption in proximal nephron. *Am. J. Physiol.* **3**, F308–F317.

Wiederhielm, C. A. (1966). Servo micropipet pressure recording technique. *Methods med. Res.* **11**, 199–201.

16
Correlation of Ultrastructure and Fluid Transport in Developing Proximal Tubules

Lars Larsson

Introduction

The postnatal development of the mammalian kidney is characterized by heterogenity of nephron maturation in such a way that the juxtamedullary nephrons are more mature than the superficial nephrons (Huber, 1905; Potter, 1972) (Fig. 1). This variation in the developmental stages of nephrons through the renal cortex implies a functional heterogenity within the maturing kidney. It is therefore not possible to obtain information about nephron function at a specific developmental stage by determining, for example, the total glomerular filtration rate of the kidney. Instead it is necessary to study the functional maturation of the nephrons at the single nephron level, but this has not previously been possible because of technical difficulties. As a consequence, knowledge about the correlation between structure and function of the nephron has also been fragmentary. However, techniques have recently been developed for analysing single tubule function both *in situ* (Horster and Valtin, 1971; Spitzer and Brandis, 1974; Aperia and Herin, 1975; Dlouha *et al.*, 1975) and *in vitro* (Horster and Larsson, 1976), and therefore correlation between structure and function is now possible. The aim of this paper is to present some structure–function correlations during nephron maturation that provide some insight into the process of proximal tubular fluid transfer.

The first part of this review deals with the general development of the proximal tubular cells and the second part with the structural development of the proximal tubular epithelium as related to fluid transfer through the proximal tubular wall.

Gross Development of the Nephron

Light microscope (Huber, 1905; Potter, 1972) and microdissection studies (Oliver, 1968; Potter, 1972) have served to clarify the structural development of the nephron. Briefly, the blind end of the collecting tubule initiates formation of nephron anlages from mesodermal cells in the lumbal region. The renal vesicle is the first clearly identifiable nephron anlage and this anlage is classified as stage I and has no connection to the collecting tubule (Fig. 1). By stage II the renal vesicle has been transformed into an S-shaped tubule, generally referred to as the S-shaped body (Fig. 1). The S-shaped body is connected to the collecting tubule and in this nephron anlage the very first glomerular anlage is recognizable (Figs 1 and 2). The S-shaped body then gives rise to the glomerulus, the proximal tubule, the loop of Henle and the distal tubule.

Ultrastructure of the Developmental Stages

Stage I
The renal vesicle is surrounded by a basement membrane. The cells are pyramidal in shape and about 15 μm in height. The nucleus is large and numerous free ribosomes are present in the cytoplasm (Fig. 3). Other cell organelles such as mitochondria, lysosomes and endocytic vacuoles occupy only a small part of the cytoplasmic volume (Fig. 3, Table I).

Stage II
In the S-shaped body the glomerular anlage is cup-shaped in three-dimensional appearance. The glomerular epithelium cells are columnar in shape and there are few capillary loops associated with the epithelial cells (Fig. 2). At this stage of nephron development no glomerular filtration seems to take place. The ultrastructural appearance of the cells in the proximal tubule anlage at stage II is very similar to that of the cells in stage I. A morphometric analysis did not demonstrate significant differences in the amounts of subcellular components between the cells of stages I and II (Table I).

FIG. 1. *Light micrograph showing a cross-section through the renal cortex of a newborn rat. The nephrogenic zone is located just below the renal capsule (RC) where, stage I, renal vesicles are observed. Deeper in the cortex one S-shaped body with its glomerular anlage (GII) and proximal tubular anlage (PII) are seen. In the lower part of the picture a glomerulus (GIII) of a stage III nephron and its corresponding proximal tubule (PIII) are seen. PIV, proximal tubule at stage IV. × 700.*

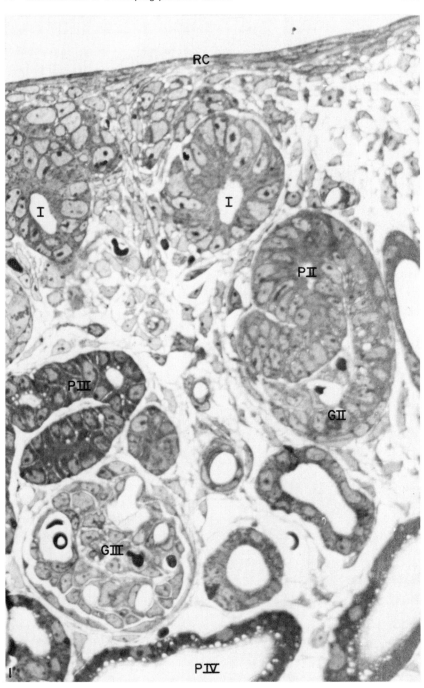

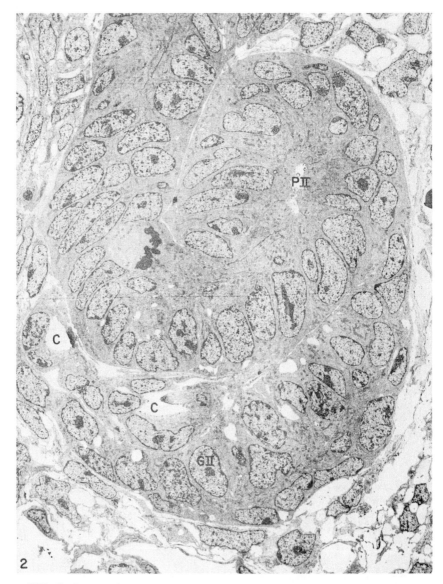

FIG. 2. *Survey electron micrograph of a stage II rat nephron (S-shaped body) showing its glomerular anlage (GII) and proximal tubule anlage (PII). A few capillaries (C) are located in close proximity to the glomerular anlage.* × 2000.

TABLE I

Morphometric analysis of subcellular components in proximal tubule cells at different developmental stages[a]

Subcellular component	Stage				
	I	II	III	IV	Adult
Nucleus (vol %)	47.0 ± 8.6	47.3 ± 5.0	42.8 ± 4.7	14.9 ± 3.4^d	9.2 ± 3.0^b
Mitochondria (vol %)	4.0 ± 0.5	4.8 ± 1.3	6.9 ± 0.5^b	13.5 ± 0.9^d	24.4 ± 6.0^d
Small endocytic vacuoles (vol %)	0.01 ± 0.01	0.01 ± 0.01	0.3 ± 0.1^c	1.0 ± 0.1^d	1.2 ± 0.6
Large endocytic vacuoles (vol %)	0	0	0.9 ± 0.6^b	2.4 ± 1.0^b	1.9 ± 0.7
Lysosomes (vol %)	0.3 ± 0.3	0.2 ± 0.2	1.9 ± 1.0^b	5.1 ± 2.0^d	6.0 ± 1.8
Surface density of basal and lateral cell membranes ($\mu m^2/\mu m^3$ cell volume)	1.07 ± 0.12	1.12 ± 0.11	1.02 ± 0.13	1.61 ± 0.44^b	2.37 ± 0.40^b

[a] Means $\pm$ s.d. Letters indicate the statistical significance of the mean in one stage as related to the previous stage ($n = 5$).
[b] $p < 0.05$.
[c] $p < 0.01$.
[d] $p < 0.001$.

The table is compiled from observations by Larsson (1975a) and Larsson and Maunsbach (1975).

Stage III

In nephrons at stage III of development the glomerulus is oval in shape (Fig. 1). The epithelial cells are still columnar and the lateral cell membranes of adjacent cells are separated by narrow intercellular spaces. A few foot processes are recognizable. In a cross-section through the equator of the glomerulus only about five capillary lumina are observed (Fig. 1). These nephrons have been demonstrated to produce glomerular filtrate (Larsson and Maunsbach, 1975), although their contribution in relation to the total glomerular filtration is probably not important.

The proximal tubule at this developmental stage has a completely different ultrastructural appearance to that in the previous stages. The tubular lumen is wider and has a diameter of about 10 μm as compared to about 5 μm during stages I and II. The cells have decreased in height to about 10 μm,

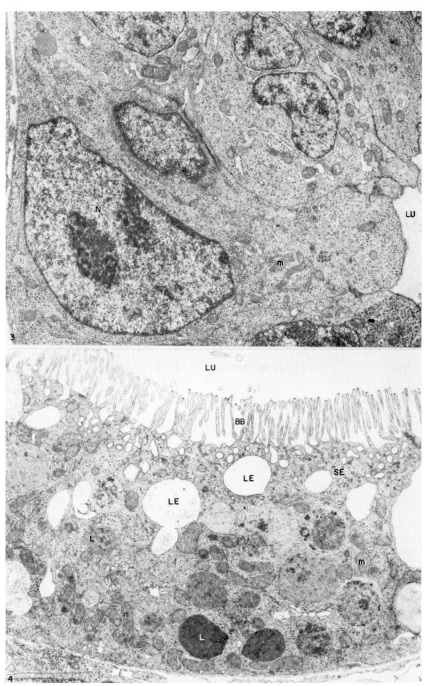

and they are characterized by an irregular brush border. The morphometric analysis of the subcellular components showed that there is an increased number of mitochondria, endocytic vacuoles and lysosomes in comparison to earlier developmental stages (Table I). The relative area (surface density) of lateral and basal cell membranes per cell volume is similar in stages I, II and III (Table I).

Stage IV
Nephrons at stage IV are responsible for nearly the total renal fluid filtration in the newborn rat. The glomerulus in this developmental stage has approximately the same structural appearance as in the adult animal, although the diameter of the glomerulus is smaller and the density of the epithelial cells per glomerular volume is higher in stage IV than in the adult glomerulus. In stage IV the structural appearance of endothelial cells, glomerular basement membrane and epithelial cells, including foot processes and slit diaphragms, is similar in stage IV to that of the adult glomerulus (Larsson, 1975a).

The proximal tubule in stage IV has approximately the same ultrastructure as the adult proximal tubule, with a regular brush border facing the tubular lumen (Fig. 4). In comparison to stage III the number of mitochondria, endocytic vacuoles and lysosomes has increased dramatically (Table I). Furthermore, the area of basal and lateral cell membranes is increased due to the development of cellular interdigitations and basal infoldings of the cell membrane (Table I). The subcellular architecture is also much more polarized in stage IV than in previous stages. Thus, the mitochondria are located in the basal part of the cells and oriented perpendicular to the tubular basement membrane in close relation to the basal and lateral cell membrane (Fig. 5). The abundant endocytic vacuoles are located in the apical part of the cytoplasm as in the adult proximal tubule cells (Fig. 4).

Adult proximal tubules
In comparison to stage IV, the cells of the adult proximal tubule contain an increased number of mitochondria and lysosomes. The cells have developed more interdigitations than in previous stages and the area of basal and lateral cell membranes has increased (Table I).

FIG. 3. *A part of the wall of a stage I rat nephron. The cells are tall and only a few cell organelles such as mitochondria (m) are seen. Nucleus (N), lumen (LU). × 7500.*

FIG. 4. *Part of the wall of a rat proximal tubule at stage IV. The cells have a regular brush border (BB) facing the tubular lumen (LU). There are many mitochondria (m), lysosomes (L), small (SE) and large endocytic vacuoles (LE). Compare Figs 3 and 4. × 11 000.*

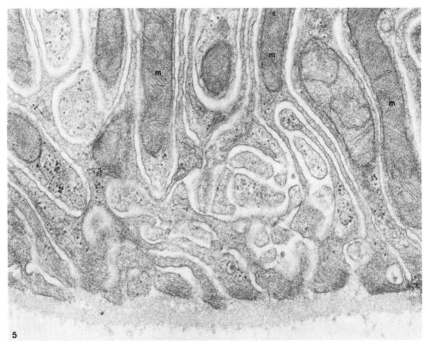

FIG. 5. *The basal part of an isolated rabbit proximal tubule. The cells show many interdigitations. Note the close proximity of the mitochondria (m) to the cell membranes.* × 30 000.

Fluid Transport: Correlation of Ultrastructure and Function

Isotonic fluid transport through many epithelia is generally considered to be due to an active sodium transport, probably mediated by the cell membrane-bound Na^+, K^+-ATPase (Skou, 1965), resulting in a flow of water and solutes through the intercellular spaces (Diamond, 1969). The structural organization of the basal and lateral cell surface of the epithelium therefore seems to play an important role in transepithelial fluid transfer. The volume flow of water and solutes in the intercellular spaces is in part directed to the contraluminal side of the epithelium due to the apical cell contacts, the tight junctions, which connect the apical parts of adjacent cells. The permeability of the tight junction is one factor determining the back-flux of water and solutes from the intercellular spaces to the luminal side of the epithelium (Boulpaep, 1971). The possible role of changes of the area of basal and lateral cell membranes, as well as changes in permeability of cell contacts for fluid transfer during proximal maturation, will therefore be considered in the following.

Ultrastructural and functional development of isolated rabbit proximal tubules
Isolated rabbit proximal tubules were perfused using the technique described
by Burg *et al.* (1966) as modified for neonatal tubules by Horster (1976).
Fluid reabsorption was determined by analysing a volume marker at the level
of the collecting pipette. Subsequent to the determination of fluid reabsorption, proximal tubules from each developmental stage were fixed by
exchanging the bath medium for a fixative solution and the tubules were
then further prepared for electron microscopy. Montages of electron micrographs covering a whole tubule cross-section were subjected to morphometric
analysis.

Fluid reabsorption in proximal tubules from day 4 to day 28 increased
from 0·26 nl/min to 1·04 nl/min or approximately by a factor of four, whereas
the area of basal and lateral cell membranes per millimetre of tubule increased
from 0.90×10^6 μm^2 to 2.33×10^6 μm^2 or approximately 2·6-fold (Larsson
and Horster, 1976).

Ultrastructural and functional development of rat proximal tubules
Fluid reabsorption in single superficial rat nephrons was determined by a
modified Gertz' (1963) split droplet technique (Aperia and Larsson, 1979).
Following the evaluation of proximal tubular fluid transfer, adjacent
proximal tubules were fixed for electron microscopy. Montages of electron
micrographs were analysed by morphometric techniques as described above.
In the rat, fluid reabsorption in superficial proximal tubules increased from
postnatal day 22 to postnatal day 45 by a factor of 2·2, whereas the area
of basal and lateral cell membranes increased 1·8-fold.

Thus, there is a concomitant increase in fluid reabsorption and area of
basal and lateral cell membranes during development both of the rat and
rabbit proximal tubules. This suggests that the increasing fluid reabsorption
may in part be the result of the increased area of basal and lateral cell
membranes. The enlarged cell surface may imply an increased number of
active sodium transporting sites per tubule length (Kyte, 1976). Further
support for this hypothesis has been obtained from a recent analysis of (Na^+,
K^+)-activated ATPase in isolated rabbit proximal tubules, which showed
an increased absolute amount of this enzyme in the proximal tubule during
development (Schmidt and Horster, 1977). This increase was proportional
to the increased area of basal and lateral cell membranes.

Cell contacts
Changes in the permeability of the tight junctions during development of
the proximal tubules were studied with different techniques. Renal tissue from
the rat was fixed by vascular perfusion with glutharaldehyde and then

incubated with colloidal lanthanum (Revel and Karnovsky, 1967) and further prepared for electron microscopy. In all developmental stages of the proximal tubule, five-layered membrane complexes, tight junctions, could be found between adjacent cells close to the tubular lumen (Figs 6 and 9). In tissue treated with lanthanum it was observed that lanthanum filled the intercellular spaces except for the region of the tight junction (Fig. 7). Lanthanum was also found in the tubule lumen (Fig. 7). In some sections where a tight junction was not observed lanthanum was located throughout the entire intercellular space (Fig. 8).

In stage III and in later developmental stages lanthanum filled the intercellular spaces but was never observed in the region of the tight junction, which appeared to resist its penetration (Fig. 9). Furthermore, deposits of lanthanum were not observed in the tubular lumen. These observations indicate that the tight junction in stages I and II do not form complete belts around the entire cells, whereas the later developmental stages when glomerular filtration occurs the tight junction appears continuous. The results suggest that during development of the proximal tubule a decrease in the permeability of the apical cell contacts occurs.

Further evidence for a decrease in permeability of the tight junction during development of the proximal tubule has been obtained in experiments where

---

FIG. 6. *Apical parts of two adjacent cells in a stage I nephron. The lateral cell membranes are in apposition and have formed a five-layered membrane complex (arrow) close to the tubule lumen (LU).* × 110 000.

FIG. 7. *Apical parts of two adjacent cells in a stage I rat nephron. The tissue was incubated with colloidal lanthanum. Lanthanum fills the intercellular space (IS) and is seen in the tubular lumen (LU). In the region where lateral cell membranes are in apposition, no deposits of lanthanum are observed (arrow).* × 70 000.

FIG. 8. *Apical parts of two adjacent cells in a stage I rat nephron. The tissue was incubated with colloidal lanthanum. Deposits of lanthanum fill the entire intercellular space (IS). Note that it is not possible to observe cell membranes in apposition in this section. Lanthanum is also seen in the tubular lumen (LU).* × 110 000.

FIG. 9. *Apical parts of two adjacent cells of a rat proximal tubule at stage IV. The tissue was incubated with colloidal lanthanum. Deposits of lanthanum are seen in the intercellular space (IS) except in the region where lateral cell membranes have formed a five-layered membrane complex (arrow). Lanthanum is not observed in the tubule lumen (LU).* × 110 000.

FIG. 10. *A portion of the wall of a rat proximal tubule at stage IV. The tubule was microperfused with microperoxidase. Microperoxidase activity is seen in the tubule lumen (LU), in close association to the brush border (BB) and in small (SE) and large endocytic vacuoles (LE). Enzyme activity is not observed in the intercellular spaces (IS). Basement membrane (BM).* × 10 000.

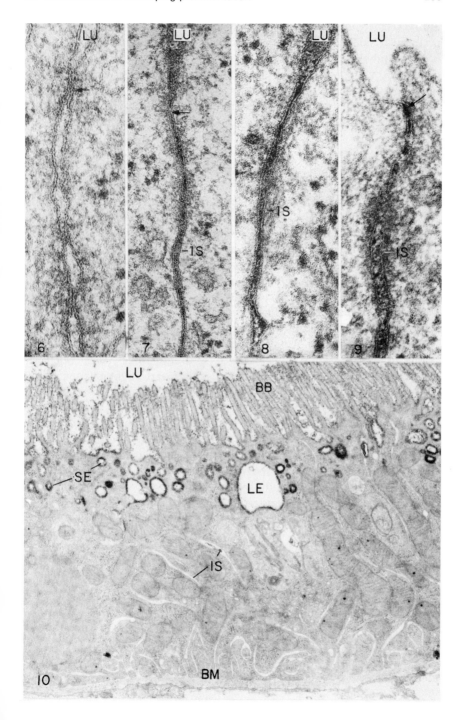

intravascularly injected horse-radish peroxidase was found to pass from the peritubular side of non-filtering rat nephron *anlages* (stages I and II) to the proximal tubular lumen (Larsson, 1975b). Passage of horse-radish peroxidase did not occur in nephrons in later developmental stages. However, when single rat superficial proximal tubules at stage IV were microperfused with microperoxidase it was not possible to demonstrate any passage of microperoxidase from the tubular lumen to the intercellular spaces (Fig. 10).

Hydraulic conductance
Hydraulic hydrostatic conductance (Lp in nanolitres per square centimetre per minute) in immature rabbit proximal tubules (postnatal day 4) was 0.037 nl cm^{-2} min^{-1} cm H$_2$O, whereas in mature rabbits (postnatal day 28) the Lp was 0.0052 (Horster and Larsson, 1976). Thus Lp in the immature tubules was sevenfold higher than in the mature tubules.

The effect of hyperoncotic serum bath medium on fluid transfer in isolated developing rabbit proximal tubules was also determined when normal serum was exchanged for hyperoncotic serum as bath solution. Immature proximal tubules at stage IV increased their capacity to transfer fluid by 67·5 per cent, whereas the increase for the mature proximal tubules was only about 25·5 per cent, when normal serum was exchanged for hyperoncotic serum as bath solution (Horster and Larsson, 1976). The decrease in Lp, as well as the change in fluid transfer after exposure of the tubules to a hyperoncotic bath, can be explained by a decrease in the permeability of the tight junction and/or the intercellular spaces during the proximal tubule maturation.

Proximal tubules from both immature and mature animals which had been perfused at high or low intratubular hydrostatic pressure were prepared for electron microscopy and the ultrathin sections were studied by electron microscope with the aid of a goniometer. This analysis failed to reveal any change in the ultrastructure of the tight junction between these experimental groups. Possible changes in the permeability of the tight junction were investigated by adding different tracers to the perfusate during the perfusion

---

FIG. 11. *A portion of the wall of an isolated rabbit proximal tubule perfused at 20 cm H₂O intratubular hydrostatic pressure with microperoxidase in the perfusate. Microperoxidase activity is observed in small (SE) and large endocytic vacuoles (LE), in the intercellular spaces (IS) and tubular basement membrane (BM). × 11 000.*

FIG. 12. *A portion of the wall of an isolated rabbit proximal tubule perfused at 20 cm H₂O intratubular hydrostatic pressure with ferritin in the perfusate. Ferritin molecules fill the tubular lumen (LU).*
Inset. *Apical parts of two adjacent cells from this tubule. Ferritin molecules are seen in the tubular lumen but not in the intercellular space (IS). Lateral cell membranes have formed a five-layered membrane complex (arrow) close to the tubular lumen. × 100 000.*

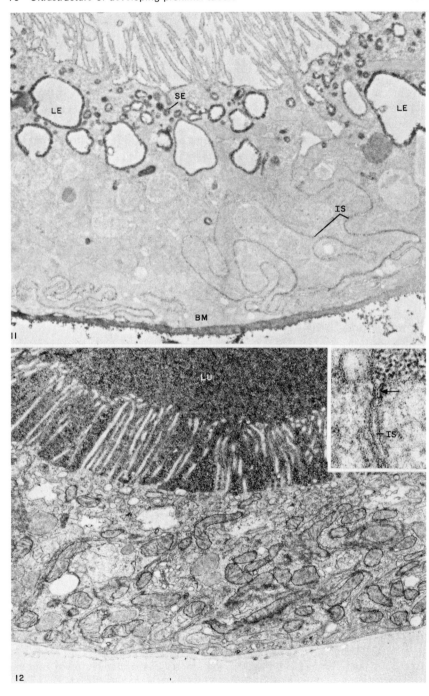

of isolated developing tubules *in vitro* at high (20 cm H_2O) or low (5 cm H_2O) intratubular hydrostatic pressure. Ferritin, horse-radish peroxidase and microperoxidase were used as tracers. It was found that microperoxidase (molecular weight about 1900 daltons), when perfused at high intratubular hydrostatic pressure in immature rabbit proximal tubules, passed from the tubular lumen to the intercellular spaces without evidence of a transcellular passage (Fig. 11) (Horster and Larsson, 1976). However, when microperoxidase was perfused at high intratubular pressure in mature tubules, it did not pass from the tubular lumen to the intercellular spaces. In both immature and mature tubules perfused at low hydrostatic pressure with microperoxidase the enzymic activity was only found in the tubular lumen and not in the intercellular spaces. None of the other tracers passed from the tubular lumen to the intercellular spaces in immature or mature tubules during perfusions at either low or high intratubular pressure (Fig. 12) (Horster and Larsson, 1976). Thus, it appears that the permeability of the tight junction to small proteins, such as microperoxidase, decreased as the tubules become mature.

Conclusions

The ability of the proximal tubules to transfer fluid increased during postnatal renal development. This increase in fluid absorption correlated to an increased area of basal and lateral cell membranes and an increased amount of (Na^+, K^+)-ATPase in the cell membrane. The decreasing permeability of the tight junction in the proximal tubule during maturation may also influence the observed changes in fluid transport during the postnatal tubule maturation. The decrease in permeability of the tight junction furthermore suggests that changes in intratubular and peritubular hydrostatic and oncotic pressure gradients affect fluid absorption in the immature tubule to a greater extent than in the mature tubules.

Acknowledgement

Support by grants from the Swedish Medical Research Council B 79–14x–05427–01.

References

Aperia, A. and Herin, P. (1975). Development of glomerular perfusion rate and nephron filtration rate in rats 17–60 days old. *Am. J. Physiol.* **228**, 1319–1325.

Aperia, A. and Larsson, L. (1979). Correlation between fluid absorption and proximal tubule ultrastructure during development of the rat kidney. *Acta physiol. scand.* **105**, 11–22.

Boulpaep, E. (1971). Permeability changes of the proximal tubule of *Necturus* during saline loading. *Am. J. Physiol.* **222**, 517–529.

Burg, M. J., Grantham, J., Abramow, M. and Orloff, J. (1966). Preparation and study of fragments of single nephrons. *Am. J. Physiol.*, **210**, 1293–1305.

Dlouha, H., Bibr, B., Jezek, J. and Zicha, J. (1975). Changing pattern of SNGFR ratios of superficial, intercortical and juxtamedullary nephrons in young rats. In *Abstracts of Free Communications, VIth International Congress of Nephrologists, Florence 1975* (S. Giovanetti, V. Bonomini and G. D'Amico, eds), Karger, Basel, Abstract 52.

Diamond, J. (1969). The coupling of solute and water transport in epithelia. In *Renal Transports and Diuretics* (K. Thurau and H. Jahrmärker, eds), Springer Verlag, Berlin, pp. 77–98.

Gertz, K. H. (1963). Transtubuläre Natriumchloridflüsse und Permebiltät für Nichtelektrolyte im Proximalen und Distalen Konvolut der Rattenniere. *Pflügers Arch. ges. Physiol.* **276**, 336–356.

Horster, M. and Larsson, L. (1976). Mechanisms of fluid absorption during proximal tubule development. *Kidney Int.* **10**, 348–363.

Horster, M. and Valtin, H. (1971). Postnatal development of renal function. Micropuncture and clearance studies in the dog. *J. clin. Invest.* **50**, 779–795.

Huber, C. G. (1905). On the development and shape of uriniferous tubules of certain of the higher mammals. *Amer. J. Physiol.* **4**, Suppl. 1.

Kyte, J. (1976). Immunoferritin determination of the distribution of $(Na^+ + K^+)$-ATPase over the plasma membranes of renal tubules. II. Proximal segment. *J. Cell Biol.* **68**, 304–321.

Larsson, L. (1975a). The ultrastructure of the developing proximal tubule in the rat kidney. *J. Ultrastruct. Res.* **51**, 119–139.

Larsson, L. (1975b). Ultrastructure and permeability of intercellular contacts of developing proximal tubule in the rat kidney. *J. Ultrastruct. Res.* **52**, 100–113.

Larsson, L. and Horster, M. (1976). Ultrastructure and net fluid transport in isolated perfused developing proximal tubules. *J. Ultrastruct. Res.* **54**, 276–285.

Larsson, L. and Maunsbach, A. B. (1975). Differentiation of the vacuolar apparatus in cells of the developing proximal tubule in the rat kidney. *J. Ultrastruct. Res.* **53**, 254–270.

Oliver, J. (1968). *Nephrons and Kidneys*, Hoeber Medical Division, Harper and Row, New York.

Potter, E. L. (1972). *Normal and Abnormal Development of the Kidney*, Yearbook Medical Publishers, Chicago.

Revel, J. P. and Karnovsky, M. J. (1967). Hexagonal array of subunits in intercellular junctions of the mouse heart and liver. *J. Cell Biol.* **33**, C7–C12.

Schmidt, U. and Horster, M. (1977). Na–K-activated ATPase: activity maturation in rabbit nephron segments dissected *in vitro*. *Am. J. Physiol.* **233**, F55–F68.

Skou, J. C. (1965). Enzymatic basis for active transport of Na^+ and K^+ across cell membrane. *Physiol. Rev.* **45**, 596–625.

Spitzer, A. and Brandis, M. (1974). Functional and morphologic maturation of superficial nephrons. Relationship to total kidney function. *J. clin. Invest.* **53**, 279–295.

17
Comparative and Functional Aspects of Thin Loop Limb Ultrastructure

Wilhelm Kriz, August Schiller, Brigitte Kaissling and
Roland Taugner

Introduction

A mammalian kidney generally contains short-looped and long-looped
nephrons. Therefore the thin limbs of Henle's loop comprise a descending thin
limb of a short loop (DTLS), a descending thin limb of a long loop (DTLL)
and an ascending thin limb (ATL), which is only present in long loops.
These segments are characterized by different epithelia. Moreover, the
epithelium of the DTLL changes in character when descending from the
outer into the inner medulla. Therefore, based on ultrastructural criteria,
this segment has to be subdivided into an upper portion (DTLL u.p.;
predominantly situated in the outer medulla) and a lower portion (DTLL l.p.;
predominantly situated in the inner medulla). Consequently, four epithelial
types must be distinguished: type I, characteristic for DTLS; type II,
characteristic for DTLL u.p., gradually transforming into type III, which is
present in DTLL l.p.; type IV epithelium generally starts a short distance
before the loop bend (in rabbit distances between 0 and 140 μm have been
found) and is characteristic for the total ATL (Fig. 1).

Previous Ultrastructural Studies

Epithelium type II was first ultrastructurally characterized in mouse (Rhodin,
1958) and has long been considered representative for all thin limb segments.
Lapp and Nolte (1962) described the epithelia type II and IV in rat. However,
since both epithelia are similiar in some respects, they came to the erroneous

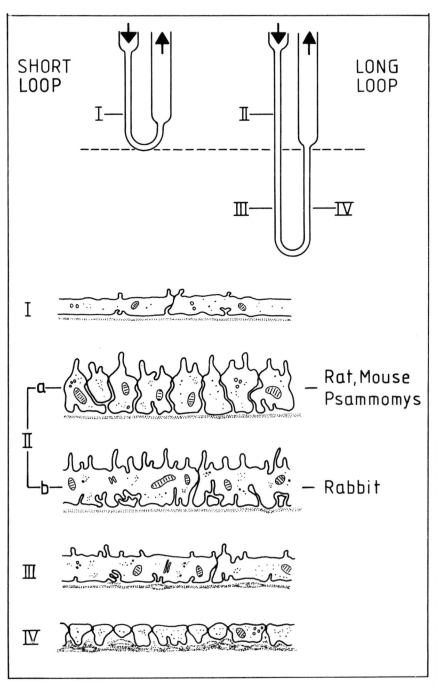

FIG. 1. *Schematic representation of the essential ultrastructural features of thin limb epithelia; the nuclear regions are not drawn.*

conclusion that epithelium IV follows after epithelium II along the descending thin limb of long loops. Bulger and Trump (1966) described the epithelia III and IV in the inner medulla of rats but they could not determine which belongs to the descending and which to the ascending limb. Also in the rat, Osvaldo and Latta (1966) clearly identified epithelium II as characteristic for the initial part of descending thin limb. However, the transition from epithelium II to IV has not been fully elucidated. Epithelium type I has first been described by Dieterich (1968) in rat; by single nephron tracing it could clearly be shown that epithelium type I belongs to the descending thin limbs of short loops, whereas epithelium type II represents the outer medullary portion of the descending thin limbs of long loops (Kriz *et al.*, 1972). Schwartz and Venkatachalam (1974) were the first to investigate systematically all thin limb segments and to describe all four epithelial types. They draw attention to differences between the cell junctions of these epithelia. Meanwhile the thin limbs have been investigated in various species: mouse (Dieterich *et al.*, 1975), *Octodon degus* (Barrett and Majack, 1977), *Psammomys obesus* (Barrett *et al.*, 1978*a, b*), rabbit (Kaissling and Kriz, 1979); preliminary data have been obtained from cat and Syrian hamster (Kriz *et al.*, 1978). In the human kidney a thin limb epithelium has been ultrastructurally described (Bulger *et al.*, 1967) which differs in some respects from the thin limb epithelia of rodents; therefore it is not possible to state to which thin limb segment it belongs. Until recently, freeze-fracture data about the tight junctions in thin limbs have been sparse (Pricam *et al.*, 1974; Humbert *et al.*, 1975). Very recently, freeze-fracture data covering all thin limb epithelia in rat have been presented (Schwartz *et al.*, 1978). We have obtained similar data and will present them in the following report.

Ultrastructure of Thin Limbs

Species differences
Before describing the different thin limb segments we must take into consideration that species differences occur. In mouse, rat and *Psammomys obesus* the descending thin limbs of short loops are spatially separated from those of long loops (the DTLS being integrated into the vascular bundles whereas the DTLL descend within the interbundle regions; Kriz *et al.*, 1976). Obviously correlated to the similar histotopographical arrangement, the thin limb segments appear to have an almost identical ultrastructural organization. These three species represent one pattern of thin limb organization which may be used as a basis for comparative considerations. A similar pattern is present in *Octodon degus*. Different patterns have been found in cat, Syrian hamster and rabbit; however, only the organization in rabbit has been thoroughly

investigated. Therefore, the thin limb organization characteristic for mouse, rat and *Psammomys* will be considered and compared to that in rabbit.

Descending thin limbs of short loops
The DTLS in rat, mouse and *Psammomys* are established by a very simple, flat and non-interdigitating epithelium (Fig. 1, type I). The tight junctions (Figs 2 and 3, Table I) consist of mostly two to four anastomosing junctional strands (Schwartz *et al.*, 1978: 3·75 strands in average). In rabbit

TABLE I
Dimensional characteristics of thin limb tight junctions[a]

	Rat		Rabbit		
	Number of junctional strands (Data from replicas)	Apical– basal depth (nm)	Number of junctional strands (Data from replicas)	Apical– basal depth (nm)	Apical– basal depth (nm) (Data from sections)
Short loops Descending	$2·3 \pm 1·0$ $(n = 21)$	$46·6 \pm 31·1$	$5·9 \pm 1·5$ $(n = 11)$	$142·5 \pm 56·8$	$119·2 \pm 42·5$ $(n = 14)$
Long loops Descending Upper portion	$1·5 \pm 0·5$ $(n = 38)$	$18·7 \pm 7·6$	$5·2 \pm 1·0$ $(n = 31)$	$98·8 \pm 43·8$	$94·6 \pm 32·0$ $(n = 53)$
Lower portion	$4·2 \pm 1·6$ $(n = 35)$	$39·2 \pm 20·2$	$3·1 \pm 1·3$ $(n = 12)$	$132·1 \pm 65·2$	$121·1 \pm 67·4$ $(n = 17)$
Ascending	$2·1 \pm 0·9$ $(n = 71)$	$23·9 \pm 17·7$	$1·6 \pm 0·7$ $(n = 36)$	$27·6 \pm 14·8$	$32·7 \pm 13·0$ $(n = 26)$

[a] This table summarizes the number of junctional strands and the apical–basal depth in the different thin limb segments. The values are means ± s.d.; *n* is the number of photographed junctions which have been used for the measurements.

FIGS 2–5. *Rat kidney, freeze-fracture replicas from the outer medulla. The replicas were prepared according to Roesinger* et al. *(1978). Figure 2 shows descending thin limb of a short loop of Henle (epithelium type I); its tight junction is shown at higher magnification in Fig. 3. Figure 4 shows upper portion of a long descending thin limb (epithelium type IIa) with its tight junction in Fig. 5. Fig. 2, × 2400; Fig. 3, × 51 000; Fig. 4, × 2600; Fig. 5, × 63 000.*

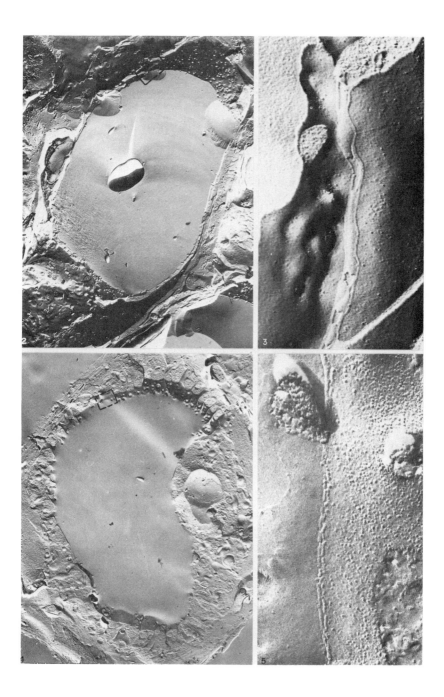

the DTLS epithelium is very similarly organized and no striking differences emerge. The tight junctions of this segment in rabbit consist of three to seven anastomosing strands and are distinctly deeper than in rat (Figs 10–13, Table I).

Descending thin limb of long loops
The DTLL u.p. in rat, mouse and *Psammomys* has a relatively high, complexly organized and heavily interdigitated epithelium with numerous apical microvilli (Fig. 1, type IIa). The numerous cell processes are linked together by very shallow tight junctions (Figs 4 and 5, Table I) which generally consist only of one or two parallel junctional strands (Schwartz *et al.*, 1978: 1 strand).

In contrast, the DTLL u.p. in rabbit are established by a non-interdigitating epithelium (Fig. 1, type IIb). It is also relatively high, bears numerous apical microvilli and has some infoldings of the basal cell membrane. The tight junctions are much deeper than in rat and consist of several anastomosing strands (Figs 14–17, Table I).

Passing down into the inner zone, the epithelium of the DTLL u.p. in all investigated species changes gradually to the simple epithelium characteristic for the DTLL l.p. The epithelial simplification shows species differences. Thus, in the rabbit the status of DTLL l.p. is reached within the lowermost part of the inner stripe, whereas in *Psammomys* or in the rat a heterogenous population of descending thin limbs is still evident in the upper parts of the inner zone. This consists of thin limbs already lined by the typical simple inner zone epithelium (type III) and others which are still lined by the more complex outer medullary epithelium (type II) in different stages of reduction.

The DTLL l.p. are very similarly organized in all investigated animals. They are again established by a flat, simple and non-interdigitating epithelium (Fig. 1, type III). The tight junctions (Figs 6, 7 and 18–21) consist of several anastomosing junctional strands (Schwartz *et al.*, 1978: in rat, 3·1 strands on average); however, the apical basal depth is clearly deeper in rabbits than in rats (Table I).

Ascending thin limb
In principle, the ATL (including the bend) are equally organized in all species investigated so far (Fig. 1, type IV). They are characterized by flat but heavily interdigitating cells. Only a few small mitochondria are encountered;

FIGS 6–9. *Rat kidney, freeze-fracture replicas from the inner medulla. Figure 6 shows lower portion of a descending thin limb of a long loop (epithelium type III) with its tight junction in Fig. 7. Figure 8 shows ascending thin limb (epithelium type IV); the corresponding tight junction is shown in Fig. 9. Fig. 6, × 3200; Fig. 7, × 32 500; Fig. 8, × 5400; Fig. 9, × 41 000.*

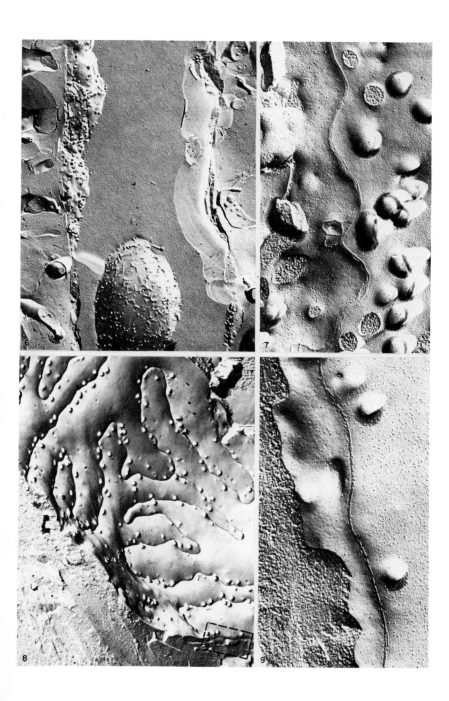

apical microvilli are scarcely present. The cells and cell processes are connected by very shallow tight junctions (Figs 8, 9 and 22–25, Table I) which consist of only one or two parallel junctional strands (Schwartz et al., 1978: in rat, 1·3 strands on average).

Functional Correlations and Conclusions

Correlating the ultrastructural organization of the epithelia with known transport and permeability properties, the following statements are possible:

(1) Due to the lack of functional membrane data no correlations concerning the DTLS can be made.
(2) In DTLL considerable species differences occur. The DTLL u.p. epithelium in rabbit (no interdigitation, deep junctions) should be expected to be much "tighter" with respect to ion permeability than the corresponding segment in rat or *Psammomys* (heavily interdigitated, shallow junctions). Whether or not the concentration of tubular fluid within the descending limbs occurs predominantly by solute addition or predominantly by water extraction may at least be partly explained by species differences in the tight junction pattern. In *Psammomys* solute addition has been found to account for a major part of the concentration increase (de Rouffignac et al., 1973; Imbert and de Rouffignac, 1976). In rabbits the increase in osmolarity is generally considered to be due to water extraction (Kokko, 1970; Kokko and Tisher, 1976).
(3) The ultrastructural organization of the ATL epithelium (heavily interdigitated, shallow junctions) fits in well with the high ion permeability of these segments in rabbit, rat and hamster (Imai and Kokko, 1974; Imai, 1977).

Acknowledgement

The investigation was supported by the Deutsche Forschungsgemeinschaft.

FIGS 10–17. *Rabbit kidney, freeze-fracture replicas and ultrathin sections from the outer medulla. The replicas have been prepared according to Roesinger et al. (1978), the sections of fixed tissue according to Kaissling and Kriz (1979). Figure 10 shows descending thin limb of a short loop (epithelium type I); the organization of the corresponding tight junction is shown in Figs 11, 12 and 13. Figure 14 shows upper portion of a long descending thin limb (epithelium type IIb) with its tight junction in Figs 15, 16 and 17. Fig. 10, × 3500; Fig. 11, × 34 000; Figs 12 and 13, × 92 000; Fig. 14, × 3400; Fig. 15, × 34 000; Fig. 16, × 92 000; Fig. 17, × 99 000.*

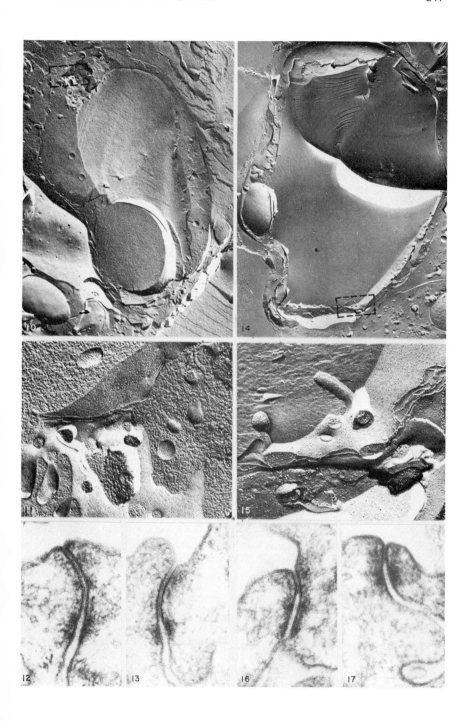

References

Barrett, J. M. and Majack, R. A. (1977). The ultrastructural organization of long and short nephrons in the kidney of the rodent (*Octodon degus*). *Anat. Rec.* **187**, 530.

Barrett, J. M., Kriz, W., Kaissling, B. and de Rouffignac, C. (1978*a*). The ultrastructure of the nephrons of the desert rodent (*Psammomys obesus*) kidney. I. Thin limbs of Henle of short-looped nephrons. *Am. J. Anat.* **151**, 487–498.

Barrett, J. M., Kriz, W., Kaissling, B. and de Rouffignac, C. (1978*b*). The ultrastructure of the nephrons of the desert rodent (*Psammomys obesus*) kidney. II. Thin limbs of Henle of long-looped nephrons. *Am. J. Anat.* **151**, 499–514.

Bulger, R. E. and Trump, B. F. (1966). Fine structure of the rat renal papilla. *Am. J. Anat.* **118**, 685–722.

Bulger, R. E., Tisher, C. C., Myers, Ch. H. and Trump, B. F. (1967). Human renal ultrastructure II. The thin limb of Henle's loop and the interstitium in healthy individuals. *Lab. Invest.* **16**, 124–141.

Dieterich, H. J. (1968). Die Ultrastruktur der Gefäßbündel im Mark der Rattenniere. *Z. Zellforsch. mikrosk. Anat.* **84**, 350–371.

Dieterich, H. J., Barrett, J. M., Kriz, W. and Bülhoff, J. P. (1975). The ultrastructure of the thin loop limbs of the mouse kidney. *Anat. Embryol.* **147**, 1–18.

Humbert, F., Pricam, C., Perrelet, A. and Orci, L. (1975). Freeze-fracture differences between plasma membranes of descending and ascending branches of the rat Henle's thin loop. *Lab. Invest.* **33**, 407–411.

Imai, M. (1977). Function of the thin ascending limb of Henle of rats and hamsters perfused *in vitro*. *Am. J. Physiol.* **3**, F201–F209.

Imai, M. and Kokko, J. P. (1974). Sodium chloride, urea and water transport in the thin ascending limb of Henle: generation of osmotic gradients by passive diffusion of solutes. *J. clin. Invest.* **53**, 393–402.

Imbert, M. and de Rouffignac, C. (1976). Role of sodium and urea in the renal concentrating mechanism in *Psammomys obesus*. *Pflügers Arch. ges. Physiol.* **361**, 107–114.

Kaissling, B. and Kriz, W. (1979). Structural analysis of the rabbit kidney. *Adv. Anat. Embryol. Cell Biol.* **56**, 1–123.

Kriz, W., Barrett, J. M. and Peter, S. (1976). The renal vasculature: anatomical-functional aspects. In *Kidney and Urinary Tract Physiology II* (K. Thurau, ed.), International Review of Science, Physiology, Series 2, Vol. 11, University Park Press, Baltimore, pp. 1–21.

Kriz, W., Schnermann, J. and Dieterich, H. J. (1972). Differences in the morphology of descending limb of short and long loops of Henle in the rat kidney. In *Recent Advances in Renal Physiology* (H. Wirz and F. Spinelli, eds), Basel, Karger, pp. 140–144.

FIGS 18–25. *Rabbit kidney, replicas and sections from the inner medulla. Figure 18 shows lower portion of a long descending thin limb (epithelium type III); the organization of the corresponding tight junction is shown in Figs 19, 20 and 21. Figure 22 shows ascending thin limb (epithelium type IV) with its corresponding tight junction morphology in Figs 23, 24 and 25. Fig. 18, × 5200; Fig. 19, × 21 000; Figs 20 and 21, × 92 000; Fig. 22, × 9500; Fig. 23, × 68 000; Figs 24 and 25, × 72 000.*

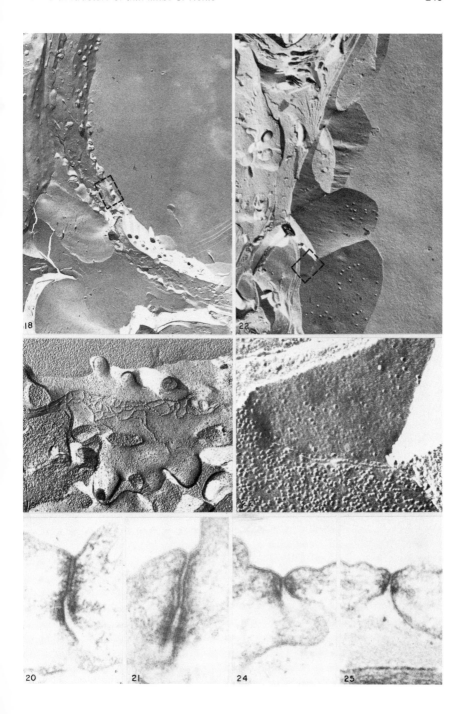

Kokko, J. P. (1970). Sodium chloride and water transport in the descending limb of Henle. *J. clin. Invest.* **49**, 1838–1846.

Kokko, J. P. and Tisher, C. C. (1976). Water movement across nephron segments involved with the countercurrent multiplication system. *Kidney Int.* **10**, 64–81.

Kriz, W., Kaissling, B. and Psczolla, M. (1978). Morphological characterization of the cells in Henle's loop and the distal tubule. In *New Aspects of Renal Function* (*Workshop Conferences Hoechst*), Vol. 6 (H. G. Vogel and K. J. Ullrich, eds), Excerpta Medica, Amsterdam and Oxford, pp. 67–78.

Lapp, H. and Nolte, A. (1962). Vergleichende elektronenmikroskopische Untersuchungen am Mark der Rattenniere bei Harnkonzentrierung und Harnverdünnung. *Frankfurt. Z. Path.* **71**, 617–633.

Osvaldo, L. and Latta, H. (1966). The thin limbs of the loop of Henle. *J. Ultrastruct. Res.* **15**, 144–168.

Pricam, C., Humbert, F., Perrelet, A. and Orci, L. (1974). A freeze-etch study of the tight junctions of the rat kidney tubules. *Lab. Invest.* **30**, 286–291.

Rhodin, J. (1958). Anatomy of kidney tubules. *Int. Rev. Cytol.* **7**, 485–434.

Roesinger, B., Schiller, A. and Taugner, R. (1978). A freeze fracture study of tight junctions in the pars convoluta and pars recta of the renal proximal tubule. *Cell Tissue Res.* **186**, 121–133.

de Rouffignac, C., Morel, F., Moss, N. and Roinel, N. (1973). Micropuncture study of water and electrolyte movement along the loop of Henle in *Psammomys* with special reference to magnesium, calcium and phosphorus. *Pflügers Arch. ges. Physiol.* **344**, 309–326.

Schwartz, M. M. and Venkatachalam, M. A. (1974). Structural differences in thin limbs of Henle: physiological implications. *Kidney Int.* **6**, 103–208.

Schwartz, M. M., Karnovsky, M. J. and Venkatachalam, M. A. (1978). Anatomic segmentation in the thin limbs of Henle's loop in the rat. In *Proceedings of an International Symposium on the Vascular and Tubular Organization of the Kidney*, Harvard Medical School, Boston, pp. 10–12.

18
Morphologic Evidence for a Transcellular Pathway via Elements of Endoplasmic Reticulum in Rat Proximal Tubules

Jørgen Rostgaard and Kjeld Møllgård

Introduction

Epithelia consist of continuous layers of cells which cover internal and external surfaces. Whether solutes traverse a given epithelium through the cells themselves (transcellular transport) or through the tight junction route (paracellular transport) is still an open question. The recently suggested classification of epithelia as "tight" or "leaky" is based on the measured transepithelial resistance of these systems (Frömter and Diamond, 1972). The principal variation in conductance appears to be the degree of paracellular permeability rather than the permeability of cell membranes, which are the principal resistive elements of the transcellular route for ion movement. Paracellular permeability, apparently not related to the active transport of ions, is largely limited by the tight junctions (Farquhar and Palade, 1963), which characteristically occur at the lumen-facing end of the epithelial intercellular space. Claude and Goodenough (1973) have attempted to correlate the physiological "tightness" of the junctions of a given epithelium with the number of sealing strands comprising the network. Some experimental evidence has been presented in which a correlation between permeability and tight junction morphology was not found (Martinez-Palomo and Erlij, 1975; Møllgård et al., 1976). Thus it is still unclear whether junctional "leakiness" and "tightness" to ions and water will prove to have morphological correlates visible in the electron microscope.

Active transport of sodium ions is presumably based on transcellular permeation from the luminal solution across the luminal cell membrane into

the cells, and then across the basolateral membrane into the lateral intercellular space and basal compartment. Thus far very little morphologic
evidence has been presented for the existence of any compartment or pathway
in the cell interior ("black box") of solute-transporting epithelial cells, which
could act as channels for ion and water transport.

In a recent study based on electron microprobe X-ray analysis of frozen-
hydrated sections of rabbit ileum some local differences in concentrations of
Na, K and Cl in the cytoplasm were measured (Gupta *et al.*, 1978). These
gradients were abolished by ouabain. Gupta *et al.* suggested that an actomyosin system localized in the cortical cytoplasm of the cells may act as a
channel in which ions are more mobile and along which Na^+ and Cl^- are
more rapidly conducted. Local differences in cytoplasmatic concentrations of
Na^+ and Cl^- have also been observed with ion-selective microelectrodes
(Zeuthen, 1977). We have recently provided ultrastructural evidence for the
presence of a continuous system of tubulo-cisternal endoplasmic reticulum
(TER) in a variety of transporting epithelia, including rabbit ileum (Møllgård
and Rostgaard, 1978). The TER abuts on apical and basolateral cell surfaces
and is localized in the periphery of the cytoplasm. It was found to be most
developed in low resistance epithelia and suggested to be implicated in
transcellular transport mechanisms.

In the present communication we have combined information provided by
thin sections with that available in replicas of freeze-fractured specimens of
rat kidneys in order to define more precisely the characteristics of the TER
of proximal tubule epithelial cells.

Methods for Visualization of the Entire Endoplasmic Reticulum

In some previous reports (Møllgård and Saunders, 1977; Møllgård and
Rostgaard, 1978) we have emphasized the use of thick sections of metal-
impregnated specimens according to the technique of Thiery and Rambourg
(1976). Thick sections are well suited for a demonstration of continuity in the
TER but less suitable for an adequate demonstration of any points of contact
between this system and the apical and basolateral cell membranes. Such
possible sites of entry into or exit from the system are better investigated in
thin sections and by freeze-fracturing. In the present communication we have
examined the detailed organization of the TER in rat proximal tubules.

Adult male rats were fixed by vascular perfusion with 2·5 per cent
glutaraldehyde in 0·1 M cacodylate buffer (pH 7·4) with 1 per cent glucose,
2 per cent polyvinylpyrolidone and 0·015 per cent $CaCl_2$ added. Small pieces
were fixed overnight and stored in the buffer.

For thin section electron microscopy small tissue blocks were postfixed 16 h at 4 °C in 1·5 per cent osmium tetroxide in 0·1 M phosphate buffer (pH 7·4). Some tissue specimens were stained 1 h at 20 °C *en bloc* in 5 per cent aqueous uranyl acetate solution. The tissue blocks were dehydrated continuously in alcohol and embedded in Epon. Thin sections were double-stained with uranyl acetate and lead citrate.

For freeze-fracturing, small blocks of kidney cortex were prepared after 12 h of fixation as described above. Following 1 h of infiltration with 25 per cent buffered glycerol at room temperature the specimens were mounted on gold disks. The tissue was then frozen in the liquid phase of partially solidified Freon 22 and stored in liquid nitrogen. Freeze-fracturing followed by carbon–platinum shadowing was performed with Balzer's apparatus (BAF 301) equipped with an electron beam gun. Specimens were fractured at a stage temperature of −115 °C and replicated with platinum–carbon without etching. The thickness of the platinum–carbon and carbon coats (approximately 2 nm and 20 nm) was controlled by a thin film monitor. Replicas were cleaned in chromic acid and chrome-sulphuric acid.

All freeze-fracture images have been mounted so that the shadow direction is from the bottom to the top of the micrograph.

The TER System—General Appearance and Terminology

A variety of sodium-transporting epithelia (frog skin, sheep choroid plexus, rabbit gallbladder and small intestine, and rat kidney) possesses a complex intracellular system of tubulocisternal endoplasmic reticulum (Møllgård and Rostgaard, 1978). The basic structural features of the system include an apical polygonal network of tortuous tubules oriented in parallel with the apical (luminal) cell membrane, some connecting elements, and a complex system of flattened cisternae along the lateral cell membrane.

In the above-mentioned study we have chosen the abbreviation TER for the system of tubulocisternal endoplasmic reticulum. In a broad sense TER may stand for transport-functioning ER, and in specialized epithelia involved in transcellular transport the TER may define a system of transcellular ER. Until these suggestions are somewhat more substantiated we use the term TER as a designation for the tubulocisternal ER (Møllgård and Rostgaard, 1978).

Metal Impregnation

The general appearance of the TER in epithelial cells of rat kidney has been described previously (Møllgård and Rostgaard, 1978). That description was

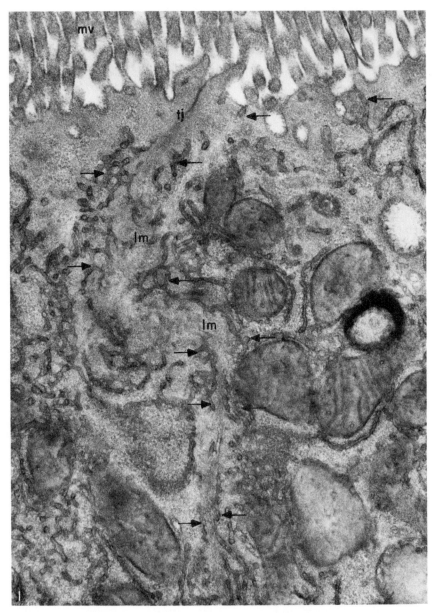

FIG. 1. *Survey picture of the luminal part of two apposing proximal tubule cells. The section passes nearly parallel to the lateral intercellular space. Microvilli (mv), tight junction (tj) and position of the lateral cell membrane (lm) are marked. Arrows mark tubular TER in the apical cytoplasm and cisternal TER apposed to the lateral cell membrane.* × *37 000.*

based on 100 kV electron microscopy of thick sections (0·2–0·4 μm) of renal tissue impregnated with metals according to the technique of Thiery and Rambourg (1976). In that study the TER was described as a highly developed system of anastomosing smooth-surfaced tubules in continuity with a complex system of flattened cisternae which were most prevalent along the basolateral cell membrane. Slender tortuous tubules or rows of vesicles connected the lateral TER system with the apical cell surface and made intimate contact with the luminal cell membrane. The TER tubules were found intermingled with the vast and well known complex system of dense apical canaliculi and associated vacuoles which characterizes the apical cytoplasm of proximal tubule cells.

Similar observations have recently been made by Thiery and Bergeron (1977), and by the use of a new block-staining technique and stereomicroscopy of thick sections these authors and their collaborators were able to visualize clearly the continuity of the entire ER. Unfortunately the metal impregnation does not provide sufficient information about the apical and lateral cell membranes in relation to the ER.

Thin Sectioning

Using electron microscopy of thin sections (60 nm) obtained from uranyl block-stained material, a much more detailed fine structural analysis of the TER can be obtained (Figs 1–3). In sections which pass nearly parallel to the lateral intercellular space and graze the lateral cell membranes of two apposing cells the anastomosing tubules and the fenestrated cisternae of the TER could be seen (Fig. 1). A major part of TER was localized in the peripheral cytoplasm in close contact with the lateral cell membrane. A minor part of the TER was situated close to mitochondria and some angular cytosomes (0·2–1 μm), interpreted in the present study as peroxisomes. Continuity with the granular endoplasmic reticulum could be demonstrated.

Serial sectioning of the apical part of the cells showed that slender tortuous tubules connect the lateral TER system with small flattened cisternae underlying the luminal cell membrane forming calyx-like structures. The calyx-like structures were positioned either at an invagination of the cell membrane or between the roots of the microvilli. The size of these cisternae was about 0·1 μm and the peripheral cisternal membrane followed the luminal cell membrane with a gap between the apposed membranes of about 10 nm (Fig. 2). The number of tubular extensions to the luminal cell membrane was estimated to be about 200 per cell or about one in every ten microvilli (in the third segment of proximal tubule).

Thin sections of the basal part of the cells showed that the fenestrated

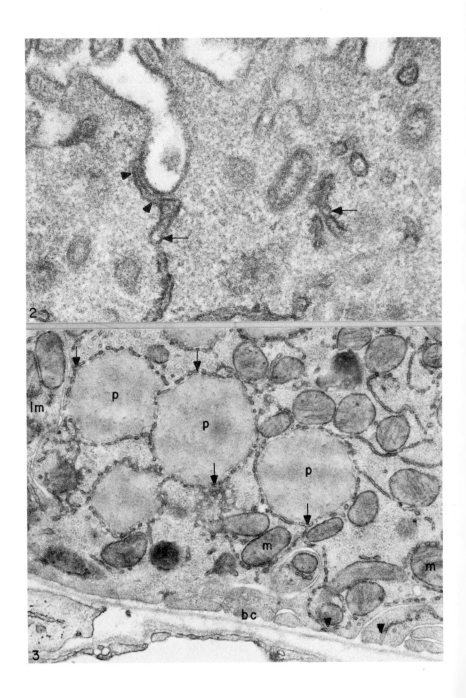

cisternae of the TER abutted on and closely followed the lateral cell membrane to the base of the cells (Fig. 3). The TER was thus interposed between the mitochondria and the basolateral cell membrane. Fenestrated cisternae of the TER extended from the main network along the basolateral cell membrane to surround mitochondria and peroxisomes (Fig. 3).

Freeze-fracture

In surveying the entire proximal tubule epithelial cell in freeze-fracture replicas (Fig. 4) it appeared that the very well developed TER system was in close apposition to apical and lateral cell membranes, the Golgi complex, peroxisomes, mitochondria and infoldings of the basal cell membrane. The elements of the TER were particularly abundant in the peripheral zone of the cytoplasm and diminishing in concentration towards the perinuclear zone. Prominent subsurface positions of the system were always encountered along the lateral cell membrane (Fig. 5) and consistently, but less frequently, along apical and basal cell membranes.

In freeze-fractured specimens the apical elements of the TER were different from other parts of the system (Fig. 5). They comprised fine membrane-bounded dilatations alternating with narrow channels arranged in a distinctive curved and angular fashion. Calyx-like extensions were closely apposed to invaginations of the apical cell membrane. Tubules of uniform diameter connected this fine apical portion to the extensive TER along the lateral cell membrane (Fig. 5). This main portion of the TER exhibited large cisternae which were closely apposed to the lateral cell membrane (Fig. 6). Elements of similar appearance followed all infoldings in the basolateral cell membrane (Fig. 7). The cisternae were usually regularly fenestrated and therefore presented some very characteristic membrane profiles in freeze-fracture replicas which facilitate their identification.

Mitochondria were easily recognized, and the organelles in the basal parts of the cells with characteristic angular shapes and a size varying from 0·2–1 μm were interpreted as peroxisomes. Mitochondria and especially peroxisomes were encaged in a network of TER elements (Fig. 8).

FIG. 2. *Luminal part of proximal tubule cell with apical tubules of TER (arrows). One tubule is seen to be connected with a small flattened cisterna apposed to the luminal cell membrane (arrowheads). × 71 000.*

FIG. 3. *Basal part of proximal tubule cell. Lateral (lm) and basal cell membrane (bc) are marked. Peroxisomes (p) surrounded by fenestrated cisternae of TER (arrows) which are connected to TER along the basolateral cell membrane (arrowheads). Mitochondria (m). × 29 000.*

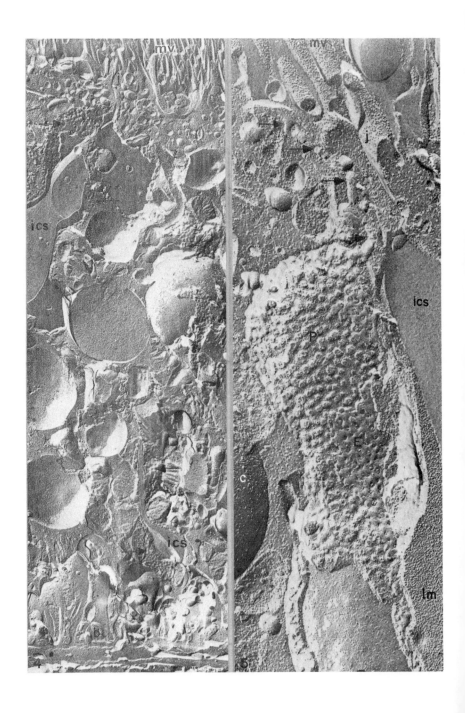

The Model

Based on the information obtained by metal impregnation, thin sectioning and freeze-fracture, a three-dimensional model of the TER in rat proximal tubule cells was produced (Fig. 9). Preliminary results have shown that the TER system in other types of isotonic solute-transporting epithelial cells is not in every detail identical to that presented in this model.

Discussion

In the present communication we have demonstrated the existence of an extensive and complex system of tubulocisternal endoplasmic reticulum (TER), which forms a continuous compartment abutting on apical and basolateral cell surfaces. Part of the TER system has been described previously. In rat kidney proximal tubule cells Ericsson (1964) has described collections of smooth-surfaced tubules and vesicles localized parallel to the lateral plasma membrane, which he named the paramembranous tubular system (PTS). These observations have been confirmed by Bulger (1965) and extended by Jacobsen and Jørgensen (1973), who found the PTS equally well developed along the entire length of the proximal tubules. Smooth-surfaced ER was characteristically found around microbodies and less frequently around mitochondria. In addition, conglomerates or single elements were scattered at random in the cytoplasm. Tisher (1976) has found the PTS to be especially well developed in rabbit kidneys.

The present study has extended the knowledge of the structure and the topography of the smooth endoplasmic reticulum in proximal tubule cells. This is mainly due to the combined use of freeze-fracture technique, serial sectioning and thick sectioning of metal-impregnated tissue, and conventional thin section electron microscopy. From the results of the present study it is clear that subsurface or paramembranous cisternae—not paramembranous tubules—underlie the lateral cell membrane all the way from the level of the tight junction to the base of the cell, and thus form a continuous compartment in the peripheral cytoplasm. Slender bending tubules connect this

---

FIG. 4 *Freeze-fracture replica of proximal tubule. Microvilli (mv), junction (j) and basal cell membrane (bc). Arrows mark fenestrated cisternae of TER apposed to the lateral cell membrane. Intercellular space (ics). × 14 000.*

FIG. 5. *Freeze-fracture replica of the apical part of proximal tubule cells. Microvilli (mv), junction (j), dilated intercellular space (ics) and cytosome (c). Fenestrated cisterna of TER with exposed P and E faces are seen along the lateral cell membrane (lm). Tubular TER (arrows). × 41 000.*

compartment with small subsurface cisternae apposed to the luminal cell membrane. Thus an intracellular, membrane-bounded channel system abuts on both the luminal and the basolateral cell membrane. Direct contact between the TER and the cell membrane has not been observed, and no gap junctions between the TER and the cell membrane have been identified in proximal tubule epithelial cells. The outer membrane of the TER cisternae is always separated from the cell membrane by a constant distance of about 10 nm, which indicates that some "spacers" may exist at this interface.

It is often argued that the localization of the mitochondria within tubule cells reflects the position of the energy-dependent pump sites along the basolateral cell membrane. If this argument is valid it is worth noting that the mitochondria are encaged within a network of cisternal ER and that the peripheral portion of the system is always interposed between the mitochondria and the basolateral cell membrane. This feature indicates that TER may be involved in energy-dependent ion transport. The ER in muscle cells is known to possess an ATP-driven calcium pump (Hasselbach, 1964), which suggests that ER in general may be involved in ion transport.

The role of the ER in synthesis, transport and storage has been thoroughly studied (for a review, see Palade, 1975). Little is known about the nature of the transport mechanism (flow) through the ER, but it has been suggested that solute transport into the ER may bring about osmotic water flow into and through the cisternae which could create a stream that carries newly synthesized protein towards the Golgi complex (cf. Oschman et al., 1974). During intestinal lipid absorption numerous droplets of triglycerides are visible in the lumen of the smooth ER in the apical portion of the cells (Cardell et al., 1967). The droplets are transported via the Golgi region to the lateral cell membrane where they are discharged as chylomicrons to the intercellular space. It is possible that a stream carries the lipid in the fluid-filled channels of the endoplasmic reticulum from the apical portion of the cells to the lateral intercellular space. In the case of nerve cell axons it is widely accepted that cholinesterase flow in the lumen of tubular ER from the perikaryon to the nerve endings (see, for example, Kreutzberg et al., 1975). (For further information about the smooth ER as a continuous intra-axonal pathway, cf. Droz et al., 1975.)

FIG. 6. *Fenestrated TER cisterna (arrows) adjacent to an infolding of the basolateral cell membrane is exposed. An angular peroxisome (p) is surrounded by cisternal TER (upper left arrows). Note the straight tubular protrusion (t) from another peroxisome. Mitochondria (m). × 37 000.*

FIG. 7. *Freeze-fracture replica showing the lateral cell membranes of two adjacent proximal tubule cells. P and E faces are marked. Fenestrated TER cisterna (arrows) apposed to the lateral cell membrane is seen. × 37 000.*

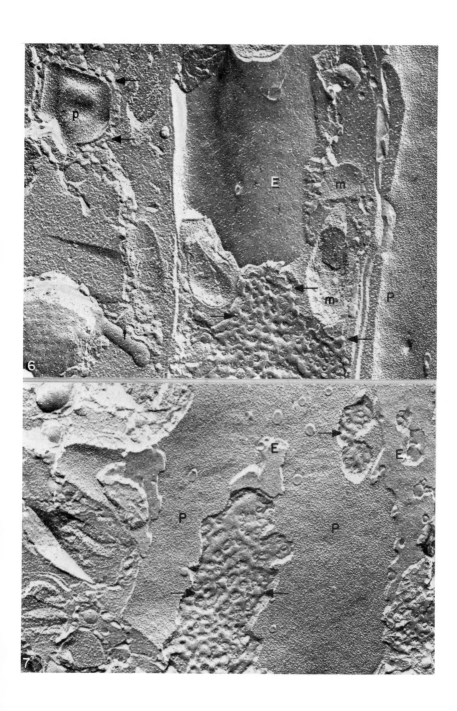

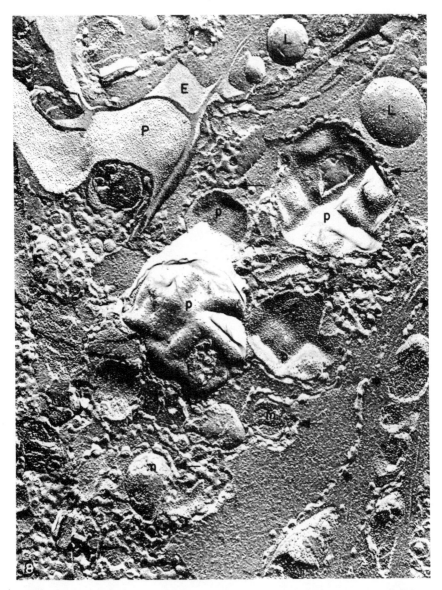

FIG. 8. *Freeze-fractured basal part of proximal tubule cells showing P and E faces of basolateral cell membranes. Cisternal TER (arrows) encages mitochondria (m) and angular peroxisomes (p) but not lysosomes (L). TER along cross-fractured lateral cell membrane is marked with stars. × 37 000.*

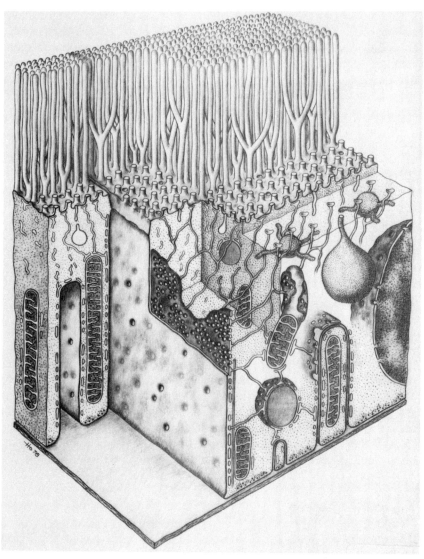

FIG. 9. *Schematic representation of the distribution of the TER, a tubulocisternal endoplasmic reticulum in rat proximal tubules. Apical tubules of the TER are confluent with calyx-like extensions closely applied to the luminal cell membrane and are also confluent with extensive cisternae of fenestrated endoplasmic reticulum apposed to the basolateral cell membrane. The TER is interposed between the mitochondria and the cell membrane in the basal infoldings. The TER is closely related to apical pinocytotic invaginations and vacuoles and in the basal part of the renal cells peroxisomes and mitochondria are surrounded by cisternae of TER.*

Recently it has been suggested that the ER is involved in transcellular sodium transport in a "tight" epithelium (Voûte et al., 1975). When isolated frog skin was exposed to a hydrostatic pressure on the inside and short-circuited, a linear relationship between active sodium transport as measured by short-circuit current and number of light microscopically observable "vacuoles" was established. Electron microscopically these "vacuoles" were identified as "scalloped sacs" and distended cisternae of ER.

No direct evidence for the involvement of ER in transepithelial solute transport in "leaky" epithelia has been presented so far. However, the findings of substantial intracytoplasmic gradients in ion concentrations by Zeuthen (1977) on epithelial cells of *Necturus* gallbladder and by Gupta et al. (1978) on rabbit ileum intestinal cells would find a natural explanation should the hypothesis that cisternal ER sequesters sodium and chloride be correct. The possibility of such an intracellular compartmentalization of ions as a function of transepithelial transport does not seem unreasonable (cf. editorial review by Civan, 1978).

Conclusion

The results of this study indicate the presence of an extensive and complex system of tubulocisternal endoplasmic reticulum (TER), which occupies a considerable part of the peripheral cytoplasm in proximal tubule epithelial cells from rat kidney, where it forms a continuous compartment abutting on apical and basolateral cell surfaces. Clearly additional study is necessary to establish the functional significance of the TER, but its potential role as the main route for transcellular movement of fluid is obvious, and a sodium-transporting system associated with this very extensive membrane compartment would be well suited for producing an isotonic transportate.

Acknowledgement

The authors are indebted to Mrs Susan Max-Jacobsen and Mr Bjarne Lauritzen for excellent technical assistance, to Mr Kjeld Stub-Kristensen for making the photographic prints, to Mr Henry Olsen for making the drawing and to Mrs Sonja Fich for typing the manuscript.

References

Bulger, R. E. (1965). The shape of rat kidney tubular cells. *Am. J. Anat.* **116**, 237–256.

Cardell, R. R., Jr, Badenhausen, S. and Porter, K. R. (1967). Intestinal triglyceride absorption in the rat. An electron microscopical study. *J. Cell Biol.* **34**, 123–155.

Civan, M. M. (1978). Intracellular activities of sodium and potassium. *Am. J. Physiol.* **234**, F261–F269.

Claude, P. and Goodenough, D. (1973). Fracture faces of zonulae occludentes from "tight" and "leaky" epithelia. *J. Cell Biol.* **58**, 390–400.

Droz, B., Rambourg, A. and Koenig, H. L. (1975). The smooth endoplasmic reticulum: structure and role in the renewal of axonal membrane and synaptic vesicles by fast axonal transport. *Brain Res.* **93**, 1–13.

Ericsson, J. L. E. (1964). Absorption and decomposition of homologous hemoglobin in renal proximal tubular cells. *Acta path. microbiol scand.* **168**, Suppl. 1, 1–121.

Farquhar, M. E. and Palade, G. E. (1963). Junctional complexes in various epithelia. *J. Cell Biol.* **17**, 375–412.

Frömter, E. and Diamond, J. (1972). Route of passive ion permeation in epithelia. *Nature new Biol.* **235**, 9–13.

Gupta, B. L., Hall, T. A. and Naftalin, R. J. (1978). Microprobe measurement of Na, K and Cl concentration profiles in epithelial cells and intercellular spaces of rabbit ileum. *Nature, Lond.* **272**, 70–73.

Hasselbach, W. (1964). Relaxation and sarcotubular calcium pump. *Fedn Proc. Fedn Am. Socs exp. Biol.* **23**, 909–912.

Jacobsen, N. O. and Jørgensen, F. (1973). Ultrastructural observations on the pars descendens of the proximal tubule in the kidney of the male rat. *Z. Zellforsch. mikrosk. Anat.* **136**, 479–499.

Kreutzberg, G. W., Schubert, P. and Lux, H. D. (1975). Neuroplasmic transport in axons and dendrites. In *Golgi Centennial Symposium: Perspectives in Neurobiology* (M. Santini, ed.), Raven Press, New York, pp. 161–166.

Martinez-Palomo, A. and Erlij, D. (1975). Structure of tight junctions in epithelia with different permeability. *Proc. natn. Acad. Sci. U.S.A.* **72**, 4487–4491.

Møllgård, K. and Rostgaard, J. (1978). Morphological aspects of some sodium transporting epithelia suggesting a transcellular pathway via elements of endoplasmic reticulum. *J. Membrane Biol.* **40**, 71–89.

Møllgård, K. and Saunders, N. R. (1977). A possible transepithelial pathway via endoplasmic reticulum in foetal sheep choroid plexus. *Proc. R. Soc. B* **199**, 321–326.

Møllgård, K., Malinowska, D. H. and Saunders, N. R. (1976). Lack of correlation between tight junction morphology and permeability properties in developing choroid plexus. *Nature, Lond.* **264**, 293–294.

Oschman, J. L., Wall, B. J. and Gupta, B. L. (1974). Cellular basis of water transport. *Symp. Soc. exp. Biol.* **28**, 305–350.

Palade, G. (1975). Intracellular aspects of the process of protein synthesis. *Science, N.Y.* **189**, 347–358.

Thiery, G. and Bergeron, M. (1977). Etudes sur coupes épaissed des polysaccharides acides de la cellule du tube contourné proximal du rein de rat. *Biologie cellul.* **30**, 279–282.

Thiery, G. and Rambourg, A. (1976). A new staining technique for studying thick sections in the electron microscope. *J. Microscopie Biol. cellul.* **26**, 103–106.

Tisher, C. C. (1976). Anatomy of the kidney. In *The Kidney* (B. M. Brenner and F. C. Rector, Jr, eds), W. B. Saunders, Philadelphia, pp. 3–64.

Voûte, C. L., Møllgård, K. and Ussing, H. H. (1975). Quantitative relationship between active sodium transport, expansion of endoplasmic reticulum and specialized vacuoles ("scalloped sacs") in the outermost living cell layer of the frog skin epithelium (*Rana temporaria*). *J. Membrane Biol.* **21**, 273–289.

Zeuthen, T. (1977). Intracellular gradients of electrical potentials in the epithelial cells of the *Necturus* gallbladder. *J. Membrane Biol.* **33**, 281–309.

Part III

Tubule: Handling of Macromolecules

19
Mechanisms of Glomerular Filtration and Tubular Uptake of Plasma Proteins in Health and Disease

Carl Erik Mogensen

Introduction

The purpose of this paper is to survey a number of factors influencing urinary protein excretion in man which have recently been studied in our laboratory. By stimulating protein excretion, information on the structure–function relationship can often be obtained with respect to renal handling of proteins in health and disease.

The pattern of proteins in the final urine is a result of two main processes in the kidney, glomerular filtration and tubular reabsorption. The factors studied are shown in Table I, according to the proposed mechanism. In order

TABLE I

Factors influencing renal handling of proteins

Glomerular filtration of proteins	Tubular reabsorption
(1) Blood pressure	(1) Dibasic amino acids and derivates
(2) Physical exercise (increased filtration pressure)	(2) Increased filtered loads of proteins
(3) Acute, heavy water drinking (wash-out effect?)	(3) Insulin
(4) Insulin	(4) Glucagon
(5) Operative and post-operative "stress"	(5) Post-operative "stress"
(6) Other "stress" situations	(6) Gentamicin

to investigate these processes, measurements using radioimmunoassay (Evrin *et al.*, 1971; Miles *et al.*, 1970) were made of the excretion of albumin, which is a marker for glomerular filtration of proteins, and of β_2-microglobulin (Phadebas® beta-micro test, Pharmacia Diagnostics), a freely filtered polypeptide molecule which is a marker for decreased reabsorption (Peterson *et al.*, 1969).

It is evident that a total inhibition of reabsorption will allow measurement of an important, unknown figure, namely the glomerular passage rate of individual plasma proteins, e.g. albumin. The discovery that certain amino acids inhibit protein reabsorption has opened new possibilities in this field (Mogensen *et al.*, 1975; Mogensen and Sølling, 1977; Sølling and Mogensen, 1977).

Effect of Dibasic Amino Acids and their Derivatives

Mechanism of initial phase in tubular reabsorption
Recently, we observed (Mogensen *et al.*, 1975) that arginine and other dibasic

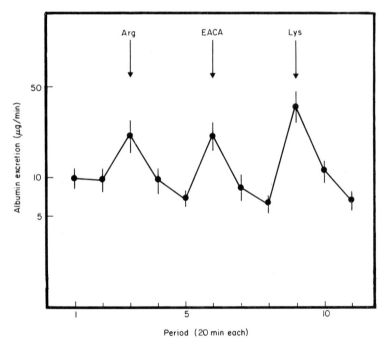

FIG. 1. *Albumin excretion after 6 g of arginine (Arg) and equimolar doses of ε-amino caproic acid (EACA) and lysine. Log scale; means ± S.E.M., n = 5.*

amino acids had a marked stimulatory effect on protein excretion, as shown in Fig. 1. In these experiments 6 g of arginine and equimolar doses of ε-amino caproic acid (EACA) and lysine were injected intravenously into five young normal male subjects at the beginning of a 20 min period.

Albumin excretion increased by a factor of two to three after arginine injection; excretion is thereafter normalized. EACA has a similar effect, whereas lysine is somewhat more effective, but normal excretion is still found in the second post-injection period.

From studies on β_2-microglobulin excretion it became clear that the effect on protein excretion of amino acids is due to inhibition of tubular protein reabsorption and not due to increased filtration, since the effect on β_2-microglobulin is much more marked than the effect on albumin excretion. As an example, Fig. 2 shows the pronounced effect after 2·4 g of ornithine. Lysine is still more effective, whereas citrulline, being a neutral amino acid,

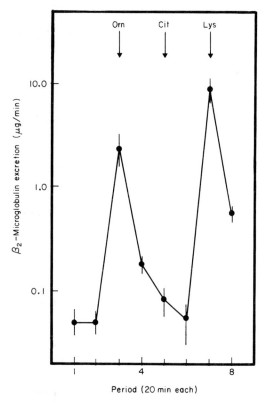

FIG. 2. β_2-Microglobulin excretion after 2·4 g of ornithine (Orn) and equimolar doses of citrulline (Cit) and lysine (Lys). Log scale; means ± S.E.M., n = 5.

has no effect. Using these rather small doses, no significant increase in albumin excretion was noted, a clear indication of an effect on the tubular cells (Mogensen and Sølling, 1977; Sølling and Mogensen, 1977).

The essentially non-metabolized, artificial amino acids EACA and cyclo-caprone, which are not (or are only slightly) reabsorbed by the tubular cells (Mogensen and Sølling, 1977), also proved to inhibit tubular reabsorption. A large number of other amino acids were tested (Mogensen and Sølling, 1977), but the only active substances turned out to ornithine, lysine, EACA, cyclocaprone and arginine. As shown in Fig. 3, these substances are charac-terized by possessing a positively charged group at physiological pH, located terminally in the molecule.

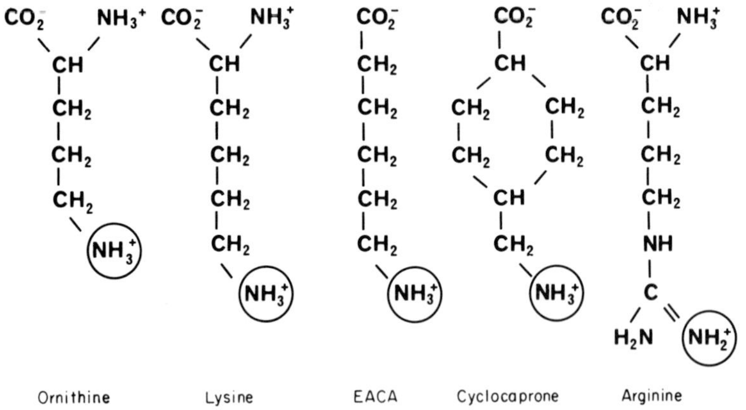

Ornithine   Lysine   EACA   Cyclocaprone   Arginine

FIG. 3. *Molecular configuration of active amino acids.*

Since the effect occurs instantaneously after injection, and since non-reabsorbed amino acids are also active, there cannot be much doubt that the effect on protein excretion is localized to the cell surface of the proximal tubular lumen, where protein reabsorption is known to take place (Mauns-bach, 1973).

On the basis of these experiments, a hypothesis regarding tubular protein reabsorption is put forward. The initial event in the normal protein reabsorp-tion is a binding between a free positively charged group of the protein molecule and a negatively charged site of the tubular cell surface. This initial event is impeded by molecules containing similarly charged groups. Thus a clear molecular structure–function relationship is proposed.

On the albumin molecule there are about 181 ionized groups at physio-logical pH, 81 positive and 100 negative (Peters, 1970). According to recent work (Geisow, 1977) on the molecular structure of albumin, the positive groups, comprising lysine and arginine residues, are located in clusters on the more accessible parts of the molecule. Such positively charged areas of the albumin molecule may therefore constitute the initial contact with the cell surface, in spite of the net negative molecular charge.

Using microperfusion techniques, Baumann *et al.* (see next chapter in this volume) recently confirmed that lysine, in contrast to alanine, exhibited a marked inhibition of tubular protein reabsorption, using labelled lysozyme as protein tracer.

Complete inhibition of protein reabsorption and measurement of glomerular of proteins

As discussed earlier, complete inhibition of tubular protein reabsorption would allow for determination of glomerular passage/rate of protein. This figure was unknown until now because no techniques for its measurement were available in man. The most active amino acid so far tested is lysine. However, complete inhibition of reabsorption can only be obtained by a special procedure (Table II).

TABLE II

Effect of rapid lysine injection on glomerular filtration rate (GFR) and β_2-microglobulin clearance (ultrashort periods)

Amount of lysine (g)	GFR (2 min period) (ml/min)	β_2-Microglobulin clearance (ml/min)	β_2-Microglobulin clearance (per cent of GFR)
5	111	49·5	45
10	102	109	107
13	119	105	88
16·5	118	105	89

Lysine was injected rapidly and intravenously during a 1 min period with subsequent short-term, very high concentration in the arterial system, including the renal arteries. Urine is then collected immediately afterwards, allowing 2 min for renal transit time, for periods of 2 min each.

In Table II is shown the effect of increasing doses of lysine. GFR is not substantially altered. β_2-Microglobulin clearance increases, but the increase levels off. It can be seen that the percentage clearance of β_2-microglobulin does not increase after 10 g of lysine, suggesting total inhibition after this dose, and consequently a clearance close to GFR.

Figure 4 shows the effect of increasing doses of lysine on albumin excretion. The curve levels off, also indicating complete inhibition of reabsorption and

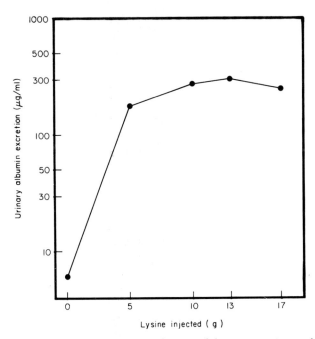

FIG. 4. *Urinary albumin excretion after rapid lysine injection and subsequent ultrashort urine collection periods (2 min).*

suggesting absence of effect on the glomerulus. It can be concluded that glomerular filtration of albumin is around 300 μg/min in this normal person. This figure is much higher than the amounts normally excreted in the final urine, namely 5–20 μg/min.

Renal Handling of Amylase in Normal Man

In a recent study the glomerular and tubular transport rate of amylase was studied by measuring the urinary excretion of this protein before and during partial inhibition of tubular protein reabsorption by lysine (Sølling *et al.*, 1979). Lysine, 0·4 g/kg body weight, was given intravenously during a 10–15 min period and urine was collected in 20 min periods (two control periods, the injection period, and seven post-injection periods). The excretion of amylase was compared with the excretion of albumin, β_2-microglobulin and free light chains of immunoglobulins. The excretion of amylase rose after lysine injection only by a factor 1·8, whereas excretion rose by a factor 28 for albumin, 1500 for β_2-microglobulin, 16 for κ chains and 8 for λ chains.

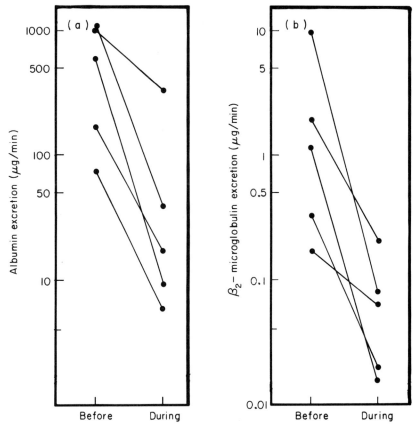

FIG. 5. (a) *Urinary albumin and* (b) β_2-*microglobulin excretion before and during treatment of severe hypertension for a mean of 3 days. Mean arterial pressure is 165–124 mm Hg.*

The molecular weight of the λ chains is 44 000 daltons, very close to that of amylase, which is about 50 000 daltons. The results show that amylase is reabsorbed by the tubular cells, but only to a very modest degree compared with the reabsorption of the other three proteins, since amylase excretion increased only very slightly after injection. In the case of amylase only about 45 per cent of the filtered molecules are reabsorbed, whereas more than 90 per cent of the filtered amount of the other molecules is reabsorbed by the tubular cells. The reason why the renal handling of amylase is so different from other proteins is not yet clarified.

Arterial Blood Pressure and Protein Excretion

Severe, untreated hypertension
Examination of the effect of acute alterations in arterial blood pressure level
on protein excretion is not feasible in normal man. However, it is possible to
work the other way round, namely to examine the relationship between
pressure levels and protein excretion in patients being treated intensively for
acute, newly diagnosed severe hypertension (Mogensen *et al.*, 1979*a*; C. K.
Christensen and C. E. Mogensen, in preparation).

Five young patients with a mean arterial blood pressure of 165 mm Hg
(diastolic pressure puls 1/3 pulse pressure) were studied before and during
intensive antihypertensive treatment for a mean of 3 days (Fig. 5). Albumin
excretion was very high and dropped considerably during treatment, clearly
indicating pressure dependency (Mogensen *et al.*, 1979*a*). Abnormal structure
is probably also involved to some extent since excretion was not normalized
in all patients. However, the major cause of the increase in albumin excretion
in newly diagnosed, untreated patients is very likely increased pressure, since
hypertensive vascular damage would not tend to be so rapidly reversible.

β_2-Microglobulin excretion was considerably increased before treatment
and dropped along with the fall in albumin excretion (Fig. 5). The high
excretion of the freely filtered β_2-microglobulin must be due to inhibition of
reabsorption, the mechanism probably being competition in the reabsorption
process from other plasma proteins, e.g. albumin, filtered due to the increased
blood pressure. Renal ischaemia may also play a role.

Moderately elevated blood pressure; effect of treatment
In earlier studies we found significantly increased albumin extraction in
Albustix-negative patients with moderately increased blood pressure.
Furthermore, a correlation between pressure levels and albumin excretion
was demonstrated. β_2-Microglobulin excretion was normal in these patients,
indicating that the increase in albumin excretion was of glomerular origin
(Parving *et al.*, 1974). It should be noted that the increase in albumin excretion
was much less pronounced than in the patients represented in Fig. 5.

In a subsequent study, a clear-cut fall in albumin excretion was found
during antihypertensive treatment for several weeks (Pedersen and Mogensen, 1976). Albumin excretion also decreased during antihypertensive treatment in patients with diabetic nephropathy and moderately increased blood
pressure (Mogensen, 1976*a*).

Protein Excretion in Diabetes Mellitus

Excretion rate in patients under average "good" diabetes control, without clinical proteinuria
As in the case of hypertension, diabetes mellitus is one of the major diseases with renal involvement, in many cases developing into renal insufficiency and uraemia. We have for some years been interested in initial phases in the development of diabetic nephropathy in order to clarify pathogenetic mechanism. The early morphological changes have been extensively studied by Østerby and co-workers, as reported elsewhere in this volume. Another line in these investigations has been to study renal function, including urinary protein excretion by sensitive techniques (Mogensen, 1976b, 1980).

Using a radioimmunoassay for albumin, it became clear that most patients under ordinary good control have normal urinary albumin excretion (Mogensen, 1971a, b, 1972, 1976a, b, c) and β_2-microglobulin excretion (Mogensen, 1980) for the first years of diabetes. Similar results were recently obtained in diabetic children (Brøchner-Mortensen et al., 1979). It should be noted that Balodimos et al. (1971) obtained somewhat different results, as discussed elsewhere (Mogensen, 1971a, b). These findings of a normal function, at least in the basal state, are surprising considering the fact that pronounced morphological changes are found early, namely a steady increase in basement membrane thickness, demonstrable after $1\frac{1}{2}$ years of diabetes (Østerby, 1975), and in some patients eventually, after many years, developing into the classical picture of late diabetic glomerulopathy. In such patients with severe, clinical proteinuria, albumin excretion may be a factor of 1000 higher than in normals (Mogensen, 1973, 1976b, c).

Provocation test using physical exercise as stimulus for protein excretion
When function is normal in the basal state it may be appropriate to use provocative tests, when abnormalities are still suspected. We have studied, among other things, the effect of physical exercise on protein excretion in normal and diabetic man (Mogensen and Vittinghus, 1975; Mogensen et al., 1979b). The main idea was to define a work-load that would not stimulate protein excretion in normal subjects but possibly in patients with early structural renal abbormalities.

First, patients were studied in two control or baseline periods, at rest in the sitting position (Fig. 6), then for two periods with exercise also in the sitting position on a bicycle ergometer, one with 450 kpm/min, that is light work, and one with 600 kpm/min, that is moderate work. Finally three post-exercise periods followed at rest. Each period lasted 20 min except for the

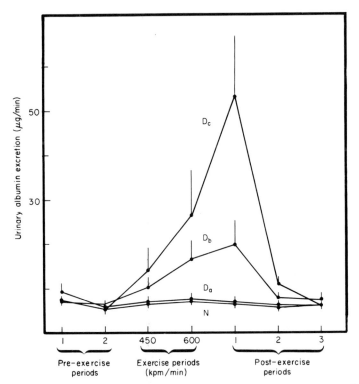

FIG. 6. *Urinary albumin excretion during exercise in 11 normals (N), six diabetics with diabetes of duration 0–1 year (D_a), 18 diabetics with diabetes of duration 2–11 years (D_b) and seven diabetics with diabetes of duration 16–20 years (D_c). Means ± S.E.M.*

600 kpm/min period, which in some cases was extended to 30 min in both normals and diabetics (Mogensen *et al.*, 1979*b*).

The lowest curve (N) on Fig. 6 shows the results of 11 normals and the next curve up (D_a) the results from juvenile diabetics with a diabetes duration of 1 year or less. No increase takes place during exercise. The next curve (D_b) shows the results of diabetics with a diabetes duration of 2–11 years. There is no difference from the normals in the baseline periods, but pronounced abnormalities emerge in these patients during exercise and the first post-exercise period. The excretion rate rose on average by a factor of three. In the third post-exercise period the excretion is again normal. The topmost curve (D_c) shows the results in diabetics with a diabetes duration of more than 15 years. Also in these patients the pre-exercise values are in the normal range and an abnormally high increase emerges in the exercise periods and the first post-exercise period.

β_2-Microglobulin excretion was unchanged in these experiments in both normal and diabetic patients, and the increase in albumin excretion must therefore be of glomerular origin (Mogensen et al., 1979b). Also, changes in the systemic circulation were unrelated to urinary albumin excretion Mogensen et al., 1979b). We therefore find it most likely that an abnormal glomerular filter, probably the basement membrane, is responsible for the abnormalities. The glomerular filter of short-term diabetic patients becomes leaky during exercise when increased glomerular filtration pressure operates. In normal subjects albumin is retained under these conditions.

These results would therefore suggest a correlation between structure and function in the development of disease, but only when a provocation test is used. Similar results were recently obtained by Viberti et al. (1978).

Increased values during bad metabolic control
In the untreated or in the insufficiently treated situation, increase in albumin excretion has been demonstrated (Mogensen, 1971a, b, 1976b; Parving et al. 1976). This increase is mainly glomerular in origin since β_2-microglobulin is only slightly increased in these patients (Parving et al., 1976). Tubular inhibition of reabsorption would induce much larger increase in β_2-microglobulin excretion at the albumin excretion level found (Mogensen and Sølling, 1977). Complete normalization is found during regulation of the metabolic derangement.

A provocation test using partial inhibition of tubular reabsorption as an index for glomerular filtration of albumin
In a recent study (Mogensen et al., 1979b), partial inhibition of tubular reabsorption was induced by lysine injection in order to investigate whether such inhibition would reveal increased glomerular passage of albumin in resting, non-exercising diabetic patients. Thirty-two young male diabetics and nine control subjects were studied by the lysine test. Lysine (0·4 g/kg body weight) was injected intravenously as described earlier.

A sharp rise in β_2-microglobulin excretion after lysine injection by a factor of about 1500 occurred in the normals, whereas albumin excretion increased by only a factor of about 30, a clear indication of inhibition of tubular protein reabsorption. No significant changes in the peak values after injection were noted in the diabetics with normal baseline albumin values, irrespective of duration of diabetes, although a few long-term diabetics had values outside the normal range. Only patients with elevated baseline values demonstrated abnormally high albumin values after lysine injection. The β_2-microglobulin and light chain responses were normal in all groups (Mogensen et al., 1979b).

Thus, evidence of an abnormal passage of albumin in the non-exercising situation was only found in patients with already elevated baseline values. It should be stressed, however, that only partial blockage was induced by the lysine dose used. Exact measurements of the glomerular passage rate of albumin as described earlier are in progress.

Hormones and Protein Excretion

Diabetes is characterized by multiple hormone abnormalities (Hansen and Lundbæk, 1976). Therefore, the effect of the hormones involved on kidney function was studied in order to clarify their possible role in the early changes in kidney function and protein excretion found in diabetes.

Insulin and protein excretion
We examined the effect of acute intravenous insulin injection on renal function in five young, male, short-term diabetic patients (Mogensen et al., 1978). Figure 7(a) and (b) shows the results of protein excretion measurements. Excretion rates were first determined in three baseline periods; thereafter, soluble insulin in a doses of 6–8 IU was given intravenously over the course of 1 min. Plasma glucose fell, but none of the patients developed hypoglycaemia.

A significant increase in albumin excretion is found. Furthermore, β_2-microglobulin excretion decreases. These changes in fact represent a unique response pattern. The results indicate that insulin in acute experiments stimulates both glomerular passage rate as indicated by increase in albumin excretion and tubular uptake of protein as indicated by the fall in β_2-microglobulin excretion. The effect on the glomerulus seems, however, to be predominately due to the noted net increase in albumin excretion in the final urine. A significant fall in both GFR and RPF was also found (Mogensen et al., 1978).

These changes must clearly be distinguished from the more long-term effect by regulation of the deranged metabolic state in diabetes, resulting in normalization of albumin and β_2-microglobulin excretion over the course of several days (Mogensen, 1971a, b; Parving et al., 1976).

Growth hormone and protein excretion
Growth hormone and glucagon have been proposed to be of importance for the development of early renal function changes in diabetes (Mogensen, 1972, 1980). However, short-term infusion of growth hormone for 3 h had no significant effect on protein excretion, as seen in Fig. 7(c) and (d) (Parving et al., 1978), and furthermore GFR and RPF were practically unchanged.

In acromegalic patients, normal albumin excretion as well as β_2-microglobulin excretion values have been found. Furthermore, treatment

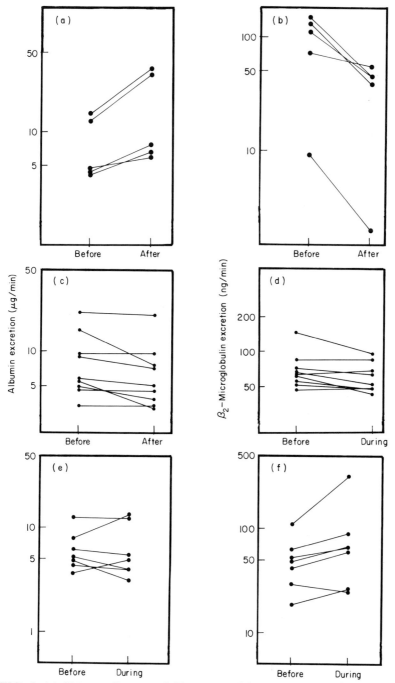

FIG. 7. (a) *Urinary albumin and* (b) β_2-*microglobulin excretion before and after intravenous insulin injection in five diabetic patients.* (c) *Urinary albumin and* (d) β_2-*microglobulin excretion before and during growth hormone infusion in nine young normal men.* (e) *Urinary albumin and* (f) β_2-*microglobulin excretion before and during glucagon infusion in seven diabetic patients.*

with Promocrotin, partially inhibiting growth hormone secretion, did not significantly alter protein excretion (Eskildsen *et al.*, 1979).

Glucagon and protein excretion

The effect of glucagon infusion on kidney function was also studied in diabetic patients (Parving *et al.*, 1980) and in normal young men (Parving *et al.*, 1977*a, b*). No effect on albumin excretion was noted, but in the case of β_2-microglobulin, a significant increase is found (Fig. 7(e) and (f)), which we also saw during metabolic derangement. GFR also increased after glucagon. Hyperglucagonaemia has been found in diabetic patients during metabolic derangement (Müller *et al.*, 1973).

Thus insulin and glucagon appear to have opposite effects on the tubular cells: insulin increases absorption, glucagon diminishes reabsorption. This reverse effect may be related to the reverse effects on sodium reabsorption of the two hormones. It is not known which morphologic structures in the tubular cells are responsible for these changes, but it may be alteration of the molecular surface structure of the proximal tubular cells.

Post-operative Protein Excretion after General Anaesthesia Compared to Epidural Analgesia in Patients Undergoing Hysterectomy

The operative and post-operative stress situation also results in a moderate increase in protein excretion (Wide and Thorén, 1972). Our recent results show that the increase is a combined effect of both increased glomerular filtration and decreased tubular reabsorption of proteins (M. Brandt, H. Kehlet and C. E. Mogensen, in preparation). A significant fall in albumin excretion is found from the first to the fourth post-operative day in patients undergoing hysterectomy during general anaesthesia (from $33\cdot3 \pm 19\cdot5$ (S.D.) $\mu g/min$ to $10\cdot9 \pm 8\cdot3$ (S.D.) $\mu g/min$, $2p < 5$ per cent) (Fig. 8). Furthermore, patients undergoing surgery during epidural analgesia showed lower albumin excretion values. In the first post-operative 24 h period, the albumin excretion was $10\cdot0 \pm 6\cdot1$ (S.D.) $\mu g/min$ versus $33\cdot3 \pm 19\cdot5$ (S.D.) $\mu g/min$ in general anaesthesia ($2p < 5$ per cent). This increase may be due to increased sympathetic nervous activity and subsequently higher catecholamine secretion during general anaesthesia (Kehlet, 1978). β_2-Microglobulin excretion tended to increase in the following post-operative days. There was a large variability in the values, and no statistically significant difference was noted between epidural analgesia and general anaesthesia.

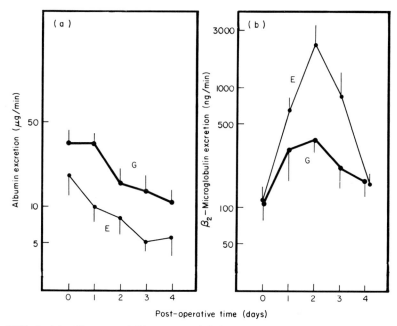

FIG. 8. (a) *Albumin and* (b) β_2-*microglobulin excretion in six patients operated on under general anaesthetic* (G) *and six patients operated on during epidural analgesia* (E) *(hysterectomy).*

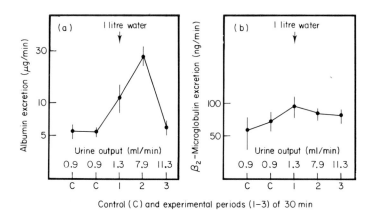

FIG. 9. (a) *Albumin excretion and* (b) β_2-*microglobulin excretion in six young normal men after drinking 1 litre of tap water in 5 min at the beginning of period 1. Mean* $\pm$ *S.E.M.*

Protein Excretion after Acute Water Loading

After drinking 1 litre of water in 5 min, a significant increase in albumin excretion is found in normal subjects in the second 30 min period after drinking, as shown in Fig. 9 (from 5.4 ± 1.9 (s.D.) μg/min to 27.2 ± 14.4 (s.D.) μg/min, $n = 6$, $2p < 0.02$). In the subsequent third period, and in the following periods, excretion rate is again normalized in spite of the fact that urine output is still higher, namely a mean of 11·3 ml/min by comparison with 7·9 ml/min in the second period and 0·9 ml/min in the control period. As shown in Fig. 9, no significant increase is found in β_2-microglobulin excretion, although the mean value tends to increase. It is not known whether this effect of acute, heavy water drinking is due to a wash-out effect or due to acute dilatation of the glomeruli with subsequent increase in albumin excretion (C. K. Christensen, G. C. Viberti and C. E. Morgensen, in preparation).

In our earlier studies, no correlation between albumin excretion and urine output was found (Mogensen, 1971a, b), but this was suggested by the findings of Jarrett et al. (1976). The results summarized in Fig. 9 indicate that it is only in the period immediately after water drinking that an increase in albumin excretion is found.

When normal subjects start to drink 250 ml of water every 20 min, as for example in clearance studies, a transient but much more moderate increase in albumin excretion is found. Excretion rate is at the baseline level $1\frac{1}{2}$ h after the start of drinking (C. K. Christensen, G. C. Viberti and C. E. Morgensen in preparation). Therefore such a lag time should be used before the start of experiments inducing alteration in albumin excretion.

Testing Possible Nephrotoxicity of Drugs by Measuring Protein Excretion

The sensitive methods for protein excretion described in the present paper should provide a method for testing early nephrotoxicity of drugs on both glomerular and tubular function. As an example, Fig. 10 shows the effect of intravenous injection of 80 mg of gentamicin in three experiments. A clear-cut increase in β_2-microglobulin excretion is found, whereas albumin excretion only exhibited a borderline increase. The effect is much more prolonged than after amino acid administration and it is present after a much smaller dose. These results suggest that the initial renal lesion or alteration after gentamicin is localized in the tubular cells. Increased β_2-microglobulin excretion may provide a very early index for testing renal nephrotoxicity of gentamicin during treatment.

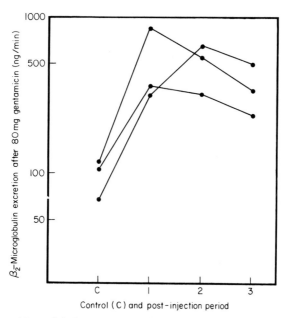

FIG. 10. *β_2-Microglobulin excretion after 80 mg gentamicin. Each period lasted 30 min.*

After conventional lithium treatment in manic-depressive patients no certain effect on protein excretion was found (Pedersen *et al.*, 1978). These patients were without symptoms of renal disorders. Abnormalities may well be found when renal symptoms are present in such patients, a topic currently under investigation in our laboratory.

Conclusions

The present survey shows that multiple factors may influence urinary protein excretion in both health and disease (see Tables III and IV). Information on such factors is of course essential when future studies on protein excretion are carried out.

The progress made in this field has depended mainly upon the newly developed radioimmunoassay for urinary protein. In turn this tool has helped to define new stimuli for protein excretion, not detectably by conventional methods of protein determination. The next step was the use of such stimuli to clarify normal physiological as well as pathophysiological processes in the kidney and their structure–function relationship. These stimuli were then used

TABLE III

Albumin and β_2-microglobulin excretion in disease

Disease or abnormality	Albumin excretion[a]	β_2-Microglobulin excretion[a]	Mechanism. Additional remarks	Reference
Diabetes mellitus, short duration, average "good" control	n	n	Generally both normal glomerular passage and tubular reabsorption	Mogensen (1971a, b, 1976a, 1980)
Diabetes mellitus, during metabolic derangement	↑	↑	Glomerular passage rate increased and to a lesser extent, tubular reabsorption diminished	Mogensen (1971a, 1976a), Parving et al. (1976)
Essential hypertension, well treated	n	n	Generally both normal glomerular passage and tubular reabsorption	Parving et al. (1974), Pedersen and Mogensen (1976)
Essential hypertension, moderately insufficiently treated (mean arterial pressure 135 mm Hg)	↑	n	Glomerular passage rate increased, tubular reabsorption undisturbed	Parving et al. (1974), Pedersen and Mogensen (1976)
Severe, newly diagnosed untreated hypertension (mean arterial pressure 165 mm Hg)	↑↑	↑	Reversible increase in glomerular passage rate. Tubular reabsorption inhibited by competition	C. K. Christensen and C. E. Mogensen (in preparation)
Acromegaly	n	n	No abnormalities found	Eskildsen et al. (1979)
Extensive skin diseases	n	n	No abnormalities found	Parving et al. (1977a)
LED, without clinical venal involvement	n	n	No abnormalities found	H. H. Parving et al. (in preparation)

[a] Symbols: n, normal; ↑, increase; ↑↑, pronounced increase.

TABLE IV

Acute alterations in urinary albumin and β_2-microglobulin excretion

Stimulus or abnormality	Albumin excretion[a]	β_2-Micro-globulin excretion[a]	Mechanism. Additional remarks	Reference
Dibasic amino acid and derivates	↑	↑↑	Normal charge-dependent tubular reabsorption inhibited	Mogensen and Sølling (1977)
Moderate exercise (in normal man)	−	−	The glomerular filter retains plasma protein during increased filtration pressure in normal man	Mogensen and Vittinghus (1975)
Moderate exercise (in diabetes)	↑	−	The glomerular filter becomes leaky in diabetics when increased filtration pressure operates	Mogensen and Vittinghus (1975)
Insulin given intravenously	↑	→	Both glomerular passage and tubular reabsorption enhanced	Mogensen et al. (1978)
Growth hormone infusion	−	−	No effect on protein excretion noted	Parving et al. (1978)
Glucagon infusion	−	↑	Glomerular passage rate unchanged, tubular reabsorption diminished	Parving et al. (1977b)
Acute water drinking (1 ℓ) in normal man	↑ (transient)	−	Transient increase in glomerular passage rate or wash-out phenomenon?	C. K. Christensen et al. (in preparation)
General anaesthesia	↑	↑	Both glomerular passage rate increased and tubular reabsorption diminished (combined effect of catecholamines and catabolism?)	Brandt et al. (in preparation)
Epidural analgesia	(↑)	↑	Both glomerular passage rate increased and tubular reabsorption diminished (combined effect of catecholamines and catabolism?) less pronounced	Brandt et al. (in preparation)
Acute gentamycin injection	(↑)	↑	Prolonged effect, primarily on the tubular cells	C. E. Mogensen (in preparation)
Long-term lithium treatment	−	−	No certain effect noted	Pedersen et al. (1978)
"Stress situations"	−	−	Observed in operating surgeons	Mogensen et al. (1979)

[a] Symbols: −, no effect; ↓, decrease; ↑, increase; (↑), increase (still doubtful); ↑↑, pronounced increase.

as the basis for the development of provocation tests for detecting the initial phases in renal disease.

Until recently the field was largely unexplored and it is still wide open for future work combining the use of sensitive methods for urinary protein excretion with the concept of stimulating protein excretion in both the normal and in the diseased state.

Acknowledgement

The very skilful work of laboratory assistant Merete Møller is gratefully acknowledged. The studies were supported by grants from The Danish Medical Research Council, The Research Fund of the University of Aarhus and Nordisk Insulin Fund.

References

Balodimos, M. C., Chlouverakis, C., Gleason, R. E., Jarrett, R. E., Kahn, R. J., Keen, H. and Soeldner, J. S. (1971). Urinary albumin excretion in the offspring of conjugal diabetics. *Lancet ii*, 239–242.

Brøchner-Mortensen, J., Ditzel, J., Mogensen, C. E. and Rødbro, P. (1979). Microvascular permeability to albumin and glomerular filtration rate in diabetic and normal children. *Diabetologia* in press.

Eskildsen, P. C., Parving, H. H., Mogensen, C. E. and Christiansen, J. S. (1979). Kidney function in acromegaly. *Acta med. scand.*, Suppl. 624, 79–82.

Evrin, P. E., Peterson, P. A., Wide, L. and Berggaard, I. (1971). Radioimmunoassay of β_2-microglobulin in human biological fluids. *Scand. J. clin. Invest.* 28, 439–443.

Geisow, M. (1977). Serum albumin structure and function. *Nature, Lond.* 270, 476–477.

Hansen, Å. P. and Lundbæk, K. (1976). Somatostatin: a review of its effects especially in human beings. *Diabete Metabolisme* 2, 203–218.

Jarrett, R. J., Verma, N. P. and Keen, H. (1976). Urinary albumin excretion in normal and diabetic subjects. *Clin. chim. Acta* 71, 55–59.

Kehlet, H. (1978). Influence of epidural analgesia on the endocrine-metabolic response to surgery. *Acta anaest. scand.* Suppl. 70, 39–42.

Maunsbach, A. B. (1973). Ultratructure of the proximal tubule. In *Handbook of Physiology*, Sect. 8, *Renal Physiology* (J. Orloff, R. W. Berliner and S. R. Geiger, eds), American Physiological Society, Washington, DC, pp. 31–79.

Miles, D. W., Mogensen, C. E. and Gundersen, H. J. G. (1970). Radioimmunoassay for urinary albumin using a single antibody. *Scand. J. clin. Lab. Invest.* 26, 5–11.

Mogensen, C. E. (1971*a*). Urinary albumin excretion in short-term and long-term juvenile diabetes. *Scand. J. clin. Lab. Invest.* 28, 183–193.

Mogensen, C. E. (1971*b*). Urinary albumin excretion in diabetes. *Lancet ii*, 601.

Mogensen, C. E. (1972). Kidney function and glomerular permeability to macromolecules in juvenile diabetes. With special reference to early changes. *Dan. med. Bull.* 19, Suppl. 3, 1–38.

Mogensen, C. E. (1973). Urinary albumin excretion and dextran clearance in the development of diabetic glomerulosclerosis. In *Protides of the Biological Fluids, 21st Colloquium* (H. Peeters, ed.), Pergamon Press, Oxford and New York, pp. 463–466.

Mogensen, C. E. (1976a). Progression in nephropathy in long-term diabetics with proteinuria and effect of initial hypertensive treatment. *Scand. J. clin. Lab. Invest.* **36**, 383–388.

Mogensen, C. E. (1976b). Renal function changes in diabetes. *Diabetes* **25**, 872–879.

Mogensen, C. E. (1976c). High blood pressure as a factor in the progression of diabetic nephropathy. *Acta med. scand.,* Suppl. 602, 29–32.

Mogensen, C. E. (1980). Pathophysiology of diabetic complications: abnormal physiological processes in kidney. In *Handbook of Diabetes Mellitus* (M. Browlee, ed.), Garland Press, New York, in press.

Mogensen, C. E. and Sølling, K. (1977). Studies on renal tubular protein reabsorption: partial and near complete by certain amino acids. *Scand. J. clin. Lab. Invest.* **37**, 477–486.

Mogensen, C. E. and Vittinghus, E. (1975). Urinary albumin excretion during exercise in juvenile diabetes. A provocation test for early abnormalities. *Scand. J. clin. Lab. Invest.* **35**, 295–300.

Mogensen, C. E., Christensen, N. J. and Gundersen, H. J. G. (1978). The acute effect of insulin on renal haemodynamics and protein excretion in diabetics. *Diabetologia* **15**, 153–157.

Mogensen, C. E., Gjøde, P. and Christensen, C. K. (1979a). Albumin excretion in operating surgeons and in hypertension. *Lancet i*, 774–775.

Mogensen, C. E., Vittinghus, E. and Sølling, K. (1975). Increased urinary albumin, light chain and β_2-microglobulin excretion after intravenous arginine administration in normal man. *Lancet ii*, 581–583.

Mogensen, C. E., Vittinghus, E. and Sølling, K. (1979b). Abnormal albumin excretion after two provocative renal test in diabetes: physical exercise and lysine injection. *Kidney Int.* **16**, 385–393.

Müller, W. A., Faloona, G. R. and Unver, R. H. (1973). Hyperglucagonemia in diabetic ketoacidosis. *Am. J. Med.* **54**, 52–57.

Parving, H. H., Jensen, H. Æ., Mogensen, C. E. and Evrin, P. E. (1974). Increased urinary albumin excretion rate in benign essential hypertension. *Lancet i*, 1190–1092.

Parving, H. H., Noer, I., Mogensen, C. E. and Svendsen, Aa. (1978). Kidney function in normal man during short-term growth hormone infusion. *Acta endocr.* **89**, 796–800.

Parving, H. H., Christiansen, J. S., Noer, I., Tronier, B. and Mogensen, C. E. (1980). The effect of glucagon on kidney function in short-term juvenile diabetes. *Diabetologia*, in press.

Parving, H. H., Worm, A. M., Knudsen, L., Mogensen, C. E. and Rossing, N. (1977a). Urinary albumin and β_2-microglobulin excretion rates in patients with extensive skin diseases. *Acta dermatovener.* **57**, 305–307.

Parving, H. H., Noer, J., Kehlet, H., Mogensen, C. E., Svendsen, P. Aa. and Heding, L. (1977b). The effect of short-term glucagon infusion on kidney function in normal man. *Diabetologia* **13**, 323–325.

Parving, H. H., Noer, I., Deckert, T., Evrin, P. E., Nielsen, S. L., Lyngsø, J., Mogensen, C. E., Rørth, M., Svendsen, P. Aa., Trap-Jensen, J. and Lassen, N. A. (1976). The effect of metabolic regulation on microvascular permeability to small and large molecules in short-term diabetes. *Diabetologia* **12**, 161–166.

Pedersen, E. B. and Mogensen, C. E. (1976). Effect of antihypertensive treatment on urinary albumin excretion, glomerular filtration rate and renal plasma flow in patients with essential hypertension. *Scand. J. clin. Lab. Invest.* **36**, 231–237.

Pedersen, E. B., Mogensen, C. E., Sølling, K., Amdisen, A. and Darling, S. (1978). Urinary excretion of albumin, β_2-microglobulin and free light chains during lithium treatment. *Scand. J. clin. Lab. Invest.* **38**, 269–272.

Peters, T. (1970). Serum albumin. *Adv. clin. Chem.* **13**, 37–113.

Peterson, P. A., Evrin, P. E. and Berggaard, I. (1969). Differentiation of glomerular, tubular and normal proteinuria: determination of urinary excretion of β_2-microglobulin, albumin and total protein. *J. clin. Invest.* **48**, 1189–1198.

Østerby, R. (1975). Early phases in the development of diabetic glomerulopathy. *Acta med. scand.* Suppl. 574, 1–80.

Sølling, K. and Mogensen, C. E. (1977). Molecular configuration and importance of charge in amino acid interference with renal tubular protein reabsorption. *IRCS med. Sci.* **5**, 30.

Sølling, K., Mogensen, C. E., Vittinghus, E. and Brock, A. (1979). The renal handling of amylase in normal man. *Nephron,* **23**, 282–286.

Viberti, G. C., Jarrett, R. J., McCartney, M. and Keen, H. (1978). Increased glomerular permeability to albumin induced by exercise in diabetic subjects. *Diabetologia* **14**, 293–300.

Wide, L. and Thorén, L. (1972). Increased urinary clearance for albumin, β_2-microglobulin, insulin and luteinizing hormone following surgical or accidental trauma. *Scand. J. clin. Lab. Invest.* **30**, 275–281.

20
Quantitative Analysis of Protein Absorption in Microperfused Proximal Tubules of the Rat Kidney

Karl Baumann, Folkert Bode, Peter D. Ottosen,
Kirsten M. Madsen and Arvid B. Maunsbach

Introduction

The kidney plays an important role in the catabolism of low molecular weight plasma proteins, including several polypeptide hormones (Rubenstein and Spitz, 1968; Mogielnicki *et al.*, 1971; Strober and Waldmann, 1974; Johnson and Maack, 1977). Such proteins are filtered in the renal glomeruli, reabsorbed from the tubule lumen by endocytosis and subsequently catabolized in the lysosomes of the proximal tubule cells (Maunsbach, 1976). Electron microscope autoradiography and tissue fractionation studies have shown that also lysozyme (molecular weight 14 400 daltons) is readily taken up by endocytosis in the proximal tubule and catabolized in the lysosomes (Christensen and Maunsbach, 1974; Ottosen *et al.*, 1979). Recent observations are consistent with all reabsorbed protein being catabolized in the lysosomes (Ottosen *et al.*, 1979; Bode *et al.*, Chapter 27 in this volume). Renal handling of lysozyme has previously been studied in whole animals (Perri *et al.*, 1964; Hansen *et al.*, 1971; Yuzuriha *et al.*, 1975; Ottosen *et al.*, 1979) and clearance experiments have shown that the uptake of lysozyme in the dog and rat kidney is a saturable process of high capacity, but with a low threshold (Maack and Sigulem, 1974; Cojocel *et al.*, 1979). However, little is known about the quantitative aspects of endocytic protein uptake, and the aim of the present study was to analyse quantitatively the protein uptake in the proximal tubule using ^{125}I-labelled lysozyme as tracer protein in microperfusion studies.

The present study demonstrates that the uptake of lysozyme in the proximal tubule is a saturable transport process and thus occurs by adsorptive endocytosis.

Methods

Microperfusion procedure
Male Wistar rats under Inactin anaesthesia were prepared in the usual manner for micropuncture experiments (Ullrich *et al.*, 1969). The tubular uptake of lysozyme was investigated quantitatively using the technique of continuous microperfusion (Sonnenberg *et al.*, 1964) as modified for the double collection of the perfusate (Loeschke and Baumann, 1969; Bode *et al.*, 1975) (Fig. 1). Lysozyme was perfused in two different pump solutions, either a Ringer's solution or a steady state solution (Gertz, 1963; Kashgarian *et al.*, 1963). The Ringer's solution, adjusted to pH 7·4, was composed of (in milliequivalents per litre) sodium 147, potassium 4, calcium 3, magnesium 1, chloride 125 and bicarbonate 30. The steady state solution, adjusted to pH 7·4, was

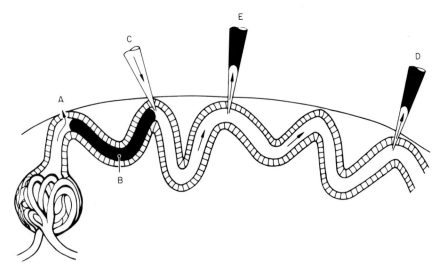

FIG. 1. *Scheme of the microperfusion method* (*Sonnenberg* et al., *1964*) *as modified for the double collection of the perfusate* (*Loeschke and Baumann, 1969; Bode* et al., *1975*). *Injected coloured oil* (*B*) *prevented the contamination of the perfusion solution with glomerular filtrate. Proximal to the oil column, the glomerular filtrate escaped through the puncture site* (*A*). *Distal to the oil column, loops of the proximal convoluted tubule were continuously microperfused via a pump pipette* (*C*). *The perfusate was collected twice, first at D and subsequently at E.*

composed of (in milliequivalents per litre) sodium 120, potassium 4, calcium 3, magnesium 1, chloride 118, bicarbonate 10, and (in millimoles per litre) raffinose 44. Both solutions contained different concentrations of non-labelled lysozyme and trace amounts of ^{125}I-labelled lysozyme.

Quantitative microperfusion studies

Single proximal convoluted tubules were continuously microperfused at a constant rate of 10 nl/min with a steady state solution containing ^{125}I-labelled lysozyme and ^{14}C-labelled inulin (no net flux of water and electrolytes). The concentration of lysozyme in the pump solution was 5·0, 0·8 and 0·032 mg/ml, respectively. The perfusion solution was collected and analysed for radioactivity, and small water fluxes were corrected by measuring changes in the concentration of ^{14}C-labelled inulin. The rate of lysozyme uptake was calculated using the perfusion rate and the decrease in ^{125}I radioactivity in the perfusate along the perfused tubular length and expressed as nanograms of lysozyme taken up per millimetre of tubular length per minute.

Many difficulties were encountered in the quantitative investigation of the protein uptake due to the low protein concentration in the perfusate and the collected samples, since a considerable fraction of the protein binds to every surface with which it comes in contact. In order to minimize the unspecific lysozyme binding, the glass surface on which the collected samples were delivered under oil were siliconized and treated for several hours with albumin (1 g per cent). The collecting pipettes were only treated with albumin, whereas the pump pipette was equilibrated with the pump solution by filling it twice for 1 h with the perfusate containing ^{125}I-labelled lysozyme.

Autoradiographic analysis of microperfused tubules

Electron microscope analysis was carried out of proximal tubules microperfused with either Ringer's solution or steady state solution containing 0·8 mg/ml lysozyme to which was added a trace amount of ^{125}I-labelled lysozyme. The perfusions were carried out exactly as in the quantitative studies and lasted for 3–20 min. When the lysozyme perfusions were completed the tubules were fixed by in vivo microperfusion for 10 min with 3 per cent glutaraldehyde in sodium cacodylate buffer. The pump pipette containing the lysozyme solution was then exchanged for a micropipette containing the fixative. In experiments with short perfusion periods a second complete microperfusion system was used for fixation. In the latter case care was taken to start glutaraldehyde perfusion while the pump filled with the lysozyme solution was still running. The fixed tubules were carefully identified on the kidney surface and partially microdissected, post-fixed and embedded for electron microscope analysis. Light microscope sections and ultrathin

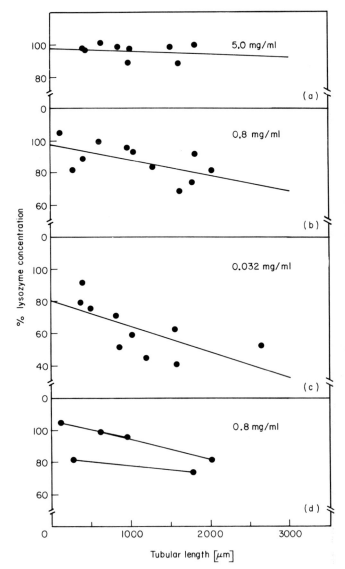

FIG. 2. *Percentage decrease of the intraluminal lysozyme concentration along microperfused proximal convoluted tubules at three different lysozyme concentrations. 100 per cent represents 5·0, 0·8 and 0·032 mg lysozyme per millilitre pump (steady state) solution in (a), (b) and (c) respectively. Each point represents the percentage lysozyme concentration in one collected perfusate. In the three upper panels the regression lines were calculated through single points. In (d) each line connects two determinations of* [125]*I-labelled lysozyme in perfusates collected at two different puncture sites in the same microperfused tubule and 100 per cent represents 0·8 mg lysozyme per millilitre.*

sections were cut and prepared for autoradiography according to methods described previously (Maunsbach, 1966).

Results and Discussion

Quantitative uptake of lysozyme in the proximal tubule
Following microperfusion with lysozyme there was a decrease of the intraluminal lysozyme concentration, demonstrating that lysozyme was absorbed in the proximal tubule. The decrease in the lysozyme concentration was dependent upon the lysozyme concentration in the pump solution. Thus, the percentage decrease was larger with low than with high lysozyme concentrations, as demonstrated in Fig. 2. The same curves also illustrate that the percentage decrease is length dependent with all concentrations used. This is also illustrated by the results from double collections from the same tubule, where the observations from the same tubules are connected to each other (Fig. 2(d)). The quantitative microperfusion studies were carried out with a steady state solution. Using this perfusion solution there is no net flux of water or solutes, which increases the accuracy in the determination of the percentage decrease in protein concentration since the inulin concentration is constant along the perfused tubular segment. When the lysozyme concentrations in the pump solution were 5·0, 0·8 and 0·032 mg/ml the calculated transport rates were equal to 1·0, 0·8 and 0·05 ng lysozyme mm^{-1} min^{-1} (Table I). These experiments indicate that the uptake of lysozyme is concentration dependent and approaches saturation at higher intraluminal lysozyme concentrations. Microperfusion studies with various intraluminal lysozyme concentrations are in progress in order to allow a complete kinetic analysis of the endocytic uptake of lysozyme.

In preliminary experiments no difference was found between the quanti-

TABLE I
Uptake of ^{125}I-labelled lysozyme in microperfused proximal convoluted tubules

Lysozyme concentration pump solution (mg ml)	Decrease of intratubular lysozyme concentration (per cent per 3 mm tubule)	Mean intratubular lysozyme concentration, S (mg ml)	Tubular lysozyme uptake rate, V (ng mm^{-1} min^{-1})
5·0	6·0	4·71	1·00
0·8	28·3	0·72	0·80
0·032	46·9	0·019	0·05

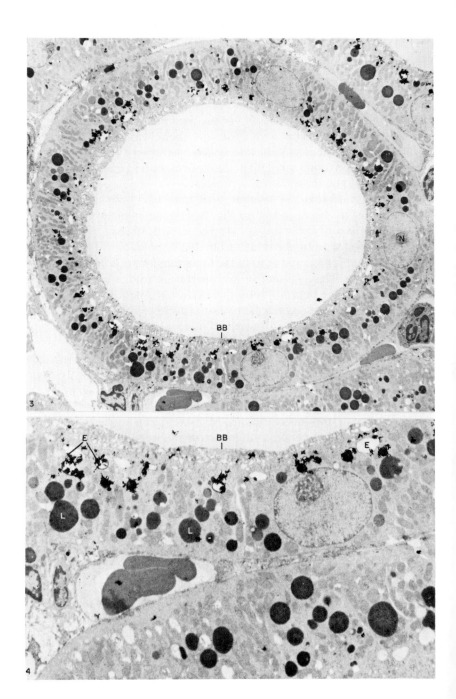

tative uptake of lysozyme in tubules perfused with Ringer's solution or the steady state solution.

Autoradiographic localization of labelled lysozyme in microperfused tubules
Following microperfusion with labelled lysozyme in either Ringer's solution or steady state solution the autoradiographic grains were initially observed over apical endocytic vacuoles and subsequently also over lysosomes (Figs 3–8). This uptake is consistent with the interpretation that the percentage decrease of the radioactivity described above is due to tubular absorption of protein. Furthermore, the autoradiographic observations demonstrate that the endocytic uptake of lysozyme starts immediately, and is a continuous cellular process that can be analysed kinetically. There was no difference between the localization of autoradiographic grains in tubules perfused with a Ringer's solution or with a steady state solution.

Mechanisms of endocytic protein uptake in the proximal tubule
The microperfusion experiments in the present study confirm earlier observations that the uptake of lysozyme in proximal tubules occurs by endocytosis. The quantitative data provide some further insight into the mechanism of the endocytic uptake. The endocytic uptake of protein in the proximal tubule cells (Maunsbach, 1976) or other types of cells (Edelson and Cohn, 1978) seems to occur in two ways: (1) adsorption or binding of molecules to the luminal cell membrane with subsequent endocytosis, which can also be referred to as adsorptive endocytosis, and/or (2) bulk uptake of macromolecules in the fluid phase of endocytic invaginations or vacuoles, also called fluid phase endocytosis. The initial step in adsorptive endocytosis is the binding of the protein to the cell surface—either to unspecific binding sites or in certain cells to specific receptors (Brown and Goldstein, 1976). When the protein is bound to specific binding sites or receptors the adsorptive endocytosis will be a saturable process, since the uptake will depend upon the affinity of the protein to the binding sites and the number of available binding sites. The present data indicate that the uptake of lysozyme is a saturable process and thus occurs mainly by adsorptive endocytosis.

FIG. 3. *Electron microscope autoradiograph of proximal convoluted tubule microperfused with Ringer's solution containing 0·8 mg ^{125}I-labelled lysozyme per millilitre for 20 min. Three minutes after the end of the perfusion with tracer, the tubules were fixed by microperfusion with 3 per cent glutaraldehyde for 10 min. BB, brush border; N, nucleus; BM, basement membrane. × 1700.*

FIG. 4. *Higher magnification from the tubule in Fig. 3. Autoradiographic grains are located over brush border (BB), endocytic vacuoles (E) and lysosomes (L). The lower right corner shows a neighbouring tubule not perfused with ^{125}I-labelled lysozyme. × 3400.*

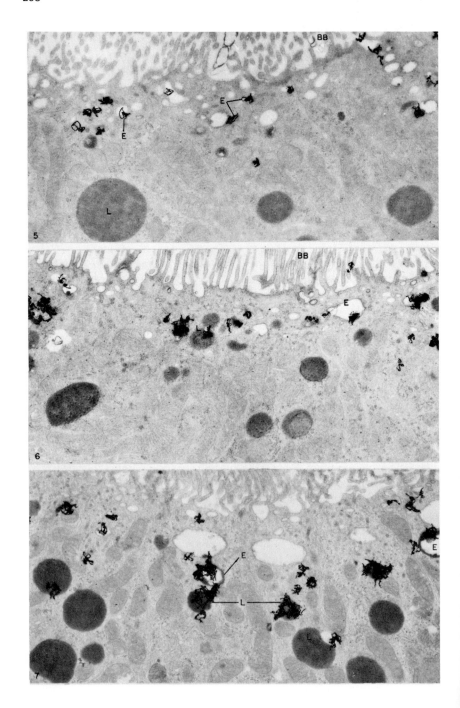

The results regarding tubular uptake of lysozyme may not apply to all other proteins since the extent of adsorptive endocytosis is determined by the affinity of proteins to the luminal cell membrane in the proximal tubule. It is likely that the cationic lysozyme with an isoelectric point of 11·5 has a much greater affinity to the cell membrane than, for example, the almost neutral horse-radish peroxidase. Indeed, Straus (1971) demonstrated that the amount of horse-radish peroxidase which accumulated in the kidney was proportional to the plasma concentration over a very wide range of concentrations. This indicates that this protein is mainly taken up by fluid phase endocytosis as in macrophages (Edelson and Cohn, 1978). Uncharged non-proteins are only reabsorbed to a very small extent. Thus, dextran T80 was almost quantitatively excreted in the urine and less than 2 per cent of the filtered dextran was absorbed by the proximal tubule cells, demonstrating that the dextran uptake probably consists of fluid-phase endocytosis (Christensen and Maunsbach, 1979).

Conclusions

(1) Protein absorption in the proximal tubule can be characterized quantitatively in microperfusion experiments.

(2) The uptake of lysozyme in the rat proximal tubule is a saturable transport process.

(3) Electron microscope analysis of microperfused proximal tubules demonstrates that the uptake of lysozyme is a continuous cellular process possible to study by kinetic analysis.

(4) The observations suggest that lysozyme uptake occurs by adsorptive rather than fluid phase endocytosis.

FIG. 5. *Proximal tubule perfused with* [125]*I-labelled lysozyme for 3 min. Autoradiographic grains are located over brush border* (*BB*) *and apical endocytic vacuoles* (*E*). *No grains are seen over the lysosomes* (*L*). × *8400.*

FIG. 6. *Proximal tubule perfused with* [125]*I-labelled lysozyme for 10 min. Autoradiographic grains are located over brush border* (*BB*), *endocytic vacuoles* (*E*) *and small lysosomes* (*L*) *in the apical part of the cell.* × *8400.*

FIG. 7. *Proximal tubule perfused with* [125]*I-labelled lysozyme for 20 min. Autoradiographic grains are located over endocytic vacuoles* (*E*) *and lysosomes* (*L*). × *8400.*

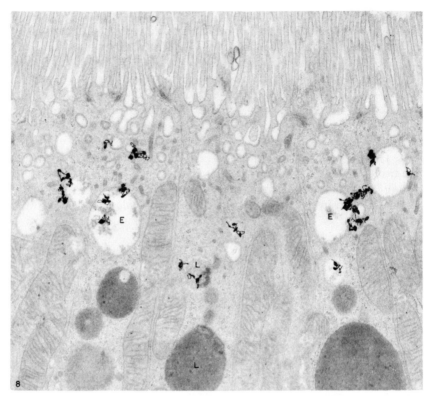

FIG. 8. *Electron microscope autoradiograph from proximal tubule microperfused with a steady state solution containing 0·8 mg ^{125}I-labelled lysozyme per millilitre for 10 min, and fixed by perfusion with 3 per cent glutaraldehyde for 10 min. Autoradiographic grains are located over endocytic vacuoles (E) and small lysosomes (L) in the apical part of the cell as in Fig. 6.* × 12 800.

References

Bode, F., Chan, Y. L., Goldner, A. M., Papavassiliou, F., Wagner, M. and Baumann K. (1975). Reabsorption of D-glucose from various regions of the rat proximal convoluted tubule: evidence that the proximal convolution is not homogenous. In *Biochemical Aspects of Renal Function. Current Problems in Clinical Biochemistry*, Vol. 4 (S. Angielski and U. C. Dubach, eds), Hans Huber Publishers, Bern, Stuttgart and Vienna, pp. 39–43.

Brown, M. S. and Goldstein, J. L. (1976). Receptor-mediated control of cholesterol metabolism. *Science, N.Y.* **191**, 150–154.

Christensen, E. I. and Maunsbach, A. B. (1974). Intralysosomal digestion of lysozyme in renal proximal tubule cells. *Kidney Int.* **6**, 396–407.

Christensen, E. I. and Maunsbach, A. B. (1979). Effects of dextran on lysosomal ultrastructure and protein digestion in renal proximal tubule. *Kidney Int.* **16**, 301–311.

Cojocel, C., Franzen-Sieveking, M., Berndt, W. and Baumann, K., (1979). Renal clearance of lysozyme in rat. *Pflügers Arch. ges. Physiol.* **379**, Suppl. R19.

Edelson, P. J. and Cohn, Z. A. (1978). Endocytosis: regulation of membrane interactions. In *Cell Surface Reviews*, Vol. 5 *Membrane Fusion* (G. Poste and G. L. Nicolson, eds), North-Holland, Amsterdam, pp. 387–405.

Gertz, K. H. (1963). Transtubuläre Natriumchloridflüsse und Permeabilität für Nichtelektrolyte im proximalen und distalen Konvolut der Rattenniere. *Pflügers Arch. ges. Physiol.* **276**, 336–356.

Hansen, N. E., Karle, H. and Andersen, V. (1971). Lysozyme turnover in the rat. *J. clin. Invest.* **50**, 1473–1477.

Johnson, V. and Maack, T. (1977). Renal extraction, filtration, absorption, and catabolism of growth hormone. *Am. J. Physiol.* **233**, F197–F200.

Kashgarian, M., Stöckle, H., Gottschalk, C. W. and Ullrich, K. J. (1963). Transtubular electrochemical potentials of sodium and chloride in proximal and distal renal tubules of rats during antidiuresis and water diuresis (diabetes insipidus). *Pflügers Arch. ges. Physiol.* **277**, 89–106.

Loeschke, K. and Baumann, K. (1969). Kinetische Studien der D-Glukose-resorption im proximalen Konvolut der Rattenniere. *Pflügers Arch. ges. Physiol.* **305**, 139–154.

Maack, T. and Sigulem, D. (1974). Renal handling of lysozyme. In *Lysozyme* (E. F. Osserman, ed.), Academic Press, New York, pp. 321–333.

Maunsbach, A. B. (1966). Absorption of ^{125}I-labelled homologous albumin by rat kidney proximal tubule cells. A study of microperfused single proximal tubules by electron microscopic autoradiography and histochemistry. *J. Ultrastruct. Res.* **15**, 197–241.

Maunsbach, A. B. (1976). Cellular mechanisms of tubular protein transport. In *Kidney and Urinary Tract Physiology II* (K. Thurau, ed.), International Review of Science, Physiology, Series 2, Vol. 11, University Park Press, Baltimore, pp. 145–167.

Mogielnicki, R. P., Waldmann, T. A. and Strober, W. (1971). Renal handling of low molecular weight proteins. I. L-Chain metabolism in experimental renal disease. *J. clin. Invest.* **50**, 901–909.

Ottosen, P. D., Bode, F., Madsen, K. M. and Maunsbach, A. B. (1979). Renal handling of lysozyme in the rat. *Kidney Int.* **15**, 246–254.

Perri, G. C., Faulk, M., Shapiro, E. and Money, W. L. (1964). Role of the kidney in accumulation of egg white muramidase in experimental animals. *Proc. Soc. exp. Biol. Med.* **115**, 189–192.

Rubenstein, A. H. and Spitz, I. (1968). Role of the kidney in insulin metabolism and excretion. *Diabetes* **17**, 161–169.

Sonnenberg, H., Deetjen, P., and Hampel, W. (1964). Methode zur Durchströmung einzelner Nephronabschnitte. *Pflügers Arch. ges. Physiol.* **278**, 669–674.

Straus, W. (1971). Comparative analysis of the concentration of injected horseradish peroxidase in cytoplasmic granules of the kidney cortex, in the blood, urine, and liver. *J. Cell Biol.* **48**, 620–632.

Strober, W. and Waldmann, T. A. (1974). The role of the kidney in the metabolism of plasma proteins. *Nephron* **13**, 35–66.

Ullrich, K. J., Frömter, E. and Baumann, K. (1969). Micropuncture and microanalysis in kidney physiology. In *Laboratory Techniques in Membrane Biophysics* (H. Passow and R. Stämpfli, eds), Springer, Berlin, Heidelberg and New York, pp. 106–129.

Yuzuriha, T., Katayama, K. and Fujita, T. (1975). Studies on biotransformation of lysozyme. II. Tissue distribution of ^{131}I-labelled lysozyme and degradation in kidney after intravenous injections in rats. *Chem. Pharmac. Bull.* **23**, 1315–1322.

21
Ultrastructural Evidence by Immunohistochemical Techniques for a Tubular Reabsorption of Endogenous Albumin and Certain Circulating Proteins in Normal Rat

Jean Bariéty, Philippe Druet, François Laliberté, Marie-France Belair, Michel Paing and Catherine Sapin

Introduction

It has been shown that autologous rat albumin, detected by immuno-peroxidase technique following *in situ* fixation, does not penetrate deeply into the glomerular basement membrane (Ryan *et al.*, 1976). In contrast, in other studies (Laliberté *et al.*, 1975) using the same technique, endogenous albumin was observed in the glomerular basement membrane and in the urinary space on the free cell coat of the epithelial foot processes. Micropuncture studies have produced direct evidence that the glomerular filtrate in the normal rat contains a small amount of albumin (Cortney *et al.*, 1970; Eisenbach *et al.*, 1975; Gaizutis *et al.*, 1972; Leber and Marsh, 1970; Oken and Flamenbaum, 1971; Oken *et al.*, 1972; Van Liew *et al.*, 1970). Such studies also demonstrate that serum albumin, which passes across the glomerular filter, is completely or to a large extent reabsorbed by the proximal tubules (Eisenbach *et al.*, 1975; Oken and Flamenbaum, 1971; Van Liew *et al.*, 1970).

The aim of this experimental study is to show that endogenous albumin (69 000 daltons), anti-peroxidase antibodies (160 000 daltons), circulating F(ab')$_2$ (100 000 daltons) and Fab fragments (50 000 daltons) of circulating heterologous anti-peroxidase are reabsorbed in the proximal tubules.

Materials and Methods

Animals
Male Wistar rats weighing 120–250 g were used.

Detection of endogenous albumin
A sheep anti-rat albumin antiserum was prepared as previously described (Bignon *et al.*, 1975). Pure antibodies were isolated using normal rat serum insolubilized with glutaraldehyde (Avrameas and Ternynck, 1969; Bignon *et al.*, 1975) concentrated to 5 mg/ml, and labelled with peroxidase (Boehring, grade I) according to the two-step technique (Avrameas and Ternynck, 1971).

Detection of the circulating anti-peroxidase antibodies and their fragments in rats
The methods used to detect circulating autologous, isologous, sheep heterologous anti-peroxidase antibodies, circulating $F(ab')_2$ and Fab fragments of heterologous anti-peroxidase antibodies are described elsewhere (Bariéty *et al.*, Chapter 3 in this volume).

Fixation
Kidneys were fixed *in situ* according to Ryan and Karnovsky (1976). The procedure used has been extensively described (Laliberté *et al.*, 1978; Ryan and Karnovsky, 1976; Ryan *et al.*, 1976). Briefly, after decapsulation, the kidney surface was fixed for 1 h by dripping a solution of 2 per cent glutaraldehyde in 0·1 M potassium phosphate buffer, pH 7·35. Sections with a maximal thickness of 1 mm were cut and immersed in the same fixative for 1 h at 4 °C.

Immunohistochemical procedure
Kidney samples were washed for 16 h with three changes of buffer. Sections 40 μm thick were then obtained with a Smith and Farquhar tissue sectioner. To detect endogenous albumin, sections were incubated with anti-rat albumin conjugate for 24 h and washed thoroughly for 48 h. To detect circulating

---

FIG. 1. *Electron micrograph of apical regions of proximal tubule cells following incubation with anti-rat albumin conjugate. The cell coat of the brush border and the invaginations are stained. A pattern of endocytosis is observed and apical tubules and endocytic vacuoles (E) are peripherally stained. × 25 000.*

FIG. 2. *Parts of proximal tubule cells fixed 5 min after injection of anti-peroxidase IgG. The brush border and apical vacuoles are negative. An intercellular space (arrow) is stained up to the tight junction. × 35 000.*

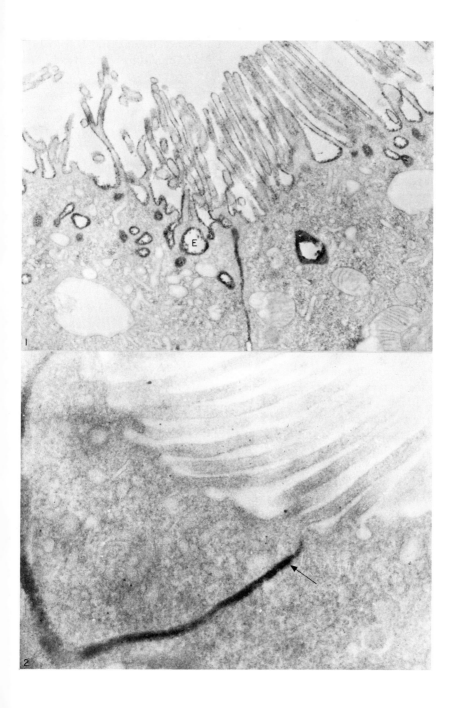

anti-peroxidase antibodies or their fragments, sections were incubated with peroxidase in phosphate buffer. All the sections were washed and the peroxidase activity was revealed as described by Graham and Karnovsky (1966). Finally, the sections were processed for electron microscopy as described elsewhere (Laliberté *et al.*, 1978).

Controls
The following controls were performed on all of the kidney samples: (1) detection of endogenous peroxidase activity by the incubation medium for peroxidase, as described by Graham and Karnovsky (1966); (2) incubation with 0·5 mg/ml of peroxidase for 1 h, followed by determination of the peroxidase activity; (3) incubation with peroxidase-labelled normal sheep IgG; (4) incubation with anti-rat albumin conjugate adsorbed on normal rat serum insolubilized with glutaraldehyde; (5) in addition some kidney samples were incubated with sheep anti-peroxidase IgG or their (Fab) or Fab fragments. After washing, the peroxidase activity was revealed as above.

Results

The present observations were made in the superficial renal cortex and only in areas where glomeruli were homogeneously filled with plasma and where the lumen of the tubules was opened.

Endogenous albumin
In the proximal tubules, diffuse labelling was observed on the cell coat of the luminal sides of the brush border projections and of the apical cell invaginations. Labelling was also observed in numerous small apical vacuoles, large apical vacuoles, and apical tubules (Fig. 1). No labelling was seen in the lysosomes.

In all of the tubules, occasional labelling was observed in the extracellular space between the cells and within the basal invaginations. The reaction product was present in the intercellular spaces up to the tight junctions and appeared to be more concentrated along the cell membranes. Sometimes, microbodies (peroxisomes) and mitochondrial cristae were slightly stained.

FIG. 3. *Proximal tubule fixed 5 min after injection of Fab. The lumen of the blood capillary, the basement membrane, the intercellular spaces (arrows), the cell coat of the brush border and the apical endocytic vacuoles (E) are stained. Lysosomes (L) are not stained. × 7000.*

FIG. 4. *Proximal tubule from same specimen as shown in Fig. 3. At this magnification it is possible to observe that the intercellular space is stained up to the apical tight junction (arrow). × 35 000.*

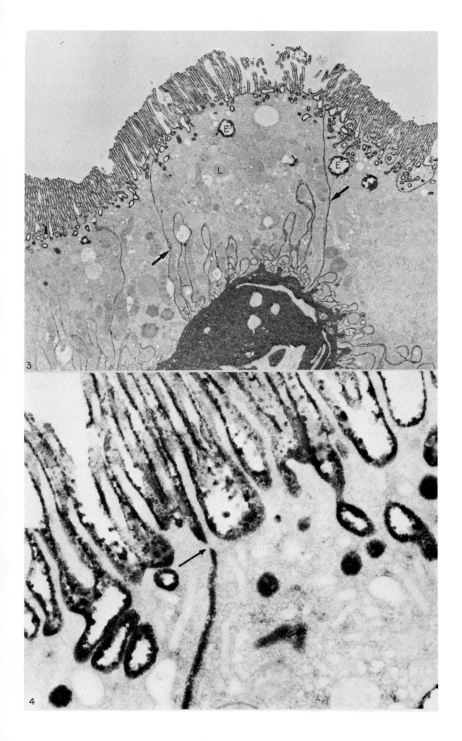

Anti-peroxidase IgG
The results were the same with heterologous, isologous or autologous anti-peroxidase antibodies. The brush border of proximal tubules and the cytoplasm of tubular cells was never stained. On the other hand, the basement membrane of interstitial capillaries, the interstitial tissue and the tubular basement membrane were always stained, although heterogeneously. Staining was also observed in the extracellular spaces between the tubular cells up to the apical tight junctions (Fig. 2) and in the basal invaginations.

Fab fragments
In the proximal tubules, when the kidney was fixed 5 min after the injection of Fab fragments, diffuse staining occurred on the cell coat of the luminal side of the brush border projections and of the apical cell invaginations. Staining was also seen on the inner side of the membrane of numerous apical vacuoles. No staining was seen in lysosomes (Figs 3, 4). When the kidney was fixed 20 min after the injection, the brush border of the proximal tubules was far less intensely stained, but apical vacuoles were stained. Numerous lysosomes appeared to be stained throughout the cytoplasm (Fig. 5). At both 5 and 20 min, staining was occasionally seen on the luminal membrane of the cells in the distal and collecting tubules, but never within the cytoplasm of the cells. The basement membrane of interstitial capillaries, the interstitial tissue and the tubular basement membrane were always homogeneously stained. In all the tubules, staining was seen in the extracellular spaces between the cells and within the basal invaginations. The reaction product was observed in the intercellular spaces, up to the tight junctions (Figs 4, 6).

F(ab′)₂ fragments
When the kidney was fixed 5 or 20 min after the injection of Fab fragments, some proximal tubules had unstained brush borders. However, in some sections, staining similar to that described for Fab fragments at 5 and 20 min (Fig. 7) was found.

Controls
All the controls were negative except for the well known endogenous

---

FIG. 5. *Proximal tubule fixed 20 min after injection of Fab. The brush border of proximal tubule shows little if any staining. Some large apical vacuoles (E) are labelled and numerous lysosomes (L) are strongly stained. ×6500.*

FIG. 6. *Distal tubule fixed 5 min after injection of Fab. Staining is seen in the basement membrane (BM), the extracellular spaces between the cells (arrow) and the basal invaginations. ×6500.*

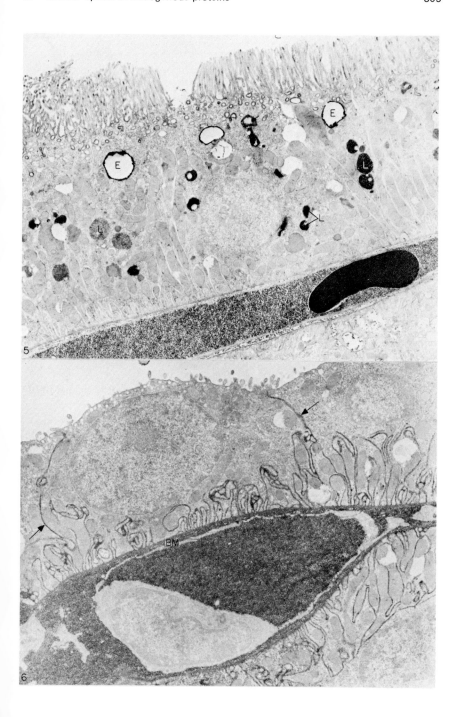

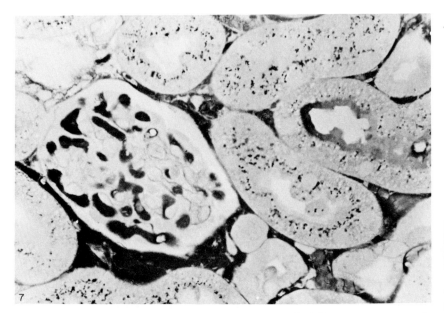

FIG. 7. *Kidney cortex fixed 20 min after injection of F(ab')₂. In some areas the brush borders of the proximal tubules are still stained. In other tubular cross-sections, the brush borders are negative but the lysosomes strongly labelled.* × 600.

activity of red blood cells, polymorphonuclear cells, and, occasionally, microbodies and mitochondrial cristae.

Discussion

In situ fixation (Pease, 1955) allows the lumens of the superficial proximal tubules to remain open. This has been shown to be the physiologic state (Hanssen, 1960; Parker *et al.*, 1962; Straus, 1964; Swann, 1960). In fact, using the *in situ* fixation procedure of Ryan and Karnovsky (1976), only the lumen of the superficial tubules remained open.

The results reported here and previously (Bariéty *et al.*, 1978) demonstrate that endogenous albumin passes across the glomerular capillary wall and is reabsorbed in superficial proximal tubules. In fact, the pattern of labelling observed is typical of endocytosis, as already described with various other proteins under different conditions (Bennet, 1956; Ericsson, 1964; Graham and Karnovsky, 1966; Graham and Kellermeyer, 1968; Horster and Larsson, 1976; Karnovsky and Rice, 1969; Laliberté *et al.*, 1975; Maunsbach, 1966*a*, *b*; Miller, 1960; Miller and Palade, 1964). No evidence for endocytosis of albumin was found in the superficial distal or collecting tubules. The proximal location of albumin reabsorption is supported by investigations on isolated perfused tubules by Bourdeau *et al.* (1972) and the micropuncture studies of Cortney *et al.* (1970). Both groups of investigators found significant uptake of homologous albumin only in the proximal convoluted tubule. It is very unlikely that the tubular endocytosis could be due to a secondary reabsorption following a tubular secretion because the tubular endocytosis was found at the very beginning of the nephron. On the other hand, no serum protein could be detected in fluid collected from single proximal tubules microperfused with protein-free solutions (Van Liew, 1970). It is also very unlikely that the tubular endocytosis could be the consequence of the reabsorption of proteins diffusing from glomeruli during the fixation because the pattern of endocytosis is detected in the most superficial tubules, and these are probably fixed very quickly.

The present study also demonstrated that 5 min after injection, Fab fragments were found diffusely distributed on the brush borders, and in the apical vacuoles of all the superficial proximal tubules, suggesting endocytosis. On the other hand, some proximal tubular sections showed a similar staining pattern when $F(ab')_2$ fragments were injected. Twenty minutes after injection of Fab or $F(ab')_2$ fragments, staining appeared in the lysosomes of the proximal tubular cells, suggesting a degradation process (Maunsbach, 1966*a*). At this time, the staining initially observed on the brush border projections was greatly reduced or had even disappeared. IgG was not detected in these structures either 5 or 20 min after injection. The staining pattern sequence was always similar in all the rats studied. This sequence clearly demonstrates that the reabsorption–degradation process is an *in vivo* phenomenon and is not due to possible glomerular diffusion of the proteins during fixation. The results reported here with Fab and $F(ab')_2$ fragments during the first stage are similar to those described for tubular reabsorption of endogenous rat albumin. However, during the final stage, two differences were found. Firstly, the lysosomes were stained when fragments were revealed, although they were not when endogenous albumin was studied. This difference was probably due to a lack of penetration of the peroxidase anti-rat albumin conjugate, although fragments were easily revealed after incubation with peroxidase alone. The second difference was the disappearance of staining on the brush border 20 min after injection of fragments. This was probably due to the fact that a small number of fragments were injected and that they were largely cleared. No staining was seen on the cell coat of the luminal part of the distal or collecting tubular cells after injection of $F(ab')_2$ fragments. Irregular staining was sometimes seen after injection of Fab fragments on the cell coat of these tubular cells. One possible explanation for this is that, under our experimental conditions, filtered whole Fab fragments were not completely reabsorbed by the proximal tubule.

The results reported here suggest that the endogenous albumin and the three other circulating proteins used as tracers diffuse from interstitial capillaries into the interstitial tissue and then into the tubular basement membranes, the intercellular spaces up to the tight junctions. This is in agreement with the results obtained *in vitro* with peroxidase (Benzel *et al.*, 1971; Ottosen and Maunsbach, 1973) and homologous albumin (Tisher and Kokko, 1974).

References

Avrameas, S. and Ternynck, T. (1969). The cross-linking of proteins with glutaralde-hyde and its use for the preparation of immunoadsorbent. *Immunochemistry* **6**, 53–66.

Avrameas, S. and Ternynck, T. (1971). Peroxidase-labelled antibody and Fab conjugates with enhanced intracellular penetration. *Immunochemistry* **8**, 1175–1179.

Bariéty, J., Druet, P., Laliberté, F., Sapin, C., Belair, M. F. and Paing, M. (1978). Ultrastructural evidence, by immunoperoxidase technique, for a tubular re-absorption of endogenous albumin in normal rat. *Lab. Invest.* **38**, 175–180.

Bennet, H. S. (1956). The concepts of membrane flow and membrane vesiculation as mechanism for active transport and ion pumping. *J. biophys. biochem. Cytol.* **2**, 99–103.

Bentzel, C. J., Tourville, D. R., Parsa, B. and Tomasi, T. B. Jr (1971). Bidirectional transport of horseradish peroxidase in proximal tubule of necturus kidney. *J. Cell Biol.* **48**, 197–202.

Bignon, J., Chahinian, P., Feldmann, G. and Sapin, C. (1975). Ultrastructural immunoperoxidase demonstration of autologous albumin in the alveolar capillary membrane and in the alveolar lining material of normal rat. *J. Cell Biol.* **64**, 503–509.

Bourdeau, J. E., Carone, F. A. and Ganote, C. E. (1972). Serum albumin uptake in isolated perfused renal tubules. *J. Cell Biol.* **54**, 382–398.

Cortney, M. A., Sawin, L. L. and Weiss, D. D. (1970). Renal tubular protein absorption in the rat. *J. clin. Invest.* **49**, 1–4.

Eisenbach, G. M., Van Liew, J. B. and Boylan, J. W. (1975). Effect of angiotensin on the filtration of protein in the rat kidney: a micropuncture study. *Kidney Int.* **8**, 80–87.

Ericsson, J. L. E. (1964). Absorption and decomposition of homologous hemoglobin in renal proximal tubular cells. An experimental light and electron microscopic study. *Acta path. microbiol. scand.* Suppl. 168, 1–121.

Gaizutis, M., Pesce, A. J. and Lewy, J. E. (1972). Determination of nanogram amounts of albumin by radioimmunoassay. *Microchem. J.* **17**, 327–334.

Graham, R. C. and Karnovsky, M. J. (1966). The early stages of absorptioɪ of injected horseradish peroxidase in the proximal tubules of mouse kidney: ultra-structural cytochemistry by a new technique. *J. Histochem. Cytochem.* **14**, 291–302.

Graham, R. C. and Kellermeyer, R. W. (1968). Bovine lactoperoxidase as a cyto-chemical protein tracer for electron microscopy. *J. Histochem. Cytochem.* **16**, 275–278.

Hanssen, O. E. (1960). Early post-mortem renal changes studied in mice with one kidney exteriorized. II. The functional and the early post-mortem morphology of the kidney. *Acta path. microbiol. scand.* **49**, 297–320.

Horster, M. and Larsson, L. (1976). Mechanisms of fluid absorption during proximal tubule development. *Kidney Int.* **10**, 348–363.

Karnovsky, M. J. and Rice, D. F. (1969). Exogenous cytochrome *c* as an ultrastructural tracer. *J. Histochem. Cytochem.* **17**, 751–753.

Laliberté, E., Sapin, C., Druet, P. and Bariéty, J. (1975). Ultrastructural study by immunoperoxidase of a rat membranous glomerulonephritis. *J. Ultrastruct. Res.* **50**, 150–158.

Laliberté, F., Sapin, C., Belair, M. F., Druet, P. and Bariéty, J. (1978). The localization of the filtration barrier in normal rat glomeruli by ultrastructural immunoperoxidase techniques. *Biologie cellul.* **31**, 15–26.

Leber, P. D. and Marsh, D. J. (1970). Micropuncture study of concentration and fate of albumin in rat nephron. *Kidney Int.* **219**, 358–363.

Maunsbach, A. B. (1966a). Absorption of I^{125}-labeled homologous albumin by rat kidney proximal tubule cells. A study of microperfused single proximal tubules by electron microscopic autoradiography and histochemistry. *J. Ultrastruct. Res.* **15**, 197–241.

Maunsbach, A. B. (1966b). Absorption of ferritin by rat kidney proximal tubule cells. Electron microscopic observation of the initial uptake phase in cells of microperfused single proximal tubules. *J. Ultrastruct. Res.* **16**, 1–12.

Miller, F. (1960). Hemoglobin absorption by the cells of the proximal convoluted tubule in mouse kidney. *J. biophys. biochem. Cytol.* **8**, 689–718.

Miller, F. and Palade, G. E. (1964). Lytic activities in renal protein absorption droplets. An electron microscopical cytochemical study. *J. Cell Biol.* **23**, 519–552.

Oken, D. E. and Flamenbaum, W. (1971). Micropuncture studies of proximal tubule albumin concentration in normal and nephrotic rats. *J. clin. Invest.* **50**, 1498–1505.

Oken, D. E., Cotes, S. C. and Mende, C. W. (1972). Micropuncture study of tubular transport of albumin in rats with aminonucleoside nephrosis. *Kidney Int.* **1**, 3–11.

Ottosen, P. D. and Maunsbach, A. B. (1973). Transport of peroxidase in flounder kidney tubules studied by electron microscope histochemistry. *Kidney Int.* **3**, 315–326.

Parker, M. V., Swann, H. G. and Sinclair, J. G. (1962). The functional morphology of the kidney. *Texas Rep. Biol. Med.* **20**, 425–445.

Pease, D. C. (1955). Electron microscopy of the tubular cells of the kidney cortex. *Anat. Rec.* **121**, 723–743.

Ryan, G. B. and Karnovsky, M. J. (1976). Distribution of endogenous albumin in the rat glomerulus: role of hemodynamic factors in glomerular barrier function. *Kidney Int.* **9**, 36–45.

Ryan, G. B., Hein, S. J. and Karnovsky, M. J. (1976). Glomerular permeability to proteins. Effects of hemodynamic factors on the distribution of endogenous immunoglobulin G and exogenous catalase in the rat glomerulus. *Lab. Invest.* **34**, 415–427.

Straus, W. (1964). Factors affecting the state of injected horseradish peroxidase in animal tissues and procedures for the study of phagosomes and phago-lysosomes. *J. Histochem. Cytochem.* **12**, 470–480.

Swann, H. G. (1960). The functional distension of the kidney: a review. *Texas Rep. Biol. Med.* **18**, 566–583.

Tisher, C. C. and Kokko, J. P. (1974). Relationship between peritubular oncotic pressure gradients and morphology in isolated proximal tubules. *Kidney Int.* **6**, 146–156.

Van Liew, J. B., Buentig, W., Stolte, H. and Boylan, J. W. (1970). Protein excretion: micropuncture study of rat capsular and proximal tubule fluid. *Am. J. Physiol.* **219**, 299–305.

22
The Renal Handling of Low Molecular Weight Polyvinylpyrrolidone and Inulin in Rats

August Schiller and Roland Taugner

Introduction

Polyvinylpyrrolidone (PVP) was introduced as the first synthetic non-toxic plasma substitute by Hecht and Weese (1943). After reports of considerable storage of PVP in the reticuloendothelial system (Ammon and Braunschmidt, 1949), and with the introduction of dextran, the clinical use of PVP as a plasma substitute declined rapidly. In experimental medicine PVP was used to determine the permeability of biological membranes, e.g. the glomerular wall, and is nowadays of interest as a constituent of drug formulations.

Working with polyvinylpyrrolidone of a relatively low mean molecular weight, Hespe *et al.* (1977) observed a rapid renal excretion and, in whole-body section autoradiographs, a preferential storage in the kidneys of rats.

The aim of this study was to investigate the renal handling of freely filterable PVP of low mean molecular weight in comparison with inulin. Inulin seemed to be the most suitable macromolecule for such comparative studies because its renal handling is well known from both animal experiments and clinical application. Our results suggest that the renal handling of PVP and inulin, if their filtration rates are equal, does not differ significantly even at widely varying dosage and different diuretic conditions: PVP, like inulin, is only filtered and not transported in the tubule.

As to the quantitites and kinetics and renal accumulation, our results show that both inulin and PVP are again identically handled: both substances are stored by endocytosis in the proximal tubule, the prolonged retention in the kidney being due to their chemical stability.

Preliminary observations suggest that the non-selective endocytosis and relatively long intrarenal accumulation of inulin and PVP may be utilized to calculate the rate of endocytic fluid uptake by the renal tubules.

Materials and Methods

Animals
The experiments were performed on male Wistar rats generally of 150–170 g body weight. In the clearance experiments the animals weighed 190–200 g.

Materials
Inulin ^{14}C-labelled carboxylic acid (13 mCi/mmol) and ^{3}H-labelled inulin (900 mCi/mmol) were provided by Amersham-Buchler. The specific activity and inulin dosage, respectively, were varied by addition of unlabelled inulin (Inulin reinst, Serva, Heidelberg). ^{14}C-labelled PVP with the following specifications was kindly supplied by BASF, Ludwigshafen, Germany: Kollidon 12, mean number molecular weight 1000, mean weight molecular weight 1700 daltons, inhomogeneity $MW/MN = 1.7$, components of molecular weight $> 14\,900 = 0.1$ per cent (all data determined by gel-permeation chromatography); specific activity 3·66 mCi/g. Specific activity and dosage, respectively, of PVP were also varied by addition of unlabelled PVP of identical chemical composition.

Uptake, clearance and storage experiments
For measurements of the renal uptake of ^{14}C-labelled inulin and ^{14}C-labelled PVP the doses shown in Fig. 3 dissolved in 0·5 ml Tyrode solution were injected into the tail vein. The activities injected amounted to 80–400 μCi/kg of ^{14}C-labelled inulin and 18–550 μCi/kg of ^{14}C-labelled PVP-K12. Three rats under Nembutal anaesthesia were used for each time and dosage shown in Figs 2 and 3. Blood was taken from the carotid artery. Finally the kidneys were removed, decapsulated, weighed and homogenized.

In the clearance experiments, dosages of PVP-K12 were used as shown in Fig. 1. The glomerular filtration rate (GFR) was determined with inulin; the priming dose contained 100 mg inulin/kg body weight; the dosage of continuously infused inulin was 450 mg kg^{-1} h^{-1}. The ^{14}C activities injected with PVP-K12 amounted, in this case, to 75–150 μCi. After intraperitoneal injection of 50 mg Nembutal/kg the animals were placed on a heating pad, and trachea, carotid artery and jugular vein were cannulated; urine was collected using urether catheters. Inulin concentrations in plasma and urine were colorimetrically determined with the anthron method.

In special storage experiments with three rats anaesthetized with Nembutal,

150 mg/kg of ^{14}C-labelled PVP-K12 were administered intravenously, and the urine collected. Fifteen minutes after injection the aorta was cannulated and the kidneys were perfused with isotonic saline and mannitol solutions, respectively, for 30 min.

For activity counting the samples were centrifuged, and 50–500 µl plasma and 50 µl urine, respectively, dissolved in Unisolve (Zinsser, Frankfurt). The kidneys were homogenized, 50–200 µl of homogenate dissolved in TS 1 solubilizer (Zinsser) and mixed with Dimilume (Packard). The samples were then counted in a Betaszint BF 5000 (Frieseke and Hoepfner, Germany).

Autoradiography

For frozen-section autoradiography, one of the kidneys was removed at 15 min and 6, 12, 24 and 72 h after intravenous (i.v.) injection of labelled inulin or PVP-K12. Near the hilus a disk of about 3 mm thickness was excised perpendicularly to the long axis of the kidney and frozen in liquid nitrogen. Frozen-section autoradiographs were prepared according to Taugner and Wagenmann (1958). The dose of PVP or inulin in these experiments amounted to 150 mg/kg, the activity to 350–450 µCi/kg. For electron microscope autoradiography 150 mg ^{3}H-labelled inulin/kg and 2·730 mg ^{14}C-labelled PVP-K12/kg (activities 8·3 and 0·9 mCi/kg respectively) were injected. After 6 h the animals were fixed by vascular perfusion through the abdominal aorta according to Forssmann *et al.* (1977). Ilford L4 emulsion was applied to ultrathin sections using the technique described by Caro and Tubergen (1962). The autoradiographs were studied in a Zeiss EM10 electron microscope.

Results

Clearance, plasma disappearance and renal uptake of inulin and PVP

The ratio clearance PVP-K12/clearance inulin (C_{PVP}/C_{IN}) at various plasma concentrations in a range of 3·5 orders of magnitude is shown in Fig. 1. For PVP-K12 the ratio C_{PVP}/C_{IN} was independent of the plasma level; its mean value in 121 clearance periods amounts to $0·994 \pm 0·115$. The ratio C_{PVP}/C_{IN} was independent of diuresis and showed insignificant variation at urine flow rates between 5 and 100 µl/min.

The plasma disappearance curves of PVP-K12 and inulin after i.v. injection (Fig. 2) initially showed a multi-exponential decrease. After 12 h the plasma regression of both substances approximated a single-exponential slope with a half-time of about 20 h. The kidney concentrations of inulin and PVP-K12 initially decreased rapidly, resulting in practically constant levels after 6 h. At faster declining plasma levels, the final ratio kidney concentration/plasma concentration of PVP and inulin was in the range 300–400.

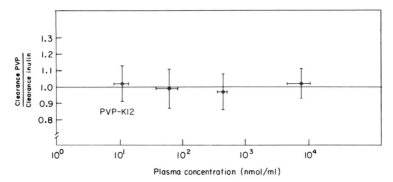

FIG. 1. *Ratio clearance PVP/clearance inulin plotted against the plasma concentration. The clearance of PVP-K12 does not differ significantly from the inulin clearance and is independent of widely varying plasma concentrations.*

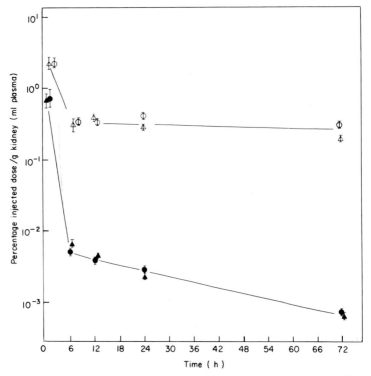

FIG. 2. *Plasma disappearance curve and kidney content of labelled PVP-K12 and inulin plotted against time after intravenous administration.* ○, *Kidney inulin;* △, *kidney PVP-K12;* ●, *plasma inulin;* ▲, *plasma PVP-K12.*

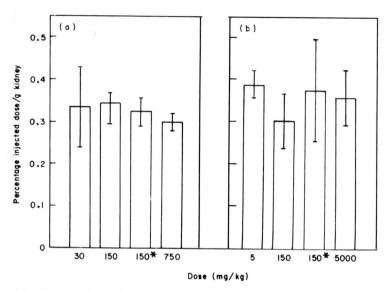

FIG. 3. *Uptake of inulin* (a) *and PVP-K12* (b) *into the kidney 6 h after i.v. injection. With dosages varying 25-fold* (inulin) *and 1000-fold* (PVP-K12) *the retention amounts constantly to 0·3–0·4 per cent of the injected dose. At the dosages marked with asterisks a pre-injection of 750 mg/kg of the unlabelled substance was given 6 h prior to the test dose.*

As shown in Fig. 3, the fractional, dosage-related renal uptake of inulin did not differ significantly 6 h after i.v. injection of 30, 150 or 750 mg/kg. Similar results were obtained with PVP-K12 dosages varying between 5 and 5000 mg/kg. Pre-injections of 750 mg unlabelled PVP/kg 6 h prior to the test dose did not influence the fractional renal uptake of the labelled substance. The same result was obtained with inulin.

Autoradiography
The intrarenal distribution of inulin and PVP-K12 was revealed using auto-radiographic techniques. Figure 4 shows a frozen section autoradiograph of a kidney removed 15 min after i.v. injection of ^{14}C-labelled PVP-K12. High concentrations of the labelled substance in the cortical collecting tubules and collecting ducts can be traced through the medullary rays down to the depth of the renal medulla. The highest grain densities were found over the papilla. The same distribution was obtained with inulin.

In Fig. 5 the intrarenal distributions of ^{14}C-labelled PVP-K12 15 min after i.v. injection is demonstrated. In contrast to Fig. 4 this kidney was subsequently perfused with isotonic mannitol–NaCl solution to eluate the tubular fluid. This autoradiograph demonstrated that much activity was

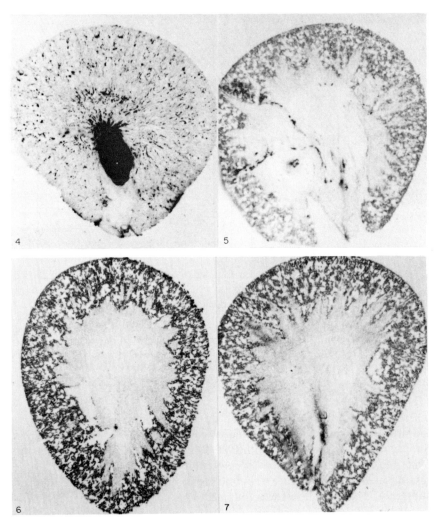

FIG. 4. *Frozen-section autoradiograph of rat kidney obtained 15 min after i.v. injection of* [14]*C-labelled PVP-K12. The label is located mainly in collecting tubules and in the papilla. Ilford G5 nuclear plate, exposure 12 days.* ×9.

FIG. 5. *Frozen-section autoradiograph obtained with* [14]*C-labelled PVP-K12 15 min after i.v. injection. In contrast to Fig. 4 the kidneys were perfused, in this experiment, with isotonic mannitol-NaCl solution for 30 min to elute the activity of the tubular lumina. Excepting some obviously obturated nephrons, the label is located in proximal tubular epithelia. Ilford G5, exposure 2 months.* ×9.

FIGS 6 and 7. *Frozen-section autoradiographs obtained 6 h after i.v. administration of* [14]*C-labelled inulin (Fig. 6) and PVP-K12 (Fig. 7). After this time, most of the activity is located in proximal tubular cells of the renal cortex. Only faint blackening is seen over the medulla. Ilford G5, exposure 1 month.* ×10.

already localized in the epithelium of the proximal tubule after 15 min.

In Figs 6 and 7 the intrarenal distribution of ^{14}C-labelled inulin and PVP-K12 6 h after i.v. injection is demonstrated. In each of these experiments high activities were found in the cortical labyrinth; only low activity was seen in the medullary rays and outer zone of the medulla. In the inner stripe and inner zone of the medulla the autoradiographic blackening was minimal. Distribution patterns as shown in Figs 6 and 7 are characteristic of a preferential uptake of labelled substances into the proximal convolutions.

The higher resolution of electron microscope autoradiography allowed the localization of labelled inulin and PVP in large lysosome-like bodies which are frequently observed after administration of macromolecular compounds.

Discussion

The results of our clearance measurements show that the renal handling of the low-molecular PVP-K12 is very similar to the handling of inulin. The constant C_{PVP}/C_{IN} ratio at plasma levels varying by several orders of magnitude shows that the renal excretion of PVP is obviously due to glomerular filtration; active tubular reabsorption or secretion can be excluded. Furthermore, there is no indication of back-diffusion in the renal tubules since the C_{PVP}/C_{IN} ratio does not change significantly when the urine flow varies up to 20-fold.

In accordance with identical clearance values of PVP-K12 and inulin, no differences between the plasma regression curves of the two substances were found within the first 6 h after i.v. injection (Fig. 2). Plasma kinetics and renal elimination of PVP-K12 and inulin suggest not only identical renal handling but also identical distribution of both substances in the body fluid spaces: PVP-K12 and inulin obviously do not enter the intracellular compartment, except by endocytosis in very small amounts which do not affect their acute plasma regression due to renal excretion. In the following period, between 6 and 72 h after i.v. injection, the slope of the plasma regression of both substances is considerably reduced. This retarded decrease cannot simply be explained by continuous clearing of the extracellular space by glomerular filtration, but rather by redistribution phenomena from intracellular storage sites. The release of very small amounts of intracellularly stored, probably endocytosed, material can be expected to become evident only after several hours, when plasma levels are already low.

Earlier studies of White and Rolf (1957) on nephrectomized rats had already shown that inulin enters the intracellular space. Hespe et al. (1977) reported uptake of low molecular weight ^{14}C-labelled PVP into different organs in rats. Most of the activity was found in the kidney, some also in liver, spleen, pancreas, skin, bone marrow and connective tissue. From such findings it seems to be characteristic of inulin and low molecular weight PVP to be stored preferentially in the kidney, while higher molecular weight PVP is avidly phagocytosed by the reticuloendothelial system. The results of our storage experiments, and the observations with the light and electron microscope, substantiate the retention of PVP and inulin in the kidney, the bulk of which was found in lysosomes of the proximal tubule.

There are many observations indicating endocytic uptake of numerous substances into the proximal tubular epithelium (Maunsbach, 1969). Endocytic uptake was reported for horse-radish peroxidase (Straus, 1962, 1964, 1971; Graham and Karnovsky, 1966), haemoglobin (Miller, 1960; Ericsson, 1964; Neustein, 1967), albumin (Maunsbach, 1966a), ferritin (Maunsbach, 1966b), insulin (Cortney et al., 1970), ribonuclease (Cortney et al., 1970), lysozyme (Maack and Sherman, 1974; Pruzanski and Wilson, 1977), aprotinin (Just, 1975), cytochrome c (Christensen, 1976), micro-globulin (Maunsbach and Christensen, 1976), adrenocorticotrophin analogues (Baker et al., 1977), growth hormone (Johnson and Maack, 1977), parathyroid hormone (Kau and Maack, 1977) and also for inulin (Gayer et al., 1960, 1961; Falbriard et al., 1967; Lanning and Post, 1968). Although the storage of all endocytosed substances is identical in the lysosomal system of the proximal tubule, there are remarkable differences in the fractional storage, i.e. the tubular uptake in relation to the injected dose or filtered load. As demonstrated in Fig. 3, the rate of endocytic uptake of PVP is independent of the dosage and identical with that of inulin. Pre-injections of these substances prior to the test dose did not decrease the endocytic uptake. From these findings it can be concluded that the endocytic mechanism involved in the tubular uptake of PVP is very similar to (or identical with) that of inulin; together with the observed lack of saturation phenomena and the absence of preload influence, it is tempting to speculate that the endocytosis of PVP and inulin is closely related to a fundamental cellular transport process. This assumption is supported by the fact that the renal endocytosis of PVP and inulin, under all conditions tested, amounts to a constant, very small value of only 0·3–0·4 per cent of the filtered load (see below), which, in long-term experiments, is identical with the injected dose, since PVP-K12 and inulin are almost completely excreted by glomerular filtration (Brode, 1977).

Several other filterable macromolecular substances are endocytosed to a much greater extent, e.g. insulin, ribonuclease to 30–50 per cent of the injected load, albumin to 0–20 per cent (Cortney et al., 1970), peroxidase to 4·5–6 per cent (Straus, 1971), aprotinin to 60 per cent (Just et al., 1975), cytochrome c to 37 per cent (Christensen, 1976), lysozyme to 50–70 per cent (Pruzanski and Wilson, 1977), growth hormone to 30 per cent (Johnson and Maack,

1977) and parathormone to 70 per cent (Kau and Maack, 1977). Although freely filterable, PVP and inulin are endocytosed at a much lower rate than peptides and proteins, some of which are only poorly filterable, e.g. albumin, indicating considerably different tubular handling, on the one hand, of proteids and, on the other hand, of inert macromolecular compounds like PVP and inulin.

For the endocytic uptake of many of the larger peptides and proteins more or less specific interactions of the transported molecules and the luminal brush border membrane are assumed, e.g. by electrostatic binding of positively charged molecules to special receptor sites of the membrane (Ryser, 1968; Just and Habermann, 1973; Just, 1975). Our findings of a small constant fractional absorption of PVP and inulin without saturation or inhibitory and stimulating effects, respectively, suggest that no specific interaction of these substances occurs with the endocytic apparatus of the proximal tubule.

From our results it could therefore be concluded that such inert substances as PVP and inulin are taken up unselectively in relation to the bulk endocytosis of tubular fluid; this would explain why their endocytic uptake is at the lowest rate known at present. If so, both substances would be suitable for the determination of the rate of tubular endocytosis, i.e. the volume of tubular fluid which is captured by bulk endocytosis per tissue unit and time, together with its content of solutes.

The quantitative aspects of the endocytic volume are poorly known and have so far been investigated mainly in primitive cells and tissue cultures (Williams et al., 1975). The endocytic rate of the proximal tubule might be calculated with inulin or PVP from the ratio substrate stored/substrate filtered. To relate the tubular storage directly to the filtered load, some special experiments, including urine collection, were performed. They showed that 2 h after administration of PVP and inulin, used as markers of the endocytic volume, about 0·3–0·4 per cent of the filtered load is stored in the kidney. In other experiments (see Fig. 7) urine was collected within 15 min after injection of PVP and inulin, respectively. Then the kidneys were perfused with isotonic solution, and the excreted plus the eluted activity measured in relation to the activity stored in the kidney tissue. In these short-term experiments also, about 0·3 per cent of the filtered (and excreted) activity was stored in the kidney.

For calculations of the rate of endocytosis the concentration of the marker of the endocytic volume in the tubular fluid has to be known.

If we assume a mean ratio tubular fluid/plasma of two along the whole proximal tubular length, and if 0·3 per cent of the filtered load is stored by endocytosis, then the rate of endocytosis can be calculated to be about 0·15 per cent of the glomerular filtration rate. In this estimation it is assumed that a stable pool of endocytosed material exists, and re-entry into the circulation or exocytosis into the tubular lumen does not occur. For more precise information on the rate of endocytosis and the turnover of the endocytosed material, experiments with isolated tubules under well defined conditions would be necessary.

Summary

Renal handling and intrarenal distribution of ^{14}C-labelled polyvinyl-pyrrolidone (PVP) of low molecular weight (1700 daltons) and of inulin were studied in Wistar rats using scintillation counting and autoradiographic techniques. The clearance of PVP-K12 is identical with the inulin clearance and is independent of plasma concentrations between 5 and 10 000 nmol PVP/ml; furthermore, the clearance of PVP does not change significantly when diuresis is varied. From these results it can be concluded that PVP excretion is solely carried out by glomerular filtration.

In addition to the equal clearance values, the intrarenal distributions of PVP and inulin are identical. For both substances intrarenal storage was found to be localized mainly in the lysosomal system of the proximal tubule; this uptake is obviously by endocytosis. The endocytic uptake of PVP and inulin into proximal tubules amounts to a constant fraction of 0·3–0·4 per cent of the i.v. injected dose or filtered load respectively, without signs of saturation. Preloading did not influence the intrarenal storage.

The endocytic uptake of PVP and inulin is very small when compared with other macromolecular compounds, suggesting that the uptake of both substances is proportional to the endocytic absorption of water into the tubular cells. If so, PVP and inulin would be suitable for the determination of the rate of endocytic fluid uptake.

References

Ammon, R. und Braunschmidt, G. (1949). Das Schicksal des Peristons im Organismus. *Biochem. Z.* **319**, 370–379.
Baker, J. R., Bennet, H. P., Christian, R. A. and McMartin, C. (1977). Renal uptake and metabolism of adrenocorticotrophin analogues in the rat; an autoradiographic study. *J. Endocr.* **74**, 23–35.
Brode, E. (1977). Excretion von PVP-K12 und PVP-K17 bei weiblichen Ratten. Projektbericht Fa. BASF, Biologische Forschung und Entwicklung.
Caro, L. G. and Tubergen, R. P. van (1962). High-resolution autoradiography. I. Methods. *J. Cell Biol.* **15**, 173–188.

Christensen, E. J. (1976). Rapid protein uptake and digestion in proximal tubule lysosomes. *Kidney Int.* **10**, 301–310.

Cortney, M. A., Sawin, L. L. and Weiss, D. D. (1970). Renal tubular protein absorption in the rat. *J. clin. Invest.* **49**, 1–4.

Ericsson, J. L. E. (1964). Absorption and decomposition of homologous hemoglobin in renal proximal tubular cells. An experimental light and electron microscopic study. *Acta path. microbiol. scand.* Suppl. 168, 1–121.

Falbriard, A., Busset, R. and Zender, R. (1967). Rétension intrarénale d'une faible fraction d'inuline. *Helv. physiol. pharmac. Acta* **25**, 123–133.

Forssmann, W. G., Ito, S., Weihe, E., Aoki, A., Dym, M. and Fawcett, D. W. (1977). An improved perfusion fixation method for the male genital tract. *Anat. Rec.* **188**, 307–314.

Gayer, J. and Barthelmai, W. (1960). Inulinextraktion und Inulinverteilungsvolumen der Nieren bei erniedrigten arteriellen Drucken. *Klin. Wschr.* **5**, 231.

Gayer, J., Graul, E. H. and Hundeshagen, H. (1961). Autoradiographical detection of tritium-labelled inulin in the kidney. *Nature, Lond.* **189**, 500.

Graham, R. C., Jr and Karnovsky, M. J. (1966). The early stages of absorption of injected horseradish peroxidase in the proximal tubules of mouse kidney: ultra-structural cytochemistry by a new technique. *J. Histochem. Cytochem.* **141**, 291–302.

Hecht, G. and Weese, H. (1943). Periston, ein neuer Blutflüssigkeitsersatz. *Münch. med. Wschr.* **90**, 11.

Hespe, W., Meier, A. M. and Blankwater, Y. J. (1977). Excretion and distribution studies in rats with two forms of ^{14}carbon-labelled polyvinylpyrrolidone with a relatively low mean molecular weight after intravenous administration. *Drug Res.* **27**, 1158–1162.

Johnson, V. and Maack, Th. (1977). Renal extraction, filtration, absorption, and catabolism of growth hormone. *Am. J. Physiol.* **233**, F185–F196.

Just, M. and Habermann, E. (1973). Interactions of a protease inhibitor and other peptides with isolated brush border membranes from rat renal cortex. *Naunyn-Schmiedeberg's Arch. Pharmac.* **280**, 161–176.

Just, M. (1975). *In vivo* interaction of the Kunitz protease inhibitor and of insulin with subcellular structures from rat renal cortex. *Naunyn-Schmiedeberg's Arch. Pharmac.* **287**, 85–95.

Just, M., Röckel, A., Stanjek, A. and Bode, F. (1975). Is there any transtubular reabsorption of filtered proteins in rat kidney? *Naunyn-Schmiedeberg's Arch. Pharmac.* **289**, 229–236.

Kau, S. T. and Maack, Th. (1977). Transport and catabolism of parathyroid hormone in isolated rat kidney. *Am. J. Physiol.* **233**, F445–F454.

Lanning, J. T. and Post, R. S. (1968). Inulin and albumin in centrifugates from rat cortex. *Fedn Proc. Fedn Am. Socs exp. Biol.* **27**, 245.

Maack, Th. M. and Sherman, R. L. (1974). Proteinuria. *Am. J. Med.* **56**, 71–82.

Maunsbach, A. B. (1966a). Absorption of ^{125}I-labelled homologous albumin by rat kidney proximal tubule cells. A study of microperfused single proximal tubules by electron microscopic autoradiography and histochemistry. *J. Ultrastruct. Res.* **15**, 197–241.

Maunsbach, A. B. (1966b). Absorption of ferritin by rat kidney proximal tubule cells. Electron microscopic observations on the initial uptake phase in cells of micro-perfused single proximal tubules. *J. Ultrastruct. Res.* **16**, 1–12.

Maunsbach, A. B. (1969). Functions of lysosomes in kidney cells. In *Lysosomes in*

Biology and Pathology, Vol. 1 (J. T. Dingle and H. B. Fell, eds), North Holland, Amsterdam, pp. 115–154.

Maunsbach, A. B. and Christensen, E. I. (1976). Uptake and digestion of low molecular weight protein in rat kidney tubules. In *Proceedings of the VIth International Congress of Nephrologists, Florence 1975* (S. Giovanetti, V. Bonomini and G. D'Amico, eds), Kager, Basel, pp. 387–391.

Miller, F. (1960). Hemoglobin absorption by the cells of the proximal convoluted tubule in mouse kidney. *J. biophys. biochem. Cytol.* **8**, 689–718.

Neustein, B. H. (1967). Hemoglobin absorption in the proximal tubules of the kidney in the rabbit. *J. Ultrastruct. Res.* **17**, 565–587.

Pruzanski, W. and Wilson, D. R. (1977). Renal handling of endogenous lysozyme in man. *J. Lab. Clin. Med.* **90**, 61–67.

Ryser, H. J.-P. (1968). Uptake of protein by mammalian cells: an underdeveloped area. *Science, N.Y.* **159**, 390–396.

Straus, W. (1962). Cytochemical investigation of phagosomes and related structure in cryostat sections of the kidney and liver of rats after intravenous administration of horseradish peroxidase. *Exptl Cell Res.* **27**, 80–94.

Straus, W. (1964). Cytochemical observations on the relationship between lysosomes and phagosomes in kidney and liver by combined staining for acid phosphatase and intravenously injected horseradish peroxidase. *J. Cell Biol.* **20**, 497–507.

Straus, W. (1971). Comparative analysis of the concentration of injected horseradish peroxidase in cytoplasmic granules of the kidney cortex, in the blood, urine and liver. *J. Cell Biol.* **48**, 620–632.

Taugner, R. and Wagenmann, U. (1958). Serienmäßige Herstellung von Gefrierschnitt-Autoradiogrammen mit optimalem Kontakt. *Naunyn-Schmiedeberg's Arch. exp. Path. Pharmak.* **234**, 336–342.

White, H. C. und Rolf, D. (1957). Whole body and tissue inulin and sucrose spaces in the rat. *Am. J. Physiol.* **188**, 151.

Williams, K. E., Kidston, E. M., Beck, F. and Lloyd, J. B. (1975). Quantitative studies of pinocytosis. I. Kinetics of uptake of ^{125}I-polyvinylpyrrolidone by rat yolk sac cultured *in vitro*. *J. Cell Biol.* **64**, 113–122.

23
Renal Tubular Transport and Catabolism of Small Peptides

Frank A. Carone, Darryl R. Peterson,
Suzanne Oparil and Theodore N. Pullman

Introduction

It is clearly established that the kidney plays an important role in the metabolism of a number of protein, polypeptide, and small peptide molecules. Absorption, transport, and/or degradation of proteins or peptides are functions of the proximal tubule; there is little evidence that other segments of the nephron have the mechanisms for uptake or transport of these substances. Indirect and direct studies indicate that a variety of proteins and polypeptides filtered at the glomerulus are absorbed by the proximal tubule by luminal endocytosis and hydrolyzed by lysosomal enzymes. Our recent studies suggest that small linear peptides, consisting of 8–10 amino acids, are handled by the proximal tubule by a different mechanism. We have demonstrated that small linear peptides microinfused into proximal tubules are hydrolyzed at the luminal surface of the brush border, which is rich in a variety of enzymes, by the process of membrane or contact digestion with reabsorption of most of the breakdown products.

The kidney has been shown to degrade circulating angiotensin II (AII) rapidly. Although 40–70 per cent of ^{14}C-labeled angiotensin II (^{14}C-AII) infused into the renal artery is extracted by the dog kidney, little labeled material appears in the urine. The high extraction ratio suggests that renal handling involves more than glomerular filtration alone (Bailie *et al.*, 1971). Similar studies have shown that 75 per cent of all ^{14}C-AII is metabolized in a single passage through the kidney, and 98·7 per cent of injected radio-labeled material is recovered in renal venous blood (Oparil and Bailie, 1973). These findings indicate that extensive renal hydrolysis occurs, and that tissue sequestration of ^{14}C-AII or its metabolites is not prolonged. Thus, renal hydrolysis of AII allows for the rapid return of cleavage products to the general circulation.

Methods

Recently, we have assessed the role of individual nephrons or isolated nephron segments in the transport and hydrolysis of radiolabeled angiotensin I (AI), AII, bradykinin (BKN), and oxytocin (OT). The techniques for *in vivo* micro-infusion of surface tubules in rats (Gottschalk *et al.*, 1965) and *in vitro* microperfusion of isolated rabbit nephron segments (Burg *et al.*, 1966) were employed. Reabsorption of radiolabeled material was measured, and the intact peptide or its metabolites were identified and quantified in urine, or bathing medium and collection fluid (Carone *et al.*, 1976). In addition, peptides were incubated in the presence of isolated membrane preparations to localize a probable cellular site of hydrolysis. Characterization of labeled material was accomplished by two-dimensional peptide mapping involving high voltage paper electrophoresis in combination with descending paper chromatography (Pullman *et al.*, 1975) or high voltage paper electrophoresis alone. Standard peptide fragments were generated by digesting labeled peptide in the presence of several purified enzymes.

Tubular Handling of Angiotensin II

^{14}C-AII labeled in the fifth position on isoleucine (Fig. 1) was microinfused *in vivo* into individual surface nephrons of the rat kidney. Following proximal infusion, 11 per cent of ^{14}C label was recovered in the urine, and most (95 per cent) of this was present as metabolites, including the carboxyl terminal tetrapeptide as the principal hydrolytic end-product. In contrast, recovery of

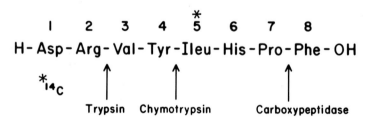

FIG. 1. *Angiotensin II labeled at fifth position with* ^{14}C. *Digestion with trypsin, chymotrypsin and carbopeptidase A (arrows) yielded standard breakdown products. (From Peterson* et al. *(1977).)*

[14]C label was 95 per cent when distal tubules were infused and virtually all was intact AII. The data suggest that the peptide is rapidly hydrolyzed and reabsorbed in the proximal tubule but not in the distal tubule.

Effect of Amino Acids on Tubular Handling of Angiotensin II

In order to examine further the proximal tubular handling of small peptides, we have attempted to dissociate the processes of enzymic degradation and tubular reabsorption by microinfusing excess unlabeled constituent amino acids together with ^{14}C-AII. For these studies we selected L-isoleucine (Ile), which occupies the fifth position of ^{14}C-AII as well as carrying the radioactive label, and L-aspartic acid (Asp), the amino-terminal amino acid and first residue to be cleaved by an aminopeptidase. We reasoned that the individual amino acids might compete for reabsorption with those derived from enzymic breakdown. Furthermore, there is evidence to indicate that under some circumstances aspartic acid is a potent inhibitor of a renal aminopeptidase (Pfleiderer, 1970), whereas isoleucine is a weak one. In addition, since aspartic acid is dicarboxylic and isoleucine monocarboxylic, they would not be expected to share a common reabsorptive mechanism (Bergeron and Morel, 1969; Ward et al., 1976; Webber, 1963).

When ^{14}C-AII was microinfused into proximal nephrons with excess unlabeled L-Ile (Pullman et al., 1978), urinary recovery of ^{14}C label greatly exceeded that seen with ^{14}C-AII alone, and increased directly with distance of the infusion site from the glomerulus (Fig. 2). Since ^{14}C-labeled Ile appeared as the predominant labeled material in urine and only 5 per cent of the labeled material excreted was in the form of intact AII, these results suggest that excess unlabeled Ile interfered with the reabsorption of labeled Ile derived from AII. However, when it is considered that the total recovery of radiolabeled material was much greater when isoleucine was infused with ^{14}C-AII than when ^{14}C-AII was infused alone, the 5 per cent of radioactivity as unaltered AII assumes greater prominence. Thus, suppression of the reabsorption of labeled Ile by excess unlabeled Ile was the predominant effect and overshadowed the inhibition of hydrolysis of AII by excess unlabeled Ile.

When aspartic acid was administered with ^{14}C-AII (Pullman et al., 1978) into the proximal five-sixths of the proximal convolution, total urinary recovery of the ^{14}C-labeled material was unchanged but percentage of recovery as ^{14}C-AII increased; with infusion into the distal one-sixth of the proximal convolution, total urinary recovery of the ^{14}C-label increased (Fig. 3). The data suggest that aspartic acid interfered with the enzymic hydrolysis of ^{14}C-AII and reabsorption of isoleucine. In distal tubules the ^{14}C-label was almost completely recovered as intact ^{14}C-AII in all protocols. The results

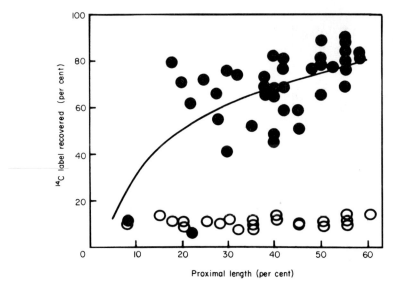

FIG. 2. *Percentage recovery of* [14]*C-AII as a function of tubular length.* ●, *Infusion of* [14]*C-AII plus unlabeled isoleucine in molar ratio of 1:2000;* ○, *infusion of* [14]*C-AII alone.* (*From Pullman* et al. (*1978*).)

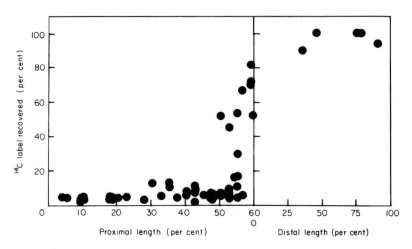

FIG. 3. *Percentage recovery of* [14]*C label from microinfused* [14]*C-AII as a function of proximal and distal tubular length. All depicted points represent recoveries after infusion of a solution of* [14]*C-AII plus unlabeled aspartic acid in a molar ratio of 1:1500.* (*From Pullman* et al. (*1978*).)

show that free amino acids influence proximal tubular handling of small linear peptides.

Tubular Handling of Angiotensins by Isolated Tubular Segments

In vitro microperfusion of rabbit proximal straight nephron segments with ^{14}C-AII or ^{14}C-AI provided direct evidence for proximal hydrolysis of the peptide, accompanied by rapid and extensive reabsorption of ^{14}C-labeled material across the tubular epithelium (Peterson *et al.*, 1977). When AII was microperfused, approximately 30 per cent of perfused ^{14}C label was reabsorbed per millimeter of tubular length over a broad range of delivery rates (Fig. 4). Most of the labeled material was rapidly transported across the tubular epithelium into the bathing medium, and less than 1 per cent of perfused label remained sequestered by the tubular cells following the 35 min perfusion period. Electrophoresis of collected perfusate demonstrated that

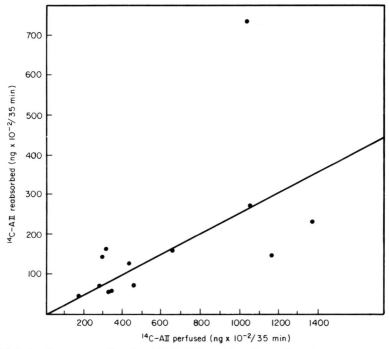

FIG. 4. *Nanograms of perfused ^{14}C-AII (per 35 min) are plotted against nanograms reabsorbed. Line was fitted to data points by linear regression analysis, and correlation coefficient indicates a positive correlation at $p = 0.02–0.05$ level of significance. (From Peterson* et al. *(1977).)*

[14]C-AII was hydrolyzed to ^{14}C-labeled Ile. When AI was microperfused (Peterson *et al.*, 1978), transport of ^{3}H label into the bathing medium varied linearly with time during 30 min of perfusion, and 12·4 per cent of perfused radiolabel was reabsorbed per millimeter of tubule length (Fig. 5), ^{3}H-labeled leucine appeared as the only hydrolytic end-product in the collection fluid and bathing medium, accompanied by little or no intact ^{3}H-AI.

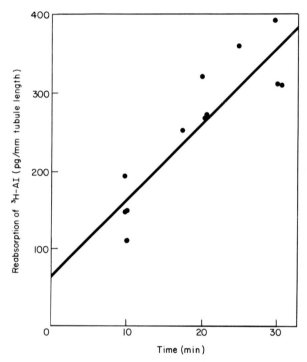

FIG. 5. *Reabsorption of* [3]*H label from proximal straight tubular segments microperfused with* [3]*H-AI as a function of time. Reabsorption is expressed as picograms* [3]*H-AI per millimeter of tubular length. (From Peterson* et al. *(1977).)*

Hydrolysis of Angiotensins by Isolated Brush Border Membranes

The foregoing data indicate that AII and AI are quickly degraded upon passage through the renal proximal tubule, and suggest that cleavage occurs at the level of the tubular luminal membrane. This hypothesis was strengthened by incubations of ^{14}C-AII or ^{14}C-AI directly in the presence of isolated membranes from rabbit renal brush border (Peterson *et al.*, 1978).

Incubation of ^{3}H-AI and ^{14}C-AII in the presence of isolated renal brush border membranes yielded ^{3}H-labeled leucine and ^{14}C-labeled isoleucine, respectively. These data indicate that ^{3}H-AI and ^{14}C-AII are hydrolyzed at the brush border of the renal proximal tubule, followed by reabsorption of hydrolytic end-products.

Tubular Handling of Bradykinin

It is not known if the rapid enzymic cleavage of AI or AII in the proximal tubule applies only to these peptides or affects other small polypeptides. To investigate this problem further, renal tubular handling of ^{3}H-labeled bradykinin (^{3}H-BKN) was studied and, in addition, tubular transit studies of simultaneously microinfused ^{3}H-BKN and ^{14}C-labeled inulin (^{14}C-In) were also determined (Carone et al., 1976). Surface nephrons in the rat kidney were microinfused in vivo with ^{3}H-BKN labeled in the second position on proline.

Following microinjection of labeled bradykinin into proximal tubules, 76 per cent of labeled material was absorbed and 24 per cent of labeled material was recovered in the urine, mostly as metabolites of bradykinin. Peptide characterization revealed that 81 per cent of labeled material in the urine was ^{3}H-labeled Pro, 4 per cent was the 1–5 peptide, and 15 per cent was intact bradykinin. Distal infusions resulted in recovery of 98 per cent of ^{3}H label, all of which appeared in the urine as intact ^{3}H-BKN. The capacity of the rat proximal tubule for handling bradykinin is large since over 95 per cent of a dose microinfused at 2×10^3 times physiologic plasma concentration was absorbed and/or metabolized during a single passage. In contrast, injection of labeled bradykinin into distal tubules resulted in essentially complete recovery of label in the urine in the form of intact bradykinin. Thus, tubular handling of bradykinin is similar to that of AI or AII. These findings suggest that this mechanism may be a nonspecific process for the tubular handling of a number of small polypeptides. Several indirect studies support this concept (Bailie et al., 1971; Oparil and Bailie, 1973; Walter and Shank, 1971).

Our finding of extensive degradation and reabsorption of angiotensin I, angiotensin II, and bradykinin by the proximal tubule suggests that a tubular mechanism contributes to the metabolic fate of these materials in the kidney. This rapid, high capacity, proximal tubular mechanism can degrade and reabsorb these peptides in concentrations thousands of times in excess of those normally found in plasma. This provides an additional mechanism for prompt inactivation of circulating vasoactive peptides, a requirement for hormones which have a rapid and precise regulatory function.

Tubular Transit of Bradykinin and Inulin

[3]H-BKN and ^{14}C-In were simultaneously infused into proximal and distal
surface nephrons, and recovery of the respective labels was plotted as a
function of time at 30 s intervals following microinfusion (Fig. 6). For both
proximal and distal tubules, the urinary concentration–time curves for [3]H
label derived from ^{3}H-BKN did not differ appreciably from those for ^{14}C-In
(Fig. 6). Since ^{3}H label represents both intact ^{3}H-BKN and hydrolytic

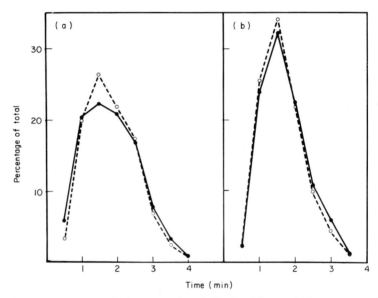

FIG. 6. *Appearance of (a) proximal and (b) distal* [3]*H and* [14]*C in urine plotted
against time.* [3]*H and* [14]*C are quantified as percentages of total excretions of each isotope,
respectively. Isotopes were simultaneously microinfused into rat tubules as* [3]*H-labelled
bradykinin and* [14]*C-labelled inulin.* ○---○, [3]*H;* ●——● [14]*C. (From Carone* et al.
(1976).)

products in varying proportions, depending upon the site of microinfusion,
tubular transit time for the metabolites of ^{3}H-BKN is essentially as rapid
as that of ^{14}C-In or intact ^{3}H-BKN. These data suggest that cleavage of
[3]H-BKN in the proximal tubule is a rapid process and favor the interpretation that ^{3}H-BKN, like ^{3}H-AI or ^{14}C-AII, is hydrolyzed at the luminal
brush border membrane.

Concept of Membrane Digestion

The concept of membrane or contact digestion has been developed to explain the hydrolysis and absorption of peptides and other substrates by cell membranes, particularly the mucosa of small bowel (Ugolev, 1965; Ugolev and DeLacy, 1973). In this scheme, peptides are digested completely by enzymes in the brush border and their constituent amino acids transported toward the serosa by carriers closely associated with the hydrolytic enzymes. An alternative explanation for peptide absorption is that polypeptides are partially digested to di- and tripeptides within the lumen or at the brush border and that these oligopeptides are taken up at the brush border by specific active transport mechanisms and further hydrolyzed within mucosal cells (Matthews, 1975; Newey and Smyth, 1960, 1962). Several lines of evidence, including competition studies between amino acids and peptides for mucosal uptake, absorption studies with nonhydrolyzable peptides, and studies of subcellular distribution of intestinal peptide hydrolases support the latter explanation for peptide absorption in the small intestine (Fijita et al., 1972; Kim et al., 1972; Matthews, 1975). Similar information is not yet available for the epithelium of the proximal tubule, and it is uncertain to what extent mechanisms of peptide absorption in kidney resemble those in the small bowel.

Effect of Peptides on Tubular Handling of Bradykinin

It is not known whether different species of small peptides share common mechanisms of enzymic degradation and uptake into proximal tubular cells or whether the hydrolytic and degradative processes are highly specific. These questions have been examined in other systems using experiments in which the competition among various peptides for transport and hydrolysis was studied (Matthews, 1975; Payne, 1975). To examine further the mechanisms of hydrolysis and reabsorption of small peptides from the proximal tubule of the rat nephron, we microinfused unlabeled BKN or AI in several hundred-fold molar excess with ^{3}H-BKN (Oparil et al., 1976). AI was selected for competition studies with ^{3}H-BKN because it is a well characterized linear peptide of comparable molecular weight but different sequence which is not vasoactive. When ^{3}H-BKN was administered with BKN or AI, urinary recovery of ^{3}H-labeled material was increased in a manner directly proportional to tubular length, suggesting that reabsorption of ^{3}H-BKN is related to extent of tubular contact (Fig. 7). BKN and AI were equally effective in inhibiting the reabsorption of ^{3}H-BKN and its metabolites from proximal

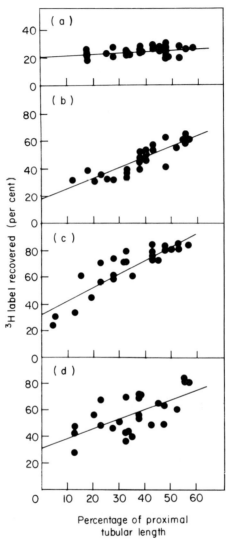

FIG. 7. *Percentage recovery of ³H-labeled material from microinfused ³H-BKN as a function of proximal tubular length:* (a) *³H-BKN alone;* (b) *³H-BKN plus unlabeled BKN in a molar ratio of 1:390;* (c) *³H-BKN plus unlabeled BKN in a molar ratio of 1:780; and* (d) *³H-BKN plus unlabeled AI in a molar ratio of 1:780.* (*From Oparil* et al. (*1976*).)

tubular fluid. In contrast, BKN (but not AI) effectively inhibited the enzymic hydrolysis of ^{3}H-BKN in the proximal tubule. The data suggest that the proximal tubular mechanism for reabsorbing BKN and its metabolites is of high capacity but not high specificity, and that the mechanisms for enzymic cleavage and reabsorption of BKN and its metabolites may have different specificities and capacities.

Tubular Handling of Nonlinear Peptides

A nonlinear molecular configuration may restrict the hydrolysis and uptake of small peptide hormones at the luminal membrane of the proximal tubule. Oxytocin (OT) (Fig. 8) and vasopressin both contain a disulfide bridge.

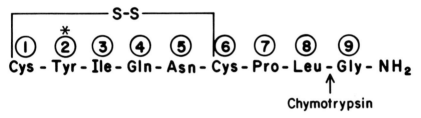

FIG. 8. *Molecular structure of oxytocin labeled with ^3H in the second position (asterisk) demonstrating the disulfide bridge between cysteines in the one and six positions.*

Although the kidney has been implicated in the hydrolysis of both peptides (Walter and Bowman, 1973; Walter and Shank, 1971), *in vitro* microperfusion of ^{3}H-OT (labeled in second position of tyrosine) (Fig. 8) through rabbit proximal straight nephron segments resulted in no detectable hydrolysis, and the reabsorption rate of labeled material was low compared to corresponding measurements for ^{14}C-AII under similar conditions (Peterson *et al.*, 1977). *In vivo* microinfusion of ^{125}I-labeled arginine vasopressin in rat nephrons yielded similar results (Lindheimer, 1977).

Conclusions

Collectively, these studies demonstrate that small linear peptides are cleaved in the proximal tubule of the rat and rabbit kidney when presented to the luminal aspect of proximal tubular cells. The mechanism for tubular handling appears to involve enzymic hydrolysis at the brush border, followed by

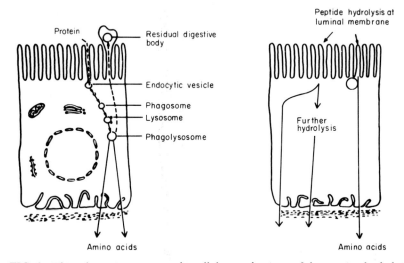

FIG. 9. *This schematic compares the cellular mechanisms of the proximal tubule for reabsorption and catabolism of protein or large polypeptide molecules to that described in our laboratory for small, linear peptides.* (a) *Protein is taken up by endocytic vesicles which fuse to form phagosomes into which primary lysosomes empty their hydrolytic enzymes. Enzymic cleavage of proteins occurs in the phagolysosomes and liberated amino acids diffuse into the interstitium and return to the renal circulation.* (b) *Tubular handling of small, linear peptides. Hydrolysis occurs at the site of enzymes associated with the brush border of the proximal tubule. Liberated amino acids are rapidly transported across the epithelium, probably involving active amino acid pumps located at the apical cell membrane. Partially hydrolyzed peptide fragments may be reabsorbed intact or undergo further intracellular cleavage prior to reabsorption.* (*From Carone* et al. (*1979*).)

rapid reabsorption of metabolites (Fig. 9). It is reasonable to believe that amino acids released by hydrolysis at the luminal membrane are actively reabsorbed by amino acid pumps known to exist there. The distal tubule appears to lack this property. Furthermore, the mechanism of this process appears to differ from that for the proximal reabsorption of proteins and large peptides, which involves endocytosis and lysosomal digestion (Fig. 9). It remains to be determined whether these larger molecules are partially degraded at the luminal membrane of the proximal tubule prior to or during the endocytic process.

Our studies indicate that the proximal tubules of the mammalian kidney possess a high capacity mechanism for the rapid hydrolysis of small linear peptides. This mechanism may be important biologically to (1) conserve amino acids, (2) inactivate toxic peptides, and (3) help regulate the circulating levels of small peptide hormones, since there is evidence that serum levels of these hormones are determined more by rates of degradation than synthesis.

References

Bailie, M. D., Rector, F. C., Jr and Seldin, D. W. (1971). Angiotensin II in arterial and renal venous plasma and renal lymph in the dog. *J. clin. Invest.* **50**, 119–126.

Bergeron, M. and Morel, F. (1969). Amino acid transport in rat renal tubules. *Am. J. Physiol.* **216**, 1139–1149.

Burg, J., Grantham, J., Abramow, M., and Orloff, J. (1966). Preparation and study of fragments of single nephrons. *Am. J. Physiol.* **210**, 1293–1298.

Carone, F. A., Pullman, T. N., Oparil, S. and Nakamura, S. (1976). Micropuncture evidence of rapid hydrolysis of bradykinin by rat proximal tubule. *Am. J. Physiol.* **230**, 1420–1424.

Fijita, M., Parsons, D. S. and Wojnarowska, F. (1972). Oligopeptides of brush border membranes of rat small intestinal mucosal cells. *J. Physiol., Lond.* **227**, 377–394.

Gottschalk, C. W., Morel, F., and Mylle, M. (1965). Tracer micro-injection studies of renal tubular permeability. *Am. J. Physiol.* **209**, 173–178.

Kim, Y. S., Birtwhistle, W. and Kim Y. W. (1972). Peptide hydrolases in the brush border and soluble fractions of small intestinal mucosa of rat and man. *J. clin. Invest.* **51**, 1419–1430.

Lindheimer, M. D., Reinharz, A., Grandchamp, A. and Vallotton, M. B. (1977). Fate of arginine vasopressin (AVP) perfused into nephron of Wistar (W) and Brattleboro (DI) rats. *Clin. Res.* **25**, 595A.

Matthews, D. M. (1975). Intestinal absorption of peptides. *Physiol. Rev.* **55**, 537–608.

Newey, H. and Smyth, D. H. (1960). Intracellular hydrolysis of dipeptides during intestinal absorption. *J. Physiol., Lond.* **152**, 367–380.

Newey, H. and Smyth, D. H. (1962). Cellular mechanisms in intestinal transport of amino acids. *J. Physiol., Lond.* **164**, 527–551.

Oparil, S. and Ballie, M. D. (1973). Mechanism of renal handling of angiotensin II in the dog. *Circulation Res.* **33**, 500–507.

Oparil, S., Carone, F. A., Pullman, T. N. and Nakamura, S. (1976). Inhibition of proximal tubular hydrolysis and reabsorption of bradykinin by peptides. *Am. J. Physiol.* **231**, 743–748.

Payne, J. W. (1975). Transport of peptides in microorganisms. In *Peptide Transport in Protein Nutrition* (D. M. Matthews and J. W. Payne, eds), Associated Scientific Publishers, Amsterdam, pp. 283–364.

Peterson, D. R., Chrabaszcz, G., Peterson, W. R. and Oparil, S. (1978). Renal hydrolysis of angiotensin I and II at the tubular luminal membrane and reabsorption of end-products. *Fedn Proc. Fedn Am. Socs exp. Biol.* **37**, 467.

Peterson, D. R., Oparil, S., Flouret, G. and Carone, F. A. (1977). Handling of angiotensin II and oxytocin by renal tubular segments perfused *in vitro*. *Am. J. Physiol.* **232**, F319–F324.

Pfleiderer, G. (1970). Particle-bound aminopeptidase from pig kidney. *Methods Enzymol.* **19**, 514–521.

Pullman, T. N., Oparil, S. and Carone, F. A. (1975). Fate of labeled angiotensin II microinfused into individual nephrons in the rat. *Am. J. Physiol.* **229**, 747–751.

Pullman, T. N., Carone, F. A., Oparil, S. and Nakamura, S. (1978). Effects of constituent amino acids on tubular handling of micro-infused angiotensin II. *Am. J. Physiol.* **234**, F325–F331.

Ugolev, A. M. (1965). Membrane (contact) digestion. *Physiol. Rev.* **45**, 555–595.

Ugolev, A. M. and DeLacy, P. (1973). Membrane digestion. A concept of enzymatic hydrolysis on cell membranes. *Biochim. biophys. Acta* **300**, 105–128.

Walter, R. and Bowman, R. H. (1973). Mechanism of inactivation of vasopressin and oxytocin by the isolated perfused rat kidney. *Endocrinology* **92**, 189–193.

Walter, R. and Shank, H. (1971). *In vivo* inactivation of oxytocin. *Endocrinology* **89**, 990–995.

Ward, P. E., Erdos, E. G., Godney, C. D., Dowben, R. M. and Reynolds, R. C. (1976). Isolation of membrane-bound renal enzymes that metabolize kinins and angiotensins. *Biochem. J.* **157**, 643–650.

Webber, W. A. (1963). Characteristics of acidic amino acid transport in mammalian kidney. *Can. J. Biochem. Physiol.* **41**, 131–137.

24
Digestion of Protein in Lysosomes of Proximal Tubule Cells

Erik Ilsø Christensen and Arvid B. Maunsbach

Introduction

It is well established that proteins located in the lumen of the proximal tubule are taken up by endocytosis and transported to lysosomes of the tubule cell (for a review, see Maunsbach, 1976) and it has been known since the pioneering work by Straus (1954) that lysosomes isolated from kidney cortex contain enzyme(s) capable of digesting protein. Furthermore, there is ultrastructural evidence that absorbed protein can be digested in proximal tubule cells (Miller and Palade, 1964; Ericsson, 1964). However, evidence obtained by biochemical methods of an intralysosomal protein digestion in intact proximal tubule cells has been lacking, and very little is known about different physiological or experimental factors that influence the uptake, transport and intralysosomal digestion of protein.

The aim of the present study was to provide biochemical evidence for intralysosomal digestion of protein in intact proximal tubule cells. As an experimental model we used renal cortical slices from rats previously injected intravenously with iodinated proteins of low molecular weight. In addition we studied the digestion of labelled proteins with lysosomal enzymes isolated from kidney cortex and determined the effects on renal protein handling of intravenous administration of dextran and sodium maleate.

Methods for Determination of Lysosomal Catabolic Activity

Isolated lysosomal enzymes
The digestive ability of lysosomal enzymes from rat kidney cortex was

investigated by incubating isolated lysosomal enzymes with iodinated proteins as substrates (Maunsbach, 1970). The lysosomal enzymes were obtained from kidney cortex of male Wistar rats, 2–6 months of age. The lysosomes were isolated from a cortical homogenate by differential centrifugation (Maunsbach, 1974) and the lysosomal enzymes released from the lysosomes by freezing and thawing. Lysozyme, cytochrome c and β_2-microglobulin (molecular weights 14 400, 12 400 and 11 800 daltons respectively) were used as substrates following iodination with ^{125}I (specific activities 0·2–0·4 mCi/mg of protein), using the iodine monochloride method (McFarlane, 1958; Izzo et al., 1964). The labelled proteins were incubated and digested in a sodium acetate buffer, pH 4·5, at 37 °C. The digestion was determined by precipitation of non-degraded protein with trichloroacetic acid (TCA) and expressed as TCA-soluble radioactivity in the incubation medium as a percentage of total radioactivity. The nature of the radioactive digestion products was determined by ascending paper chromatography (Maunsbach, 1970).

Cortical slices
Digestion of protein in lysosomes of intact tubule cells was demonstrated in renal cortical slices (Christensen and Maunsbach, 1974). Labelled proteins were injected intravenously in rats and after different time intervals slices were removed by a Stadie–Riggs-type microtome and incubated in a bicarbonate–saline solution (Maude, 1968) with the addition of 1 mM non-radioactive monoiodotyrosine. Protein digestion was measured as TCA-soluble radioactivity in the incubation medium and the cortical slices and expressed as a percentage of total radioactivity. The radioactive digestion products were identified by ascending paper chromatography.

Electron microscope methods
The subcellular localization of the radioactive protein prior to removal of the slices, as well as during the incubation of slices, was determined by electron microscope autoradiography. For this purpose intact kidneys were fixed with 1 per cent glutaraldehyde by retrograde perfusion through the aorta and then further fixed either in the same fixative or in 3 per cent glutaraldehyde. Cortical slices were fixed by immersion in 3 per cent glutaraldehyde. Tissue from kidneys fixed *in vivo* or from cortical slices was postfixed in 1 per cent osmium tetroxide, dehydrated and embedded in Epon 812 or Vestopal. Thin sections were either left unstained or stained with uranyl acetate and lead citrate. For electron microscope autoradiography Ilford L4 emulsion was applied to ultrathin sections by a wire loop method (Maunsbach, 1966a) and exposed for 1–3 months before development and analysis in the electron microscope (Siemens Elmiskop 1A, Jeol 100 B or 100 C).

In some experiments lysosomes were identified in the tissue by electron

microscope histochemistry. Tissue fixed in glutaraldehyde as described above
was incubated for acid phosphatase in the Gomori medium as modified by
Barka and Andersson (1962) at 37 °C for 10–20 min and then prepared for
electron microscopy as described above.

Digestion of Protein with Isolated Lysosomal Enzymes

The incubation of iodinated protein with isolated lysosomal enzymes leads
to a digestion of the labelled protein, as demonstrated by the appearance of
TCA-soluble radioactivity in the incubation medium (Maunsbach, 1968). The
rate of digestion of protein *in vitro* is dependent both upon pH and temperature, and the TCA-soluble radioactivity consists largely of mono-iodotyrosine
(Maunsbach, 1970).

During incubation of β_2-microglobulin with lysosomal enzymes there was

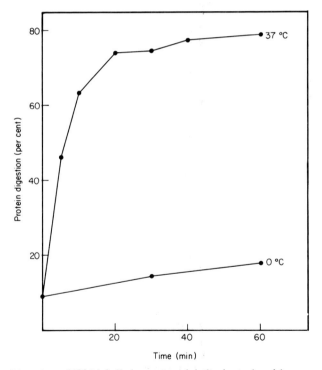

FIG. 1. *Digestion of* [125]*I-labelled* β_2-*microglobulin by isolated lysosomal enzymes
from proximal tubule lysosomes. Digestion occurs at 37 C, but not at 4 C, and is
determined as the release of TCA-soluble radioactivity.*

an initial rapid degradation of the protein and after 60 min of incubation about 80 per cent of the protein had been digested (Fig. 1). The amount of labelled protein decreased from 64 to 15 per cent and the amount of mono-iodotyrosine increased from 14 to 67 per cent (Fig. 2).

Since the major digestion product of iodinated proteins is mono-iodotyrosine, the labelled proteins are, at least in part, digested to the amino acid level. There are small differences in the pH optimum for the lysosomal digestion of different proteins. Thus, the pH optimum is 4·8 for albumin

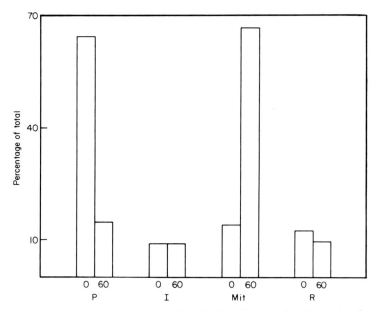

FIG. 2. *Distribution of digestion products, before (0) and after 60 min incubation of* ^{125}I-labelled β_2-microglobulin with lysosomal enzymes from proximal tubules. During digestion there is a decrease in the amount of labelled protein (P), and an increase in labelled mono-iodotyrosine (MIT), but no change in free iodine (I) and remaining activity in the chromatogram (R).

(Maunsbach, 1970), 3·5–5·0 for β_2-microglobulin (Maunsbach and Christensen, 1976), 4·5 for cytochrome c and 5·0–6·0 for lysozyme. Furthermore, differences exist in the susceptibility to digestion between different proteins. Whereas all radioactivity can be released as TCA-soluble radioactivity following digestion of iodinated homologous albumin, and consists predominantly of mono-iodotyrosine (Maunsbach, 1970), even prolonged incubation of iodinated lysozyme (Christensen and Maunsbach, 1974) leaves some of the radioactivity precipitable with TCA. In addition, similar concentrations of enzyme digest proteins at different rates and, for example, labelled egg-white albumin is only digested very slowly. Since denaturation of a protein may be a prerequisite for its digestion by lysosomal enzymes (Coffey and de Duve, 1968), it is possible that the ability of lysosomal enzymes to digest the substrate proteins is dependent upon their susceptibility to denaturation at an acid pH *in vivo* or *in vitro*.

Since the isolated lysosomes from which the enzymes were obtained almost exclusively originate from proximal tubule cells (Maunsbach, 1966*b*), the *in vitro* experiments demonstrate that proximal tubule lysosomes contain enzymes capable of catabolizing a variety of iodinated proteins.

Intracellular Digestion of Protein in Renal Cortical Slices

Autoradiographic localization of labelled protein in slices.
Investigations using a variety of protein tracers (for a review, see Maunsbach,

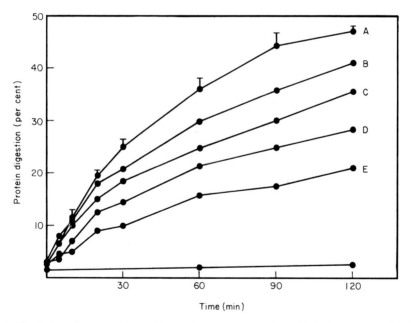

FIG. 3. *Catabolism of* [125]*I-labelled lysozyme in renal cortical slices removed 1 h after intravenous injection of trace amount of labelled lysozyme (curve A). Curves B, C, D and E demonstrate decreased protein digestion in the slices when 25, 50, 75 and 100 mg of non-labelled lysozyme was injected intravenously 10 min before the labelled lysozyme. Protein catabolism was measured as TCA-soluble radioactivity in slices and medium as the percentage of total radioactivity. Lowest curve is control at 4 °C.*

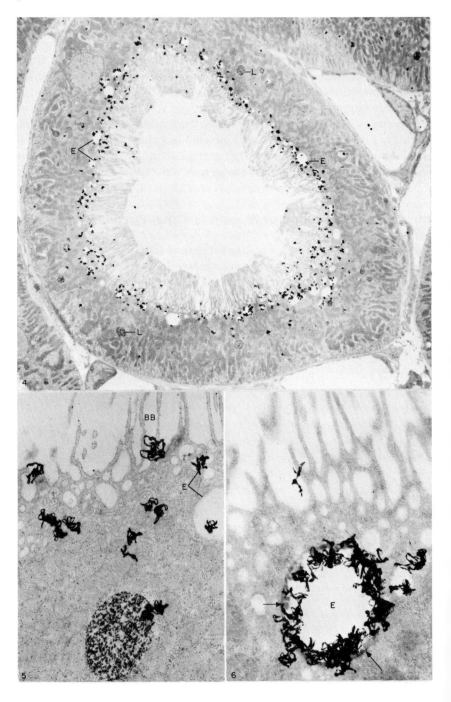

1973) have demonstrated that protein is absorbed from the lumen of the proximal tubule by way of plasma membrane invaginations, in which sections of membrane are pinched off and form endocytic vacuoles (Figs 4–6), and that the endocytic vacuoles subsequently transfer the protein to the lysosomes (Fig. 7). When slices were removed from the kidney cortex and incubated *in vitro*, intracellular transport of protein to the lysosomes continued (Christensen and Maunsbach, 1974). In slices removed from rats 1 h after intravenous injection of labelled lysozyme and incubated *in vitro* for 2 h, almost all autoradiographic grains were located directly over or very close to the lysosomes of the proximal tubule cells (Fig. 8). This localization of the protein suggests that protein digestion during incubation (Fig. 3) takes place within the lysosomes.

Ultrastructure of proximal tubule cells in slices
As observed by electron microscopy the proximal tubule cells in incubated renal cortical slices were usually well preserved even after 2 h of incubation (Fig. 8). However, in most cells there was an increase in the number of small vesicles in the apical parts of the cells, and in the central parts of the slices many cells appeared swollen and the mitochondria enlarged in size (Christensen and Maunsbach, 1974; Martell-Pelletier *et al.*, 1977). The increased number of small vesicles in the apical parts of the cells during incubation is somewhat similar to the alterations caused by sodium maleate (compare Figs 8 and 9) and experimental ischaemia (Reimer *et al.*, 1972), and indicates that there is a decreased fusion of endocytic vesicles both with each other and with the lysosomes due to lack of energy in the cells. The ultrastructure of the lysosomes is essentially unchanged (Fig. 8).

Digestion of protein in slices
During incubation of renal cortical slices removed 1 h after intravenous

---

FIG. 4. *Electron microscope autoradiograph of proximal tubule from rat injected with* [125]*I-labelled cytochrome c. The kidney was fixed after 3 min by glutaraldehyde perfusion and lysosomes located by acid phosphatase cytochemistry. Labelled cytochrome c is almost exclusively located over the apical cytoplasm, which contains endocytic vacuoles* (E), *while the lysosomes* (L) *deep in the cells are unlabelled.* × 2300.

FIG. 5. *High magnification of apical region from same experiment as in Fig. 4. Autoradiographic grains which represent labelled cytochrome c are located over the brush border* (BB) *and endocytic vacuoles* (E) *as well as over apical lysosomes* (L). × 15 000.

FIG. 6. *Apical part of proximal tubule cell from kidney fixed 5 min after injection of labelled cytochrome c. The labelled protein is present in an endocytic vacuole* (E) *and appears preferentially associated with the inner side of its limiting membrane* (arrows). × 26 500.

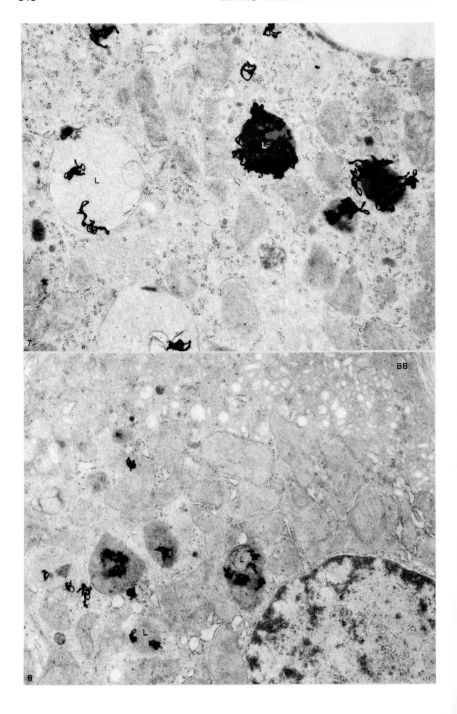

injection of ^{125}I-labelled lysozyme there was a gradual release of TCA-soluble radioactivity, demonstrating the digestion of labelled lysozyme within the slices (Fig. 3). Since the labelled lysozyme was shown by electron microscope autoradiography to be situated in the lysosomes (Fig. 8), it is concluded that the digestion observed in the slices occurred within the lysosomes. About 70 per cent of the radioactive digestion products in the incubation medium consisted of mono-iodotyrosine provided 1 mM non-radioactive mono-iodotyrosine was added to the incubation medium (Christensen and Mauns-bach, 1974). If cold mono-iodotyrosine was not present in the incubation medium, the main radioactive digestion product was iodine. The effect of the addition of cold mono-iodotyrosine to the incubation medium is probably due to the presence of a mono-iodotyrosine deiodinase in the kidney tissue (Stanbury, 1957).

When rats were injected with 25, 50, 75 or 100 mg non-radioactive lysozyme 10 min before the injection of the labelled lysozyme, there was a dose-dependent decrease in the digestion of the protein (Fig. 3). Thus, after 2 h of incubation the digestion in slices from an animal that received 100 mg cold lysozyme was only 21 per cent, as compared to 47 per cent in controls, probably due to a decreased transport of protein from the endocytic vacuoles to the lysosomes and/or a decreased intralysosomal digestion due to a high concentration of substrate (lysozyme) in the lysosomes.

The total accumulation of lysozyme in the kidneys was also decreased in animals that received large doses of non-radioactive lysozyme prior to the radioactive tracer. In animals receiving 10 mg of cold lysozyme 5 min before injection of labelled lysozyme, the renal accumulation of lysozyme 30 min after the injection was only 17·5 per cent, as compared to 40·0 per cent in controls. Instead, the urinary excretion increased to 16·9 per cent, as compared to 0·3 per cent of the injected dose in controls. These observations are consistent with the demonstration by Straus (1962) that pre-injection of egg-white into rats decreased the subsequent uptake of peroxidase by the proximal tubule cells to about 10–25 per cent of controls.

The decreased renal accumulation of labelled lysozyme after injection of 10 mg of non-radioactive lysozyme was due to a decreased tubular uptake, since the glomerular filtration of labelled lysozyme (urinary excretion + renal

FIG. 7. *Part of proximal tubule cell from animal injected 15 min before fixation with labelled cytochrome c. Most absorbed protein, located by electron microscope autoradiography, is present in lysosomes (L) × 15000.*

FIG. 8. *Part of proximal tubule cells in renal cortical slice incubated for 2 h in* vitro. ^{125}*I-labelled lysozyme was injected in the animal 1 h before removal of the cortical slice. The labelled protein is predominantly located in the lysosomes (L).* **BB** = *brush border.* × 11500.

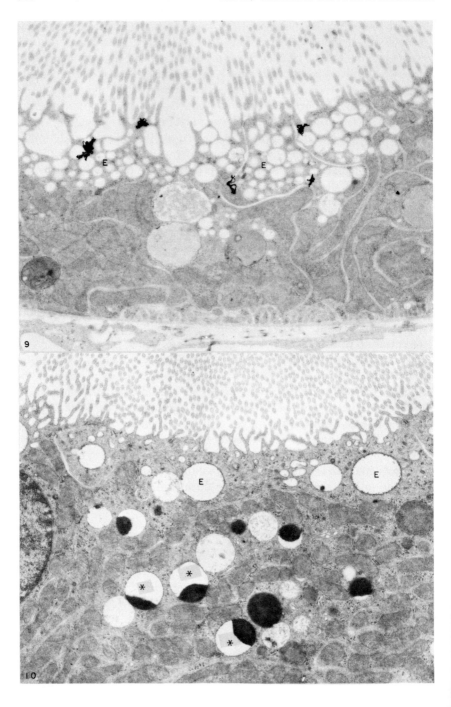

accumulation) was only decreased to 86 per cent of the amount filtered in controls (17·5 + 16·9 per cent as a percentage of 40·0 + 0·3 per cent). Thus, in animals preloaded with non-radioactive lysozyme, about 50 per cent of the filtered radioactive protein was reabsorbed and 50 per cent excreted in the urine.

Rate of Protein Uptake and Intracellular Transport

The rate of endocytic protein uptake and transport of absorbed protein to the lysosomes varies for different proteins. All proteins seem to be present in the lysosomes within half an hour or less after exposure of the proximal tubule cells to the tracers, but it is not known when the lysosomal protein catabolism starts. When ^{125}I-labelled cytochrome c was injected intravenously into rats, some of the labelled proteins absorbed by the proximal tubule cells were observed by autoradiography in apical lysosomes 3 min after injection (Fig. 5). A quantitative analysis of the grain distribution revealed that the accumulation of label over the lysosomes was statistically higher than over the cytoplasm of the proximal tubule cells (Christensen, 1976). Fifteen minutes after injection of labelled cytochrome c, grains were abundant over the lysosomes in the tubule cells (Fig. 7). In parallel experiments a significant digestion of labelled cytochrome c was demonstrated in renal cortical slices 13 min after intravenous injection of the protein (Christensen, 1976). The autoradiographic demonstration of cytochrome c within lysosomes during the time interval when the tracer starts to be digested provides evidence that cytochrome c is digested in the lysosomes.

A very rapid digestion of low molecular peptides has been demonstrated in the proximal tubule (Carone *et al.*, 1976). This digestion probably occurs in the tubule lumen and is effected by peptidases known to be located in the brush border of the proximal tubule cells (Booth and Kenney, 1976). However, all peptides are not degraded by brush border peptidases and large protein molecules might be more or less unaffected by the brush border peptidases.

FIG. 9. *Proximal tubule from rat injected with sodium maleate and 5 min later with* ^{125}*I-labelled lysozyme. After 1 h the kidney was fixed by perfusion. The labelled protein is present in the apical cytoplasm, which shows an accumulation of small endocytic vacuoles (E). × 10 000.*

FIG. 10. *Proximal tubule from dextran-resistant rat which was infused with dextran T-40 for 3 h before perfusion fixation. The lysosomes contain seemingly empty regions (*). Some endocytic vacuoles (E) and lysosomes are enlarged but other cell organelles appear unchanged. × 8000.*

Experimental Modifications of Protein Uptake, Transport and Digestion in Proximal Tubule Cells

Effects of sodium maleate

Sodium maleate, a strong inhibitor of α-ketoacid oxidation in mitochondria (Angielski and Rogulski, 1975) has been shown to cause pronounced urinary excretion of protein (Frederiksson and Peterson, 1975) simultaneously with an increase in the number of endocytic vacuoles in the proximal tubule cells (Worthen, 1963; Rosen *et al.*, 1973). The mechanism of the proteinuria was investigated in rats, which received an intravenous injection of 400 mg/kg body weight of sodium maleate. After 5 min ^{125}I-labelled lysozyme was given intravenously, and 15 min later cortical slices were removed and incubated *in vitro*. In separate experiments the kidneys of similarly treated animals were fixed by perfusion with 1 per cent glutaraldehyde, and in some experiments the total urinary excretion and total renal uptake of labelled lysozyme was determined.

The injection of sodium maleate rapidly caused an increase in the number of endocytic vacuoles in the proximal tubule cells. In rats that received labelled lysozyme intravenously 5 min after maleate injection it was observed by autoradiography that the protein remained within the cytoplasmic region containing the vacuoles even 60 min after injection (Fig. 9). Furthermore, there was a decrease in the renal accumulation of lysozyme and an increase in the urinary excretion of protein 1 h after injection. Thus, the renal accumulation in maleate-treated rats was 7·7 per cent of the injected dose as compared to 34·3 per cent in controls, and the urinary excretion of lysozyme was 7·5 per cent in maleate-treated rats and 0·2 per cent in controls. These results demonstrate that in addition to a tubular decrease in the reabsorption of protein, there was also a decreased glomerular filtration of protein.

In maleate-treated rats the digestion of labelled lysozyme was reduced in renal cortical slices removed 60 min after intravenous injection of the labelled protein. In comparable experiments, the digestion after 2 h of incubation was 19 per cent in maleate-treated animals as compared to 49 per cent in controls (Fig. 11). Furthermore, electron microscope autoradiography revealed that the transport of protein into the lysosomes of the proximal tubule cells was much reduced. A quantitative analysis of the grain distribution showed that 1 h after injection of labelled protein about 70 per cent of the label in controls was located over lysosomes (or within 0·5 μm from the lysosomal membrane) as compared to 8 per cent in maleate-treated rats. These results suggest that the decreased digestion of lysozyme in renal cortical slices is due to a decreased transport of protein from the endocytic vacuoles to the lysosomes,

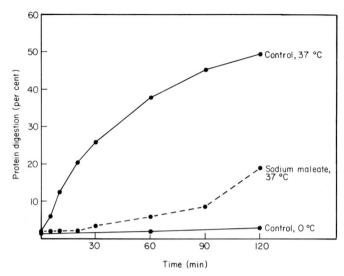

FIG. 11.   *Digestion of* ^{125}I-*labelled lysozyme in renal cortical slices from rat injected with labelled protein and sodium maleate 1 h before preparation of slices. The protein digestion is much reduced in slices from sodium maleate-treated animals.*

probably as a consequence of decreased fusion of endocytic vacuoles with each other and with the lysosomes.

In the exocrine pancreas the vesicular transport of protein from the endoplasmic reticulum to condensing vacuoles is an energy-dependent process (Jamieson and Palade, 1968). The energy requirements for the vesicular transport of protein to lysosomes in proximal tubule cells are not known. However, since sodium maleate inhibits cellular ATP synthesis (Kramer and Gonick, 1970), it is possible that the effects of sodium maleate on the vacuolar system in proximal tubule cells are due to decreased production of cellular energy.

Effects of dextran infusions

The infusion of dextran and several other carbohydrates has been shown to cause pronounced ultrastructural changes of the vacuolar system in the proximal tubular cells (Maunsbach *et al.*, 1962; Engberg and Ericsson, 1969; Diomi *et al.* 1970). However, little is known about the functional changes that accompany the apparent accumulation of foreign substances in the lysosomes.

In the present study we used male Wistar rats of a strain showing no anaphylactoid reaction to dextrans (Harris and West, 1963) to investigate the proximal tubular handling of reabsorbed protein following dextran infusion. The rats were infused intravenously for 2 h with dextran T-40 (10 per cent in saline) to a total of 5 g/kg body weight. Immediately after the infusion the rats received a single intravenous injection of ^{125}I-labelled lysozyme, and 1 h later slices were removed from the renal cortex and incubated *in vitro* for the analysis of protein digestion. The other kidney was fixed by perfusion with glutaraldehyde and the tissue prepared for electron microscopy.

Following dextran infusion, lysosomes were increased in size and seemingly empty spaces were present within the lysosomal matrix (Fig. 10). However, when the kidney was fixed *in vivo* by dripping a lead-containing fixative (Simionescu *et al.*, 1972) on the kidney surface, dextran was visualized as a fine precipitate in endocytic vacuoles and lysosomes (Figs 12 and 13), in agreement with the observation by Caulfield and Farquhar (1976). The dextran was located in those parts of the lysosomes that appeared empty after conventional fixation (compare Figs 10 and 12). The observations provide evidence that dextran is taken up and transported into the lysosomes by endocytosis by way of the same route as proteins. However, dextran was always evenly distributed within the endocytic vacuoles without association to the limiting membrane of the vacuoles. This indicates that dextran is taken up merely as a solute in the tubular fluid enclosed in endocytic invaginations and later in endocytic vacuoles, in contrast to many proteins which are bound to the plasma membrane before and during endocytosis (compare Figs 6 and 13). The uptake of dextran is a typical example of a substance taken up by so-called fluid-phase endocytosis.

The inefficiency of the uptake mechanism for dextran is further underlined when the uptake is analysed from a quantitative point of view. When rats were injected intravenously with ^{3}H-labelled dextran T-80, the total urinary excretion was 43 per cent and the renal accumulation about 1 per cent of the total injected dose (Christensen and Maunsbach, 1979). Since 30 per cent of the dextran accumulated in the kidney was located in the renal medulla, the cortical uptake was only about 1·4 per cent of the filtered amount of dextran, a value which contrasts sharply with the efficient uptake of labelled lysozyme,

---

FIG. 12. *Proximal tubule from dextran-resistant rat infused for 3 h with dextran and then fixed* in vivo *with the lead-containing fixative of Simionescu* et al. *(1972). The lysosomes (L) are enlarged but the seemingly empty regions within the lysosomes observed in Fig. 10 now contain an electron-dense precipitate (arrows) representing dextran absorbed by endocytosis from the tubule lumen.* × *15 000.*

FIG. 13. *Higher magnification of apical region of proximal tubule cells from similar preparation as in Fig. 12. Dextran precipitate can be visualized in the tubule lumen around the microvilli of the brush border (BB), in apical endocytic invaginations (arrow) and in endocytic vacuoles (E) in the apical cytoplasm. Note that dextran is also located in the centre of the vacuoles (compare Fig. 6).* × *37 500.*

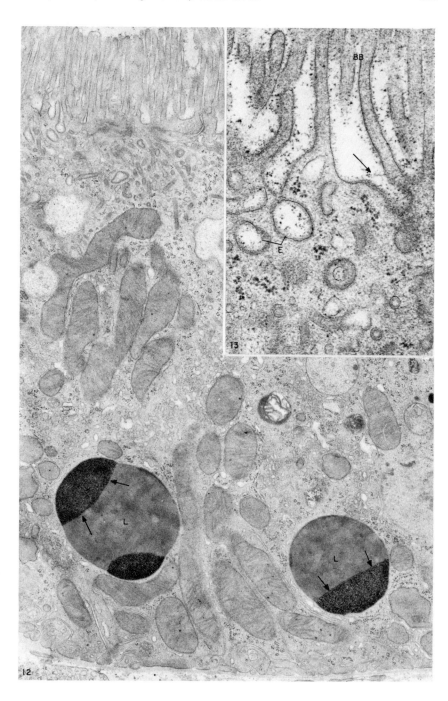

which under comparable experimental conditions was about 40 per cent of the injected amount and more than 99 per cent of the filtered load.

The pronounced ultrastructural changes of the lysosomes observed after dextran administration were not associated with alterations in the lysosomal digestion of protein in renal cortical slices following intravenous injection of labelled lysozyme (Fig. 14). The dextran precipitate was more dense in the lysosomes than in endocytic vacuoles, indicating an accumulation of dextran within the lysosomes. Such a concentration requires that the membrane

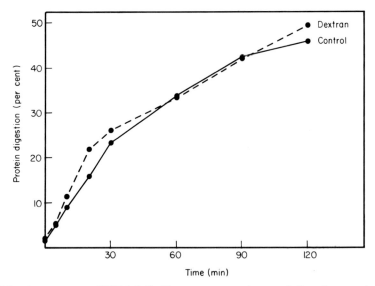

FIG. 14. *Digestion of* [125]*I-labelled lysozyme in renal cortical slices from rat infused with dextran and injected with labelled protein 1 h before preparation of slices. Protein digestion is not influenced by dextran infusion.*

material of the endocytic vacuoles is not incorporated in lysosomal membrane, and is consistent with the possibility that endocytic membrane material is recycled to the plasma membrane either before or after the fusion between the endocytic vacuoles and lysosomes.

Conclusions

(1) Isolated lysosomal enzymes from rat kidney cortex digest different iodinated proteins, in part to the amino acid level.

(2) Renal cortical slices from rats previously injected with labelled low

molecular proteins can be used to demonstrate the digestion of proteins in proximal tubule cells.

(3) Protein digestion in renal cortical slices occurs predominantly in proximal tubule lysosomes, which contain almost all absorbed tracer protein.

(4) The intralysosomal digestion in proximal tubule cells proceeds in part to the amino acid level and is retarded by previous injection of unlabelled protein.

(5) Sodium maleate induces a pronounced proteinuria and a decreased protein catabolism in proximal tubular lysosomes due to decreased endocytosis and impaired fusion of endocytic vacuoles and lysosomes.

(6) Intravenously administered dextran causes pronounced ultrastructural alteration of the lysosomal system, but the ability of the altered lysosomes to digest absorbed protein is unchanged.

References

Angielski, S. and Rogulski, J. (1975). Metabolic studies in experimental renal dysfunction resulting in experimental renal dysfunction resulting from maleate administration. In *Current Problems in Clinical Biochemistry*, Vol. 4, *Biochemical Aspects of Renal Function* (S. Angielski and U. C. Dubach, eds), Hans Huber Publisher, Bern, pp. 86–100.

Barka, T. and Anderson, J. (1962). Histochemical methods for acid phosphatase using hexazonium pararosanilin as coupler. *J. Histochem. Cytochem.* **10**, 741–753.

Booth, A. G. and Kenny, A. J. (1976). Identification of protein subunits in the kidney microvillus membrane. *Biochem. Soc. Trans.* **4**, 348–350.

Carone, F. A., Pullman, T. N., Oparil, S. and Nakamura, S. (1976). Micropuncture evidence of rapid hydrolysis of bradykinin by rat proximal tubule. *Am. J. Physiol.* **230**, 1420–1424.

Caulfield, J. P. and Farquhar, M. G. (1974). The permeability of glomerular capillaries to graded dextrans. Identification of the basement membrane as the primary filtration barrier. *J. Cell Biol.* **63**, 883–903.

Christensen, E. I. (1976). Rapid protein uptake and digestion in proximal tubule lysosomes. *Kidney Int.* **10**, 301–310.

Christensen, E. I. and Maunsbach, A. B. (1974). Intralysosomal digestion of lysozyme in renal proximal tubule cells. *Kidney Int.* **6**, 396–407.

Christensen, E. I. and Maunsbach, A. B. (1979). Effects of dextran on lysosomal ultrastructure and protein digestion in renal proximal tubule. *Kidney Int.* **16**, 301–311.

Coffey, J. W. and de Duve, C. (1968). Digestive activity of lysosomes. I. The digestion of proteins by extracts of rat liver lysosomes. *J. Biol. Chem.* **243**, 3255–3263.

Diomi, P., Ericsson, J. L. E., Matheson, N. A. and Shearer, J. R. (1970). Studies on renal tubular morphology and toxicity after large doses of dextran-40 in the rabbit. *Lab. Invest.* **22**, 355–360.

Engberg, A. and Ericsson, J. L. E. (1969). Effects of dextran 40 on proximal renal tubule. *Acta chir. scand.* **135**, 263–274.

Ericsson, J. L. E. (1964). Absorption and decomposition of homologous hemoglobin in renal proximal tubular cells. An experimental light and electron microscopic study. *Acta path. microbiol. scand.* Suppl. 168, 1–121.

Frederiksson, Å. and Peterson, P. A. (1975), Effects of renal dysfunction on β_2-microglobulin metabolism. *Scand. J. Urol. Nephrol.* Suppl. 26, 61–76.

Harris, J. M. and West, G. B. (1963). Rats resistant to the dextran anaphylactoid reaction. *Br. J. Pharmac.* **20**, 550–562.

Izzo, J. L., Bale, W. F., Izzo, M. J. and Roncone, A. (1964). High specific activity labeling of insulin with [131]I. *J. biol. Chem.* **239**, 3742–3748.

Jamieson, J. D. and Palade, G. E. (1968). Intracellular transport of secretory proteins in the pancreatic exocrine cell. IV. Metabolic requirements. *J. Cell Biol.* **39**, 589–603.

Kramer, H. J. and Gonick, H. C. (1970). Experimental Fanconi syndrome. I. Effect of maleic acid on renal cortical Na, K-ATPase activity and ATP levels. *J. Lab. clin. Med.* **76**, 799–808.

McFarlane, A. S. (1958). Efficient trace labeling of proteins with iodine. *Nature, Lond.* **182**, 53.

Maude, D. L. (1968). Stop-flow microperfusion of proximal tubules in rat kidney cortex slices. *Am. J. Physiol.* **214**, 1315–1321.

Martell-Pelletier, J., Guérette, D. and Bergeron, M. (1977) Morphologic changes during incubation of renal slices. *Lab. Invest.* **36**, 509–518.

Maunsbach, A. B. (1966*a*). Absorption of ^{125}I-labeled homologeous albumin by rat kidney proximal tubule cells. A study of microperfused single proximal tubules by electron microscopic autoradiography and histochemistry. *J. Ultrastruct. Res.* **15**, 197–241.

Maunsbach, A. B. (1966*b*). Isolation and purification of acid phosphatase containing autofluorescent granules from homogenates of rat kidney cortex. *J. Ultrastruct. Res.* **16**, 13–24.

Maunsbach, A. B. (1968). Role of lysosomes during protein absorption by proximal tubule cells. *Annls Acad. Sci. Fenn. A IV* **128**, 23–28.

Maunsbach, A. B. (1970). Ultrastructure and digestive activity of lysosomes from proximal tubule cells. In *Proceedings of the IVth International Congress of Nephrologists, Stockholm 1969*, Vol. I (N. Alwall, F. Berglund and B. Josephson, eds), Karger, Basel, pp. 102–115.

Maunsbach, A. B. (1973). Ultrastructure of the proximal tubule. In *Handbook of Physiology*, Sect. 8, *Renal Physiology* (J. Orloff and R. W. Berliner, eds), American Physiological Society, Washington, DC, pp. 31–79.

Maunsbach, A. B. (1974). Isolation of kidney lysosomes, 32. *Methods Enzymol.* **31**, 330–339.

Maunsbach, A. B. (1976). Cellular mechanisms of tubular protein transport. In *Kidney and Urinary Physiology II* (K. Thurau, ed.), International Review of Science, Physiology, Series 2, Vol. 11, University Park Press, Baltimore, pp. 145–167.

Maunsbach, A. B. and Christensen, E. I. (1976). Uptake and digestion of low molecular weight protein in rat kidney tubules. In *Proceedings of the VIth International Congress of Nephrologists, Florence 1975* (S. Giovannetti, V. Bonimini and G. D'Amico, eds), Karger, Basel, pp. 387–391.

Maunsbach, A. B., Madden, S. C. and Latta, H. (1962). Light and electron microscopic changes in proximal tubules of rats after administration of glucose, mannitol, sucrose, or dextran. *Lab. Invest.* **11**, 421–432.

Miller, F. and Palade, G. E. (1964). Lytic activities in renal protein absorption droplets. An electron microscopical cytochemical study. *J. Cell Biol.* **23**, 519–552.

Reimer, K. A., Ganote, C. E. and Jennings, R. B. (1972). Alterations in renal cortex following ischemic injury. III. Ultrastructure of proximal tubules after ischemia or autolysis. *Lab. Invest.* **26**, 347–363.

Rosen, V. J., Kramer, H. J. and Gonick, H. C. (1973). Experimental Fanconi syndrome. II. Effect of maleic acid on renal tubular ultrastructure. *Lab. Invest.* **28**, 446–455.

Simionescu, N., Simionescu, M. and Palade, G. E. (1972). Permeability of interstitial capillaries. Pathway followed by dextrans and glycogens. *J. Cell Biol.* **53**, 365–392.

Stanbury, J. B. (1957). The requirement of monoiodotyrosine deiodinase for triphosphopyridine nucleotide. *J. biol. Chem.* **228**, 801–811.

Straus, W. (1954). Isolation and biochemical properties of droplets from the cells of rat kidney. *J. biol. Chem.* **207**, 745–755.

Straus, W. (1962). Colorimetric investigations of the uptake of an intravenously injected protein (horseradish peroxidase) by rat kidney and effects of competition by egg white. *J. Cell Biol.* **12**, 231–246.

Worthen, H. G. (1963). Renal toxicity of maleic acid in the rat. Enzymatic and morphologic observations. *Lab. Invest.* **12**, 791–801.

25
Lysosomal Degradation of Human Choriogonadotropin in the Proximal Tubule Cells of Rat Kidney

Seppo O. Markkanen and Hannu J. Rajaniemi

Introduction

The serum level of proteins and polypeptides is a function not only of the synthesis and secretion of these substances but also of their removal from the circulation. Hormonal proteins and polypeptides constitute one of the most important groups of the circulating proteins. In spite of great advances in our knowledge in chemistry and mechanism of action of these hormones, there is little information regarding their metabolic fate after their removal from the circulation by the target and non-target tissues. It has been reported that the kidneys and liver have an important role in the removal of insulin (Mirsky *et al.*, 1949; Mirsky, 1957; Weisenfeld *et al.*, 1957), gonadotropins (Rajaniemi and Vanha-Perttula, 1972; Ascoli *et al.*, 1975; Vaitukaitis *et al.*, 1971), prolactin (Rajaniemi *et al.*, 1974), parathyroid hormone (Fang and Tashian, 1972; Neuman *et al.*, 1975) and somatotropin (Mizejewski, 1973) from the circulation in the rat and mouse. Morphological studies employing light microscopic autoradiography have disclosed that the proximal tubule cells in the kidney concentrate, for example, radiolabelled insulin (Beck and Fedenskyj, 1967), parathyroid hormone (De Kretser *et al.*, 1970) and pituitary gonadotropins (De Kretser *et al.*, 1969; Rajaniemi and Vanha-Perttula, 1972), and are responsible for their degradation following the uptake. The observations obtained by electron microscopic autoradiography have suggested further that the uptake of the hormones such as insulin (Bourdeau *et al.*, 1973), corticotropin (Baker *et al.*, 1976, 1977), lutropin (Robinson *et al.*, 1977) and somatotropin (Stacy *et al.*, 1976) takes place by endocytosis and leads

subsequently to lysosomal degradation of the hormones. The general significance of the lysosomal system in degradation of proteins in renal cells has
been extensively reviewed by Maunsbach (1969).

In the present paper we report an attempt to elucidate the role of the renal
proximal tubule cells in the removal and catabolism of ^{125}I-labelled human
choriogonadotropin (^{125}I-hCG) utilizing biochemical and autoradiographic
techniques.

Materials and Methods

Materials
Highly purified hCG (11 550 IU/mg) for radioiodination and specific anti-
serum for hCG was donated by Dr A. R. Midgley, Jr, University of Michigan.
Crude hCG (Pregnyl, 2000 IU/mg) was obtained from Organon, Oss,
Holland. Highly purified α- and β-subunits of hCG, and specific antiserum
for α-subunit, were obtained from the National Institute of Arthritis,
Metabolic and Digestive Deseases, NIH, Bethesda, USA.

Adult female and male Wistar rats were used in the experiments. The
animals were housed in a room with controlled temperature, humidity and
illumination (14 h light, 10 h dark) and were fed with a standard pellet diet
with water *ad libitum*. For the experiments the rats were anaesthetized with
an intraperitoneal injection of Nembutal (sodium pentobarbital, 60 mg/kg).

Radioiodination of hCG and hCG subunits
The intact hormone and subunits (10–20 μg) were labelled carefully with
0·5–1·5 mCi carrier-free Na ^{125}I (Radiochemical Centre, Amersham,
England) for 20 s, at a low temperature (4 °C), and using minimal chlora-
mine-T concentration (10 μg) (Leidenberger and Reichert, 1972). The specific
activity averaged 30–50 μCi/μg. The fraction of labelled hCG that was capable
of binding to LH (hCG) receptor was tested by performing the receptor assay
in the absence or presence of a 1000-fold excess of unlabelled hCG and
using an excess of LH (hCG) receptor-rich particles (20 000g pellet) from
pseudopregnant rat ovarian homogenate (Rajaniemi *et al.*, 1974). The specific
binding averaged 54 per cent when the assays were conducted at 37 °C for
30 min. The labelled hormone was found to disappear from the circulation
in parallel with the unlabelled hormone, suggesting that it can be used as a
tracer for metabolic studies of hCG.

*Assessment of the disappearance of labelled hCG from the circulation and the
uptake by the kidneys*
Female rats were injected intravenously with 10^6 c.p.m. of ^{125}I-hCG (32 ng).

The animals were killed at 5 or 30 min, 1, 2, 4 or 8 h after the injection by opening the abdominal and thoracic cavities and perfusing the left heart ventricle with 150 ml of 0·9 per cent NaCl. Specimens were taken from the kidney cortex and medulla, weighed, and counted for radioactivity. A blood sample of 1 ml was drawn from each animal before perfusion. Urine was also aspirated from the bladder of each animal for determination of the excreted radioactivity.

Light and electron microscopic autoradiography
Male rats were injected with a single femoral vein injection of 10^8 c.p.m. of ^{125}I-hCG (1·9 μg). The animals were killed at 30 min, 2 or 4 h by perfusing the left heart ventricle with 15 ml of modified Tyrode's solution (Maunsbach, 1966). One kidney was removed rapidly for gel filtration analysis of the degradation products of the hormone. The perfusion was continued thereafter with an additional 200 ml of 1 per cent glutaraldehyde in modified Tyrode's solution at a constant rate of 12–15 ml/min, and specimens from the remaining kidney cortex were taken for postfixation in ice-cold 1 per cent glutaraldehyde for 2 h, followed by an additional 2 h in 1 per cent OsO_4 buffered with *s*-collidine to pH 7·3. Following postfixation, the specimens were rinsed in Tyrode's solution, stained in uranyl acetate for 15 min, dehydrated in alcohol and embedded in Spurr Epon. All blocks were trimmed and 1 μm sections were routinely taken for light microscopic autoradiography to screen the sections and test the right exposure time for electron microscopic autoradiography.

Some animals were killed by decapitation 60 min after the injection of ^{125}I-hCG, and the kidneys were fixed in Bouin's fixative, dehydrated in alcohol, embedded in paraffin and sectioned at 7 μm. Light microscopic sections were coated with Kodak NTB-3 emulsion and exposed for 2–3 weeks at −12 °C as described by Rajaniemi and Midgley (1975).

For electron microscopic autoradiography, 100 nm sections were collected on grids and stained with uranyl acetate and lead citrate, covered with a layer of carbon, and then coated with Ilford L4 emulsion by the loop method of Caro and Van Tubergen (1962). After exposure for 2 months at −18 °C the emulsion was developed in Kodak Microdol X (5 min) and fixed in Hypam Rapid Fixer (5 min). The autoradiographs were examined in an EOL 100 B electron microscope.

Analysis of the degradation products of hCG
The kidney specimens were homogenized in 5 ml of 0·5 per cent Triton X-100 in PBS using a Potter-Elvehjelm homogenizer with a Teflon pestle. To separate the solubilized radioactivity, the homogenate was centrifuged at 106 000**g** for 1 h (Sorvall OTD-2 centrifuge). An aliquot (100 000 c.p.m.) of

the supernatant was subjected to gel filtration on a Sepharose 6B column (2·6 cm × 68 cm) equilibrated and eluted with 0·5 per cent Triton X-100 in PBS at 4 °C. The elution velocity was 18 ml/h. The radioactive peaks were identified in terms of the binding capacity to LH(hCG) receptor, anti-hCG gammaglobulin Sepharose 4B and anti-α-subunit serum Sepharose 4B as described previously (Markkanen *et al.*, 1979). The partition coefficients were calculated using blue dextran, labelled hCG, α-subunit and β-subunit of hCG and radioiodine as references.

The radioactivity eluted at the total volume was further analysed by using a copper–Sephadex G-25 column standardized and eluted as described by Fazakerley and Best (1965).

Some specimens, 2 h after the hormone injection, were homogenized in 0·25 M sucrose in PBS. The organelle pellet and cytosol were separated by centrifuging at 106 000**g** for 1·5 h at 4 °C. Subsequently, the pellet was extracted with 0·5 per cent Triton X-100 as described above. The Triton extract of the organelle pellet, as well as the cytosol fraction, were further analysed for degradation products by the gel filtration on a Sepharose 6B column as described earlier.

Results

Uptake of labelled hCG by the kidney
The accumulation of radioactivity in the kidney cortex and medulla was rapid, and a maximum was observed within 0·5–2 h following the injection (Fig. 1). The total uptake in the kidney was approximately 10 per cent of the injected radioactivity at 2 h, whereas that in the liver was only 2·2 per cent and in the ovary 1·9 per cent. The other organs studied showed no concentration of radioactivity.

The increase of radioactivity in the kidney cortex and medulla within the first 2 h was accompanied by a concomitant rapid decline in blood radio-activity (Fig. 1). The urine radioactivity increased parallel to the accumu-lation of radioactivity in the kidney cortex and medulla. The total radio-activity in urine at 2 h was 1·5 per cent of the injected labelled hormone.

Cells responsible for the uptake of labelled hCG in the kidneys
Figure 2 shows an autoradiograph prepared from the kidney 1 h after the hormone injection. Most of the radioactivity was associated with tubular structures located in the kidney cortex. More detailed autoradiographs prepared from 1 μm Epon section showed that the radioactivity is located almost exclusively in the proximal tubule cells (Fig. 3).

These observations disclose that the proximal tubule cells in the kidney cortex are responsible for the uptake of radiolabelled hCG.

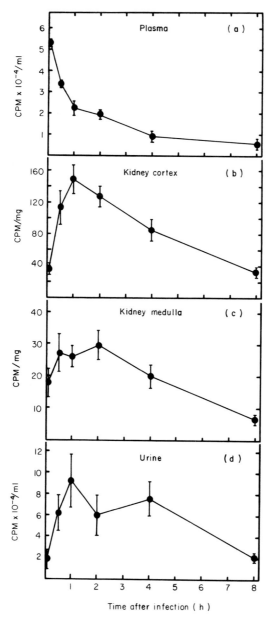

FIG. 1. *Disappearance rates of radioactivity from (a) blood of female rats and a concomitant accumulation of radioactivity in (b) the kidney cortex, (c) medulla and (d) urine, following a single intravenous injection of labelled hCG. Each point represents the mean ± S.E.M. of five animals.*

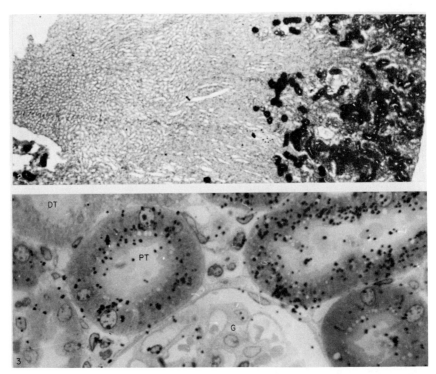

FIG. 2. *Localization of radioactivity in the kidney. Autoradiograph is prepared from 7 μm section. Note the heavy labelling over the tubular structures in the cortex region. × 460.*

FIG. 3. *Detailed localization of radioactivity in the kidney cortex. Autoradiograph is prepared from 1 μm Epon section. Note the heavy density of silver grains over the proximal tubule cells. PT, proximal tubule; DT, distal tubule; G, glomerulus. × 770.*

Degradation of labelled hCG in the proximal tubule cells

To determine whether the labelled hCG initially taken up by the proximal tubule cells undergoes some type of degradation, Triton X-100 extracts were prepared from the tissue samples and fractionated on a Sepharose 6B column. More than 85 per cent of the original radioactivity in the sample was obtained in soluble form with a single extraction. The radioactivity distributed in the gel filtration to three peaks in each experiment (Fig. 4). The first peak was chromatographically indistinguishable from the intact hCG ($K_{av} = 0.52$) and the eluted material bound specifically to anti-hCG-gammaglobulin Sepharose 4B and anti-α-subunit serum Sepharose 4B and LH(hCG) receptor. The second peak eluted coinciding with labelled α-subunit of hCG ($K_{av} = 0.71$) and also behaved identically with α-subunit in the receptor and immunolo-

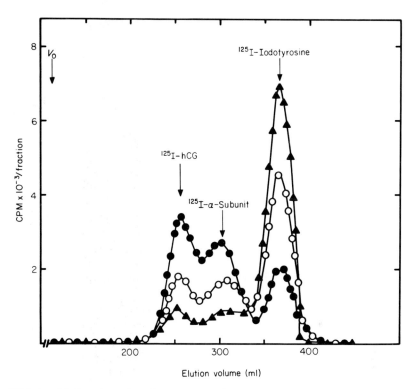

FIG. 4. *Gel filtration of renal extracts on the Sepharose 6B column. Extracts were prepared 30 min (●——●), 2 h (○——○) and 4 h (▲——▲) after the intravenous injection of* ^{125}*I-hCG.*

gical binding tests. The radioactive compound eluted in the total volume of the column was retained by the copper–Sephadex G-25 column and was eluted identically with ^{125}I-labelled iodotyrosine (Fig. 5). These analyses suggest that the first peak represents apparently intact labelled hCG, the second one labelled hCG-α-subunit and the third one free ^{125}I-labelled tyrosine. The percentage radioactivity in the first peak diminished markedly with time in association with a marked increase of the low molecular weight peak.

The division of the renal homogenate to the organelle and cytosol fractions revealed that at 2 h 78 per cent of the radioactivity was associated with the organelle fraction. The radioactivity extracted from the organelle pellet represented almost solely α-subunit of hCG (Fig. 6), while in the cytosol there was, in addition to α-subunit, also free hormone and ^{125}I-labelled iodotyrosine present.

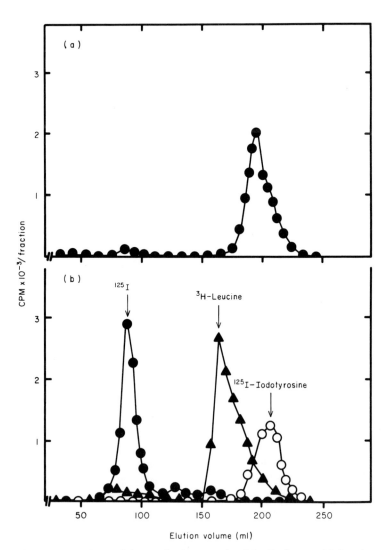

FIG. 5. (a) *Analysis of the total volume peak of the Sepharose 6B fractionation by copper–Sephadex G-25 column. The peak fractions were pooled, concentrated and applied to the column. The elution was carried out with* 0·2 N *HCl.* (b) *Radioiodine* (●──●), L-[³H]*leucine* (▲──▲) *and,* [¹²⁵I]*iodo-*L-*tyrosine* (○──○) *were used in the calibration of the column.*

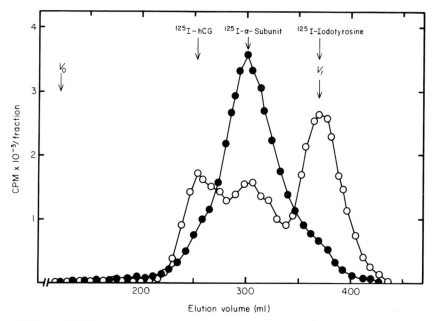

FIG. 6. *Gel filtration of the extract prepared from the 106 000g pellet of kidney homogenate (●——●) and cytosol (○——○) on the Sepharose 6B column. The kidney specimen was taken 2 h after the injection of labelled hCG.*

Subcellular site of the degradation of hCG in the proximal tubule cells
The intracellular site where the labelled hormone was degraded in the proximal tubule cells was elucidated by means of electron microscopic auto-radiography. Figure 7 shows a typical distribution of the silver grains over the kidney tubules 30 min after the injection of radiolabelled hCG. The silver grains were located almost exclusively over the luminal portion of the proximal tubule cells, while the distal tubule cells were devoid of the grains.

Detailed electron microscopic autoradiographs prepared from the proximal tubule cells showed clearly that most of the grains were associated with dense cytoplasmic bodies (lysosomes) and large apical vesicles (endocytotic vesicles) (Figs 8 and 9). The analysis of the grain distribution was carried out by the method described by Salpeter *et al.* (1978). The results of the analysis at 2 h are presented in Table I. It can be seen that the number of observed grains over the lysosomes is markedly higher than that of the expected grains ($\chi^2 = 1339{\cdot}0$). The number of observed grains also exceeds that of expected grains over the large apical vesicles ($\chi^2 = 6{\cdot}7$), while not over the mitochondria, cytoplasm and nucleus. The analysis gives a qualitative indication that the lysosomes and large apical vesicles are labelled, whereas the other organelles are not.

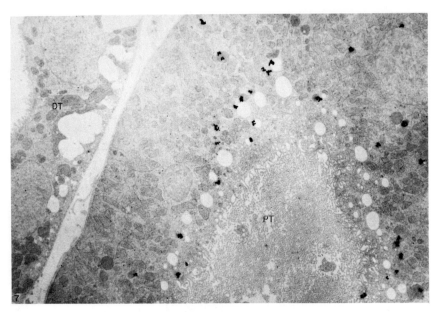

FIG. 7. *A low-power electron microscopic autoradiograph showing a cross-section from a proximal (PT) and distal tubules (DT). Note the labelling of the luminal region of the proximal tubule.* × 2700.

TABLE I

*Distribution of observed and expected grains between different cellular compartments
2 h after injection of labelled hCG*

Cellular compartment	Observed grains	Expected grains[a]	χ^2
Lysosomes	256	32	1339·0
Large apical vesicles	25	15	6·7
Small apical vesicles	11	18	2·7
Mitochondria	25	133	87·7
Nuclei	2	23	19·2
Cytoplasm	39	107	43·2
Brush border	1	27	25·0
Lumen	0	4	4·0
	359	359	$\Sigma\chi^2 = 1527·5$

[a] Statistical analysis according to Salpeter *et al.* (1978).

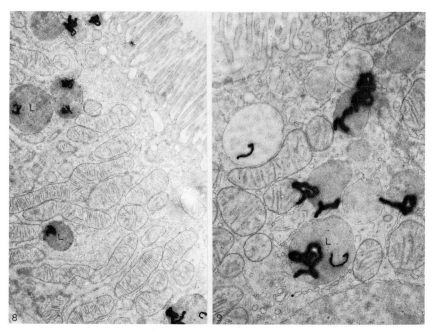

FIGS 8 and 9. *Electron microscopic autoradiograph showing a cross-section of a proximal tubule cell. The silver grains are numerous over the lysosomes (L) while the other organelles are essentially devoid of the silver grains. Fig. 8, × 8800; Fig. 9, × 15 600.*

Discussion

The biological response of the target tissue to hormonal stimulation is determined by a number of factors, including the local concentration of biologically active hormone at the site of action. This effective level of the hormone depends upon the rate of secretion as well as the removal of the hormone from the circulation. Despite accumulating evidence of the important role of the kidneys in the removal of protein and polypeptide hormones from the circulation (Rajaniemi and Vanha-Perttula, 1972; Ascoli *et al.*, 1975), there is little information available regarding the catabolic fate of the hormones in the kidneys. Our observations indicate that the kidneys are mainly responsible for the removal of labelled hCG from the circulation in the rat. The concentration of the hormone takes place in the proximal tubule cells. The gel filtration of the radioactivity extracted from the kidneys at different time intervals after the hormone injection suggested that it is rapidly split into subunits and hydrolysed to free amino acids. Similarily, ovine lutropin has been reported to undergo a degradation to oligopeptides and free amino acids in the kidney (Ascoli et al., 1976). The electron micro-scopic autoradiographs showed that the organelles significantly labelled in the proximal tubule cells following the injection of hCG were lysosomes and large apical vesicles. This suggests that the degradative processes of hCG takes place in the lysosomes and probably in the endocytotic vesicles as well.

This is also supported by the observation that the radioactivity in the organelle fraction represented almost exclusively α-subunit of the hormone. In turn, the presence of [^{125}I]iodotyrosine only in the cytosol fraction is probably due to the fact that it is rapidly transported from the lysosomes to cytoplasm (LaBadie et al., 1975). We have also found that the kidneys excrete, in addition to labelled hCG, considerable amounts of hCG subunits (Markkanen et al., 1979). This may indicate that the plasma membrane of the proximal tubule cells possess enzyme(s) capable of catabolizing of hCG.

Conclusions

The present observations indicate that the kidneys are mainly responsible for the removal of labelled hCG in the rat. The hormone appears to be concentrated by the proximal tubule cells, where it subsequently undergoes catabolic modifications leading to the cleavage of the subunits and hydrolysis to free amino acids. The degradative processes take place in the lysosomes and probably in the endocytotic vesicles.

Acknowledgements

The authors wish to thank Dr A. Rees Midgley, Jr, University of Michigan, for the gift of highly purified hCG and specific antiserum for hCG, and NIAMDD for specific antiserum for α-subunit of hCG. The authors are grateful to Miss Tuula Räisänen, Miss Arja Venäläinen and Mrs Eija Voutilainen for their skilful technical assistance and to Mrs Maija Pellikka for her expert secretarial assistance. This study was supported by grants from the National Research Council for Medical Sciences, Finland, and The Cultural Foundation of Finland.

References

Ascoli, M., Liddle, R. A. and Puett, D. (1975). The metabolism of luteinizing hormone. Plasma clearance, urinary excretion, and tissue uptake. *Molec. cellul. Endocr.* **3**, 21–36.

Ascoli, M., Liddle, R. A. and Puett, D. (1976). Renal and hepatic lysosomal catabolism of luteinizing hormone. *Molec. cellul. Endocr.* **4**, 297–310.

Baker, J. R. J., Bennett, H. P. J., Christian, R. A. and McMartin, C. (1977). Renal uptake and metabolism of adrenocorticotropin analogues in the rat; an autoradiographic study. *J. Endocr.* **74**, 23–35.

Baker, J. R. J., Bennett, H. P. J., Hudson, A. M., McMartin, C. and Purdon, G. E. (1976). On the metabolism of two adrenocorticotropin analogues. *Clin. Endocr.* **5**, Suppl., 61s–72s.

Beck, L. V. and Fedenskyj, N. (1967). Evidence from combined immunoassay and radioautography that intact insulin-^{125}I molecules are concentrated by mouse kidney proximal tubule cells. *Endocrinology* **81**, 475–485.

Bourdeau, J. E., Chen, E. R. Y. and Carone, F. A. (1973). Insulin uptake in the renal proximal tubule. *Am. J. Physiol.* **225**, 1399–1404.

Caro, L. G. and Van Tubergen, R. P. (1962). High resolution autoradiography. I. Methods. *J. Cell Biol.* **15**, 173–178.

De Kretser, D. M., Martin, T. J. and Melick, R. A. (1970). The radioautographic localization of ^{125}I-labelled bovine parathyroid hormone, *J. Endocr.* **46**, 507–510.

De Kretser, D. M., Catt, K. J., Burger, H. G. and Smith, G. C. (1969). Radioautographic studies on the localization of ^{125}I-labelled human luteinizing and growth hormone in immature male rats. *J. Endocr.* **43**, 105–111.

Fang, V. S. and Tashian, A. H., Jr (1972). Studies on the role of the liver in the metabolism of parathyroid hormone. I. Effects of partial hepatectomy and incubation of the hormone with tissue homogenates. *Endocrinology* **90**, 1177–1184.

Fazakerley, S. and Best, D. R. (1965). Separation of amino acids, as copper chelates from amino acid, protein, and peptide mixtures. *Analyt. Biochem.* **12**, 290–295.

LaBadie, J. H., Chapman, K. P. and Aronson, N. N., Jr (1975). Glycoprotein catabolism in rat liver. Lysosomal digestion of iodinated asialo-fetuin. *Biochem. J.* **152**, 271–279.

Leidenberger, F. L. and Reichert, L. E., Jr (1972). Studies on the uptake of human chorionic gonadotropin and its subunits by rat testicular homogenates and interstitial tissue. *Endocrinology* **91**, 135–143.

Markkanen, S., Töllikkö, K., Vanha-Perttula, T. and Rajaniemi, H. (1979). Disappearance of human ^{124}I-iodo chorionic gonadotropin from the circulation in the rat, tissue uptake and degradation. *Endocrinology* **104**, 1540–1547.

Maunsbach, A. B. (1966). Influence of different fixatives and fixation methods on the ultrastructure of rat kidney proximal tubule cells. I. Comparison of different perfusion methods and of glutaraldehyde and osmium tetroxide fixatives. *J. Ultrastruct. Res.* **15**, 242–282.

Maunsbach, A. B. (1969). Functions of lysosomes in kidney cells. In *Lysosomes in Biology and Pathology*, Vol. I (J. T. Dingle and H. B. Fell, eds), North Holland, Amsterdam, pp. 115–154.

Mirsky, I. A. (1957). Insulinase, insulinase-inhibitors, and diabetes mellitus. *Recent Progr. Hormone Res.* **13**, 429–465.

Mirsky, I. A., Broh-Kahn, R. H., Perisutti, G. and Brand, J. (1949). The inactivation of insulin by tissue extracts. I. The distribution and properties of insulin inactivating extracts (insulinase). *Archs Biochem.* **20**, 1–9.

Mizejewski, G. J. (1973). Tissue distribution of radioiodinated human growth hormone in the mouse. *Proc. Soc. exp. Biol. Med.* **142**, 589–594.

Neuman, W. F., Neuman, M. W., Lane, K., Miller, L. and P. J. Sammon (1975).

The metabolism of labeled parathyroid hormone. V. Collected biological studies. *Calcif. Tissue Res.* **18**, 271–287.

Rajaniemi, H. J. and Midgley, A. R., Jr (1975). Autoradiographic techniques for localizing protein hormones in target tissue. *Methods Enzymol.* **37**, 145–167.

Rajaniemi, H. and Vanha-Perttula, T. (1972). Specific receptor for LH in the ovary: evidence by autoradiography and tissue fractionation. *Endocrinology* **90**, 1–9.

Rajaniemi, H. J., Hirshfield, A. N. and Midgley, A. R., Jr (1974). Gonadotropin receptors in the rat ovarian tissue. I. Localization of LH binding sites by fractionation of subcellular organelles. *Endocrinology* **95**, 579–588.

Rajaniemi, H., Oksanen, A. and Vanha-Perttula, T. (1974). Distribution of ^{125}I-prolactin in mice and rats. Studies with whole-body and microautoradiography. *Hormone Res.* **5**, 6–20.

Robinson, J. P., Derreberry, S., Liddle, R. A., Ascoli, M. and Puett, D. (1977). Renal uptake of lutropin. Studies based on electron microscopic autoradiography and nephrectomy. *Molec. cellul. Biochem.* **15**, 63–66.

Salpeter, M. M., McHenry, F. A. and Salpeter, E. E. (1978). Resolution in electron microscope autoradiography. IV. Application to analysis of autoradiographs. *J. Cell Biol.* **76**, 127–145.

Stacy, B. D., Wallace, A. L. C., Gemmel, R. T. and Wilson, B. W. (1976). Absorption of ^{125}I-labelled sheep growth hormone in single proximal tubules of the rat kidney. *J. Endocr.* **68**, 21–30.

Vaitukaitus, J. L., Sherins, R., Ross, G. T., Hickman, J. and Ashwell, G. (1971). A method for the preparation of radioactive FSH with preservation of biologic activity. *Endocrinology* **89**, 1356–1360.

Weisenfeld, S., Jauregui, R. H. and Goldner, M. G. (1957). Inactivation of insulin by the isolated liver of the bullfrog. *Am. J. Physiol.* **188**, 45–48.

26
Kallikrein in Lysosomes and Plasma Membranes Isolated from Rabbit Kidney Cortex using Free-flow Electrophoresis

Hans-G. Heidrich, Klaus Mann and Reinhard Geiger

Introduction

In 1960 Werle and Vogel found kallikrein activity (EC 3.4.21.8) in rat kidney homogenates (Werle and Vogel, 1961) and since then several attempts have been made to locate this enzyme in the kidney. It has been found mainly in the cortical part of the kidney, either in glomeruli (Mann et al., 1976; Scicli et al., 1976a; Tyler, 1978) or in the more distal part of the nephron (Ørstavik et al., 1976; Carretero and Scicli, 1976). The precise subcellular location has not yet been unequivocally identified. Kallikrein activity has been reported to be present in the microsomal fraction (Nustad and Rubin, 1970; Ward et al. 1976), in the plasma membrane (Ward et al., 1976) and in the lysosomes (Carvalho and Dinitz, 1966; Baggio et al., 1975).

In this work several techniques of cell fractionation, such as differential pelleting, density gradient centrifugation and free-flow electrophoresis (Hannig and Heidrich, 1974), were used to separate unequivocally subcellular components from rabbit kidney cortex homogenates. We characterized the organelle fractions enzymically and morphologically and found very high kallikrein activities in lysosomes and lysosome-like organelles and a somewhat lower activity in plasma membranes containing Na^+-K^+-ATPase (non-microvillous plasma membrane).

Methods

Isolation of subcellular components

Kidneys from brown rabbits were each perfused with 70 ml of isolation (= electrophoresis) medium which was made of triethanolamine 10 mM, acetic acid 10 mM, ethylenediamine tetraacetate (EDTA) 0·25 mM, sucrose 355 mM (pH 7·4 with 2 N NaOH; osmolality 415 mosmol/kg H_2O; electric conductivity $5·2 \times 10^2$ μmho). The cortices (15 g) were removed, pressed through a tissue press and, after dilution 1:1 with medium, homogenized in a Dounce L homogenizer. The homogenate was centrifuged three times at 650g and the resulting supernatant for 5 min at 6800g. The pellet from the latter centrifugation was resuspended in 40 ml medium and then spun for 2 min at 2000g. The speed was then increased to 6800g for 5 min. Two layers were visible in the pellet: a dark layer at the bottom (lysosomal/mitochondrial layer) and a brownish/white layer at the top (mitochondrial/plasma membrane layer). The layers were separated by gentle shaking with buffer, whereby the upper fluffy layer comes away from the dark pellet.

For preparing lysosomes the dark bottom layer (16 mg total protein) was resuspended in 6 ml of medium and injected into an FF5-Apparatus (Bender and Hobein, D-8000 München) at 150 mA, $140 \pm V/cm$, buffer flow 2·0 ml per fraction per hour, 5 °C. Total protein and enzyme activities were determined in the fractions at the end of the run. 16 mg total protein injected into the apparatus resulted in 1·9 mg of lysosomal protein. For isolating lysosomes on the basis of their density a linear sucrose gradient similar to that described by Maunsbach (1974) was used (57–30 per cent w/w) for 90 min at 63 500g in an SW-rotor.

Plasma membranes were prepared from the upper layer of the differential pellet. The suspension in isolation medium (6 ml) was layered on top of three gradients and spun as described above. The white layer at the entrance of the gradient (34·1–37·9 per cent sucrose, density 1·145–1·165 g/ml) was removed (5 mg total protein), washed twice with isolation medium and run in the FF5-Apparatus. Two distinct bands were observed and the fractions were assayed for total protein and enzyme activities. Plasma membrane protein (2·2 mg) and microvilli protein (1·9 mg) were obtained from 5 mg protein injected.

Analytical procedures

Total protein was determined in a Technicon AutoAnalyzer (Heidrich, 1969). Enzyme activities were determined as described previously (Heidrich *et al.*, 1972). Kallikrein was assayed after liberation of kinins from purified HMW-kininogen using the rat uterus test (Mann *et al.*, 1976). The specifity of kallikrein was tested by inhibition of the enzyme with Trasylol and with the blood pressure test.

Results and Discussion

The results discussed in the following clearly show that lysosomes and lysosome-like particles were unequivocally separated from plasma membranes and that kallikrein activity could be assayed in both subcellular components.

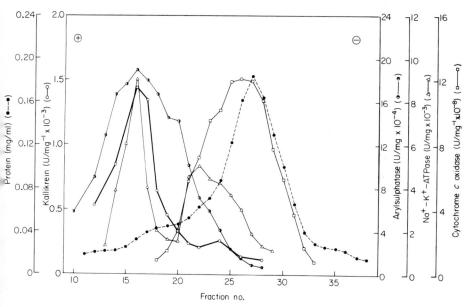

FIG. 1.   *Free-flow electrophoresis for the isolation of lysosomal particles. The sample injection was above fraction 65, i.e. all the material was deflected towards the anode.*

The electrophoretic separation of lysosomes and lysosome-like particles from rabbit kidney cortex (Fig. 1) resulted in a very heterogeneous population of organelles (Fig. 2) whose morphology, however, differed from that of the very homogenous organelles isolated by Maunsbach (1974) from rat kidney homogenates using density gradient centrifugation. That the fraction obtained using electrophoresis was highly enriched in lysosomes was proven by the very high lysosomal marker activities (see, for example, arylsulphatase in Fig. 1). Mitochondrial enzymes and enzymes from the endoplasmic reticulum (not shown) were not found in the lysosomal fractions. However,

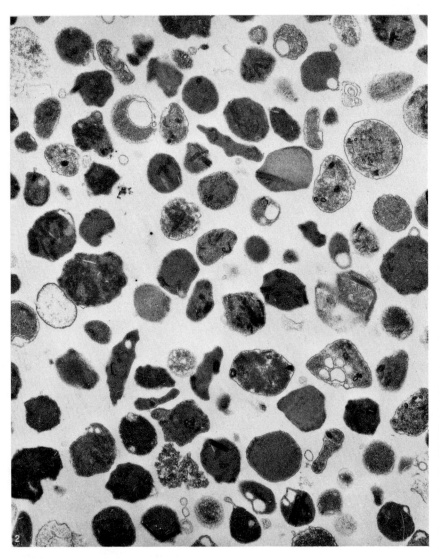

FIG. 2. *Electron micrograph of the lysosomal fraction from the electrophoresis run shown in Fig. 1 (fractions 12–22). × 21000.*

a clear but low Na^+–K^+-ATPase activity was assayed in fractions 13–18. This activity is in theory unlikely to arise from plasma membrane contamination since plasma membranes have an electrophoretic mobility different from that of lysosomes and cannot be deflected into the lysosomal region. As expected from this, plasma membranes could not be morphologically identified in these fractions. They are present in fractions 21–25 of the electrophoresis run. In order to prove that Na^+–K^+-ATPase activity did not result from plasma membrane contamination in the the lysosomal fractions, lysosomes were also prepared using sucrose density centrifugation as already reported for rat kidney, and described in detail by Maunsbach (1966, 1974).

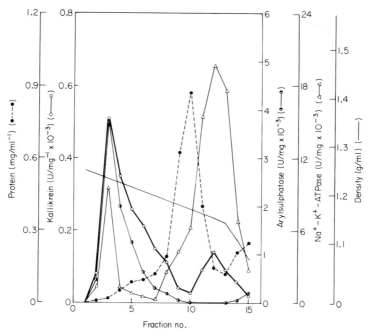

FIG. 3. *Sucrose gradient centrifugation for the isolation of lysosomal particles. The mitochondrial marker cytochrome c oxidase is not shown in the graph but is present in fractions 8–11.*

The resulting lysosomal fraction again contained almost the same specific activity of Na^+–K^+-ATPase (Fig. 3) as was found in the lysosomes isolated by electrophoresis. The plasma membrane was found in another part of the gradient (fractions 10–14 in Fig. 3).

From both experiments it must be concluded that either secondary lysosomes, or lysosome-like particles, isolated here contain membrane domains with Na^+–K^+-ATPase activity, or that subcellular particles have been isolated which possess the same physical properties as lysosomes and which are mainly derived from the plasma membrane, as suggested recently by Nustad *et al.* (1978). Since the population of the lysosomes is so heterogeneous (Fig. 2), the latter might be true. The isolated fraction of lysosomes or lysosome-like particles contains a high activity of kallikrein (Figs 1 and 3), and this activity is membrane-bound, since it could not be released from the particles after osmotic shock with distilled water. Studies are under way now to separate this lysosomal organelle fraction into sub-populations using Percoll gradients, as has been successfully carried out by Pertoft *et al.* (1978) with rat liver lysosomes. It should thus be possible to obtain the fraction containing kallikrein activity in a homogeneous form which can then be characterized.

Na^+–K^+-ATPase-containing plasma membranes from kidney cortex have a different electrophoretic mobility to that of the lysosomal organelles. The membranes from the top part of the gradient (Fig. 3; density 1·145–1·164 g/ml) show two very distinctly separated bands in the electrophoresis run,

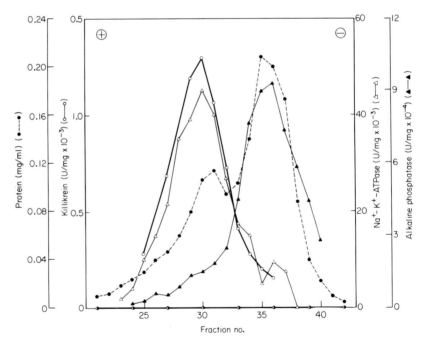

FIG. 4. *Free-flow electrophoresis for the isolation of* Na^+–K^+-*ATPase-containing plasma membrane and for microvilli membrane (alkaline phosphatase-containing). Injection was above fraction 65.*

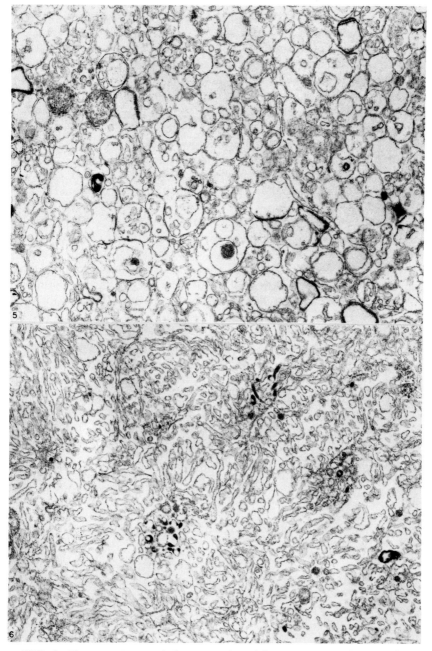

FIG. 5. *Electron micrograph from particles of fractions 27–32 of Fig. 4 showing plasma membranes containing Na^+-K^+-ATPase.* × 13 500.

FIG. 6. *Electron micrograph from particles of fractions 34–38 of Fig. 4 showing microvilli membranes containing alkaline phosphatase.* × 13 500.

and this is also expressed in the enzyme pattern of the run (Fig. 4): plasma membranes containing $Na^+–K^+$-ATPase are clearly separated from alkaline phosphatase-active microvilli membranes. The mitochondrial contamination (not shown in the graph) does not interfere with the plasma membranes, and an activity from the endoplasmic reticulum could not be found. Basically, the separation resembles the results obtained earlier from rat kidney cortex (Heidrich *et al.*, 1972). However, the morphology of the membrane fractions obtained from rabbit is different from that of rat: while long microvilli and large sheets of basolateral plasma membrane are obtained from rat, microvilli vesicles and plasma membrane vesicles are found in rabbit experiments (Figs 5 and 6).

Kallikrein activity is present in the $Na^+–K^+$-ATPase-containing plasma membranes, as has also been shown by Ward *et al.* (1976). The activity is high (Fig. 4), but somewhat lower than in the lysosomal fraction described above. No kallikrein activity was found in the microvilli. No attempts have been made yet to show how kallikrein is bound to the membrane or whether it becomes non-specifically attached to it. The latter possibility is excluded by the activation experiments carried out by Ward *et al.* (1975). The real reason why kallikrein is found in such high activities in lysosomal or lysosomal-like particles and in the $Na^+–K^+$-ATPase-containing plasma membrane of the kidney cortex, and the mechanisms by which it is brought into and by which it is released from these membranes, can be discussed only after the cell population of the tubule in which kallikrein is present has been isolated. Evidence exists that the cells lie in the distal part of the nephron (Ørstavik *et al.*, 1976; Scicli *et al.*, 1976*b*; R. Bahu, J. Pierce and F. A. Carone, personal communication), and attempts are being made to isolate this cell population (Heidrich and Dew, 1977).

References

Baggio, B., Favaro, S., Antonello, A., Zen, A., Zen, F. and Borsatti, A. (1975). Subcellular localization of renin and kallikrein in rat kidney. *Ital. J. Biochem.* **24**, 199–206.

Carretero, O. A. and Scicli, A. G. (1976). Renal kallikrein: its localization and possible role in renal function. *Fedn Proc. Fedn Am. Socs exp. Biol.* **35**, 194–198.

Carvalho, I. F. and Diniz, C. R. (1966). Kinin-forming enzyme (kininogenin) in homogenates of rat kidney. *Biochim. biophys. Acta* **128**, 136–148.

Hannig, K. and Heidrich, H.-G. (1974). The use of continuous preparative free-flow electrophoresis for dissociating cell fractions and isolation of membranous components. *Methods Enzymol.* **31**, 746–761.

Heidrich, H.-G. (1969). Isolation of pure inner and outer mitochondrial membranes in preparative scale using a new technique. In *Advances in Automated Chemistry. Proceedings of the Technicon International Congress 1969*, Vol. I, Mediated Incorporated, pp. 347–350.

Heidrich, H.-G. and Dew, M. E. (1977). Homogeneous cell populations from rabbit kidney cortex. *J. Cell Biol.* **74**, 780–788.

Heidrich, H.-G., Kinne, R., Kinne-Saffran, E. and Hannig, K. (1972). The polarity of the proximal tubule cell in rat kidney. Different surface charges for the brush-border microvilli and plasma membranes from the basal infoldings. *J. Cell Biol.* **54**, 232–245.

Mann, K., Geiger, R. and Werle, E. (1976). A sensitive kinin liberating assay for kininogenase in rat urine, isolated glomeruli and tubules of rat kidney. *Adv. exp. Med. Biol.* **70**, 65–73.

Maunsbach, A. B. (1966). Isolation and purification of acid phosphatase containing autofluorescent granules from homogenates of rat kidney cortex. *J. Ultractruct. Res.* **16**, 13–34.

Maunsbach, A. B. (1974). Isolation of kidney lysosomes. *Methods Enzymol.* **31**, 330–339.

Nustad, K. and Rubin, I. (1970). Subcellular localization of renin and kininogenase in rat kidney. *Br. J. Pharmac.* **40**, 325–333.

Nustad, K., Ørstavik, T. B., Gautvik, K. M. and Pierce, J. V. (1978). Glandular kallikreins. *Gen. Pharmac.* **9**, 1–9.

Pertoft, H., Wärmegard, B. and Köök, M. (1978). Heterogeneity of lysosomes orginating from rat liver parenchymal cells. *Biochem. J.* **174**, 309–317.

Scicli, A. G., Carretero, O. A., Oza, N. B. and Schork, A. M. (1976a). Distribution of kidney kininogenases. *Proc. Soc. exp. Biol. Med.* **151**, 57–60.

Scicli, A. G., Carretero, O. A., Hampton, A., Cortes, P. and Oza, N. B. (1976b). Site of kininogenase secretion in the dog nephron. *Am. J. Physiol.* **230**, 533–536.

Tyler, D. W. (1978). Localization of renal kallikrein in dog. *Experientia* **34**, 621–622.

Ward, P. E., Gedney, C. D., Dowben, R. M. and Erdös, E. G. (1975). Isolation of membrane-bound renal kallikrein and kininase. *Biochem. J.* **151**, 755–758.

Ward, P. E., Erdös, E. G., Gedney, C. D., Dowben, R. M. and Reynolds, R. C. (1976). Isolation of renal membranes that contain kallikrein. *Clin. Sci. molec. Med.* **51**, 267s–270s.

Werle, E. and Vogel, R. (1961) Über die Freisetzung einer kallikreinartigen Substanz aus Extrakten verschiedener Organe. *Archs int. Pharmacodyn. Thér.* **131**, 257–261.

Ørstavik, T. B., Nustad, K., Brandtzaeg, P. and Pierce, J. V. (1976). Cellular origine of urinary kallikreins. *J. Histochem. Cytochem.* **24**, 1037–1039.

27
Does Transtubular Transport of Intact Protein Occur in the Kidney?

Folkert Bode, Peter D. Ottosen, Kirsten M. Madsen and Arvid B. Maunsbach

Introduction

Renal handling of proteins has been studied intensively during recent years (Miller and Palade, 1964; Straus, 1964; Graham and Karnovsky, 1966; Maunsbach, 1966; Bourdeau and Carone, 1974; Strober and Waldmann, 1974; Maunsbach, 1976), and it is now evident that the kidney plays an important role in the catabolism of low molecular weight plasma proteins, including several polypeptide hormones (Chamberlain and Stimmler, 1967; Wochner et al., 1967; Bernier and Conrad, 1969). After glomerular filtration these proteins are reabsorbed by endocytosis in the proximal tubule and transferred to the lysosomes, where catabolism of the reabsorbed protein takes place (Maunsbach, 1969; Davidson, 1973; Christensen and Maunsbach, 1974).

Besides the pathway involving lysosomal catabolism of reabsorbed proteins, an additional transport of intact protein across the tubular epithelium has been postulated (Bulger and Trump, 1969; Maack and Kinter, 1969). Observations interpreted in favour of a transtubular transport of intact lysozyme have been presented in different experiments on flounder kidney (Maack and Kinter, 1969), mouse (Maack et al., 1971), and rat (Maack, 1975), where lysozyme has been used as a tracer. However, no evidence of transtubular transport was found in other investigations using different methods or other tracers including albumin (Maude et al., 1965; Maunsbach, 1966), insulin (Maack, 1975), growth hormone (Johnson and Maack, 1977), parathyroid hormone (Kau and Maack, 1977), lysozyme (Christensen and Maunsbach, 1974), and ferritin (Ottosen, 1976). Since transepithelial transport of intact protein is known to occur in other tissues, such as intestinal epithelium of newborn animals (Rodewald, 1973), the present paper is addressed to the question whether or not a transtubular transport of intact protein occurs in the proximal tubule.

The Cross-circulation Method in Studies on Renal Handling of Protein

Principle of the method
The blood concentration of low molecular weight protein such as lysozyme decreases rapidly following intravenous injection (Fig. 1). This decrease is in part due to renal uptake of circulating lysozyme, as indicated by the slower decrease in blood concentration in binephrectomized animals (Fig. 1). By determining the blood levels of tracer protein it is possible to analyse the influence of the kidney on small molecular weight proteins, and to evaluate the influence of experimental conditions which simulate either an increased or a decreased transtubular transport of protein. However, small differences

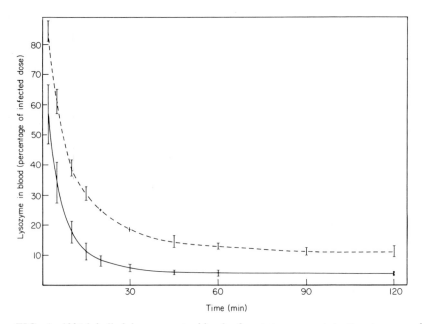

FIG. 1. ^{125}I-*labelled lysozyme in blood after intravenous injection to normal* (————) *and binephrectomized* (– – – –) *animals. The ordinate gives the total amount of* ^{125}I-*labelled lysozyme in the blood as a percentage of the injected dose. Bars give the* S.D.

in the concentration of tracer proteins in the blood are very difficult to determine, but can be studied by means of a cross-circulation method developed by Just *et al.* (1975). We have applied the cross-circulation procedure in a somewhat modified form (Ottosen *et al.*, 1979) to study the renal handling of ^{125}I-labelled lysozyme. In these experiments we injected ^{125}I-labelled lysozyme intravenously to one rat (donor) and 30 min later blood from this animal was cross-circulated to another rat (acceptor).

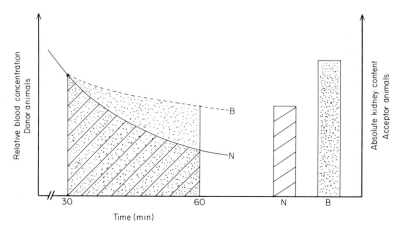

FIG. 2. *Schematic drawing showing the principle of the cross-circulation. The left part of the figure illustrates the difference in blood level of ^{125}I-labelled lysozyme between normal (N) and binephrectomized (B) donors during cross-circulation. The right part shows the corresponding difference in uptake of ^{125}I-labelled lysozyme in the kidneys of the acceptor animals. The uptake of ^{125}I-labelled lysozyme in the acceptor kidneys (stippled and hatched columns) is proportional to the area under the blood curve (stippled and hatched areas) since the acceptor kidneys will continuously accumulate a fraction of the ^{125}I-labelled lysozyme in the donors' blood.*

The amount of lysozyme taken up by the kidney of acceptor animals after 30 min of cross-circulation was then determined. This amount is proportional to the volume of blood transferred from donor to acceptor and to the concentration of lysozyme in the blood of the donor animal (Fig. 2). Since the kidneys of acceptor animals accumulate lysozyme continuously from the blood, small differences in the blood concentration of donor animals can be expected to give detectable differences in acceptor kidney content (Fig. 2).

Cross-circulation with normal donors
When a normal donor animal was cross-circulated to an acceptor animal 30 min after injection of lysozyme to the donor, the kidneys of the acceptor

animal contained $14·5 \pm 1·2$ s.e.m. $\mu g\,ml^{-1}\,min^{-1}$ ^{125}I-labelled lysozyme after 30 min of cross-circulation (Ottosen *et al.*, 1979). The blood level of lysozyme in the donor in these experiments was evidently influenced by the removal of lysozyme by glomerular filtration. In addition, it is a possibility that the blood level was influenced by transtubular transport of intact lysozyme through the wall of the proximal tubule, if such a transport exists.

Cross-circulation with binephrectomized donors
In these experiments both kidneys were removed from the donors 30 min after injection of lysozyme and immediately before start of cross-circulation. The uptake of lysozyme in the kidneys of the acceptors in five experiments was $20·9 \pm 1·1$ s.e.m. $\mu g\,ml^{-1}\,min^{-1}$ ^{125}I-labelled lysozyme, which is

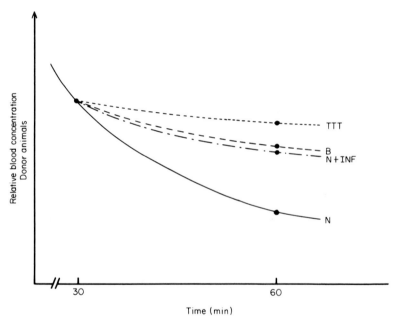

FIG. 3. *Schematic drawing illustrating the blood level of* ^{125}*I-labelled lysozyme in donors in four different conditions. N, Normal donor; B, binephrectomized donor. The blood level in the binephrectomized donor (B) decreases slower than in normal animals (N), since lysozyme is not removed from the blood by glomerular filtration. N + INF, Normal donors given a continuous infusion of* ^{125}*I-labelled lysozyme corresponding to the glomerular filtration rate for* ^{125}*I-labelled lysozyme. The blood level in this group will be equal to group B in the absence of transtubular transport of lysozyme. TTT, Normal donors given a continuous infusion of* ^{125}*I-labelled lysozyme as in N + INF, but in the presence of a hypothetical transtubular transport. Such a transport would in this condition result in a net addition of lysozyme from the kidney to the blood.*

significantly higher ($p<0.02$) than the value of 14.5 ± 1.2 s.e.m. μg ml^{-1} min^{-1} obtained with normal donor animals (Ottosen *et al.*, 1979). Thus the lysozyme concentration in the blood of binephrectomized donors is higher than in normal donors, as can be expected (Figs 2 and 3). Obviously, the blood level of lysozyme in binephrectomized animals is influenced neither by glomerular filtration nor by a hypothetical transtubular transport.

Cross-circulation with lysozyme infusion to normal donors
The removal of lysozyme by the glomerular filtration in normal donors can be compensated for by intravenous infusion of lysozyme at a rate corresponding to the glomerular filtration of lysozyme. Under these conditions a hypothetical transtubular transport of lysozyme would be detected as an increase in the blood concentration in the donor animal as compared to binephrectomized donors (Fig. 3). When an infusion was given to five normal animals at the rate corresponding to the calculated filtration of lysozyme the acceptor kidneys contained 19.5 ± 1.1 s.e.m. μg ml^{-1} min^{-1} ^{125}I-labelled lysozyme, which was not significantly different from the value obtained with binephrectomized donors (Ottosen *et al.*, 1979). These results suggest that the kidneys exclusively removed lysozyme from the blood of normal donors and do not provide any evidence for the existence of a transtubular transport of intact lysozyme. In separate experiments it was estimated that the sensitivity of the system was such that a transtubular transport of more than 9 per cent of the amount of lysozyme available for transport would have been detected.

Other Experimental Approaches to the Problem of Transtubular Transport of Protein

Autoradiography
It has repeatedly been shown by electron microscope autoradiography that labelled proteins are absorbed by the proximal tubule cells via endocytic invaginations and endocytic vacuoles and then transferred to the lysosomes (Maunsbach, 1976). However, Maack *et al.* (1971) traced intravenously injected labelled lysozyme in the kidney by light microscope autoradiography and concluded that a major part of the label was located in the cytoplasm without association to cytoplasmic bodies; they suggested that the lysozyme was transversing the cytoplasm from the tubule lumen to the peritubular space. More recent studies using electron microscope autoradiography have conclusively demonstrated that labelled lysozyme is absorbed by way of endocytic vacuoles and transferred into the lysosomes (Christensen and Maunsbach, 1974). In a quantitative analysis by means of electron micro-

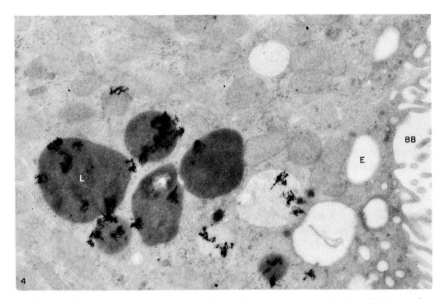

FIG. 4. *Electron microscopic autoradiograph from proximal tubule cell 30 min after intravenous injection of* [125] *I-labelled lysozyme. The grains are mainly located over the lysosomes (L). BB, brush border; E, endocytic vacuole.* × 14 000.

scope autoradiography (Fig. 4) in connection with the cross-circulation experiments, we found that the grain density over the lysosomes was almost 300 times larger than over the cytoplasm, and that in total 95 per cent of all grains were associated either with endocytic vacuoles or lysosomes 30 min after injection of the label (Table I) (Ottosen *et al.*, 1979). Furthermore, electron microscope autoradiography of single tubules microperfused with labelled lysozyme for very short periods has also demonstrated that 3 min after start of perfusion the labelled protein is located in endocytic vacuoles (Baumann *et al.*, Chapter 20 in this volume). It is therefore concluded that autoradiographic studies at the electron microscope level provide substantial evidence for protein uptake into the lysosomal system, but no evidence for transtubular transport of protein.

Tissue fractionation
Maack *et al.* (1971) used tissue fractionation to investigate the localization of lysozyme in the mouse kidney following intraperitoneal injection of the protein. The kidneys were removed 10 h after injection of the tracer and homogenized in 0·2 M KCl. After differential centrifugation, the distributions of lysozyme and lysosomal marker enzymes were determined in different subcellular fractions. Depending upon the dose, 46–63 per cent of the tracer

TABLE I

Quantitative analysis of autoradiographic grains over proximal tubule cells following intravenous injection of ^{125}I-labelled lysozyme in rats

	Number of grains	Grain density (grains/100 μm^2)[a]	Percentage of all grains[b]
Endocytic vacuoles	129	29·8	14·9
Lysosomes	686	151·3	80·1
Brush border	23	0·8	1·1
Cytoplasm	69	0·8	2·9
Cytoplasm[c]	42	0·5	0·9
Nucleus	4	0·5	0·1

[a] Not corrected for background, which was 0·4 grains/100 μm^2.
[b] After subtraction of grains originating from background.
[c] After subtraction of cytoplasmic area and grains located within 0·5 μm of endocytic vacuoles or lysosomes.

was found in the final supernatant and interpreted as originating from the "cytoplasmic sap", and representing lysozyme transversing the tubular cell cytoplasm. However, this conclusion is questionable since it is generally recognized that any tissue fractionation procedure will lead to damage and rupture of cell organelles, e.g. lysosomes, and that lysosomal contents will always be present to some extent in the final supernatant (de Duve, 1971). Furthermore, potassium chloride is not a good isolation medium when attempting the isolation of intact lysosomes. In tissue fractionation experiments carried out in parallel with the cross-circulation study of the renal handling of ^{125}I-labelled lysozyme (Ottosen *et al.*, 1979), we observed a distinct enrichment of the tracer protein in the lysosomal fraction (Table II) which was identified due to its content of the lysosomal marker acid

TABLE II

Relative specific activity of ^{125}I-labelled lysozyme in subcellular fractions from kidney cortex[a]

	Nuclear fraction	Lysosomal fraction	Mitochondrial fraction	Brush border fraction	Supernatant
In vivo[b]	1·07	4·11	1·36	1·14	0·66
In vitro[c]	1·05	0·17	0·49	1·24	1·08

[a] The subcellular fractions were isolated by differential centrifugation (Maunsbach, 1974).
[b] The subcellular fractions were isolated 30 min after intravenous injection of ^{125}I-labelled lysozyme.
[c] The subcellular fractions were isolated after addition of ^{125}I-labelled lysozyme to homogenates from non-injected animals.

phosphatase. In control experiments, when labelled lysozyme was added to renal cortical homogenates obtained from non-injected animals, we found a very low relative specific activity of the tracer in the lysosomal fraction, and the bulk of the label was recovered in the final supernatant (Table II). These experiments support the autoradiographic observations in locating absorbed lysozyme to the lysosomal system and provide no proof of other subcellular localizations.

In vitro *studies*

The suggestion that protein can be transported intact across the wall of the renal tubule was much stimulated by *in vitro* studies on flounder tubule by Maack and Kinter (1969). They found that lysozyme became concentrated in the kidney tubules after parenteral administration and that a considerable fraction of lysozyme could be released from isolated flounder kidney tubules during incubation *in vitro*. This release was taken as evidence that the lysozyme was transported intact across the tubule wall in this system. However, subsequent studies have demonstrated that isolated flounder tubules have a considerable capacity for a reversible peritubular binding of tracer protein. Thus, Ottosen and Maunsbach (1973) demonstrated that horse-radish peroxidase binds to the peritubular face of isolated flounder tubules in a reversible fashion, and furthermore that protein can be demonstrated by ultrastructural cytochemical methods in the intercellular space between the cells. In a later study, Ottosen (1978) demonstrated that ^{125}I-labelled lysozyme, with an electrophoretic mobility indistinguishable from native lysozyme, also binds reversibly to flounder tubules and even more strongly than does peroxidase. Therefore, the release of protein from flounder tubules which have been exposed *in vitro* or *in vivo* from the peritubular surface with tracer protein cannot be interpreted as evidence for transtubular transport of the tracer. The same applies to results obtained with the isolated perfused mammalian kidney where release of lysozyme was only observed following perfusion with very large doses of the tracer protein (Maack, 1975). In slices of rat kidney cortex from animals injected *in vivo* with lysozyme there was a significant release to the incubation medium of digestion products of the tracer protein, but not of intact lysozyme, suggesting that lysozyme was digested inside the lysosomes and that the lysosomes did not release their contents into the peritubular space (Christensen and Maunsbach, 1974).

Application of hydrostatic pressure gradient

Bulger and Trump (1969) injected ferritin retrograde via the ureter into the flounder kidney and found considerable amounts of the tracer in the lateral intercellular spaces. The observations were interpreted as evidence of transport of intact protein through the tubular epithelium. However, Ottosen (1976) demonstrated that such injections increase the intratubular pressure and that artefactual passage of tracers into the lateral intercellular space occurs due to localized ruptures in the tubule wall. In a further analysis of the effect of hydrostatic pressure, Ottosen injected tracer into isolated single flounder tubules under pressure control. When the intraluminal pressure was not elevated there was no transtubular passage of protein, but elevation of the intraluminal pressure led to extensive passage of tracer through the tubule wall due to ruptured cells and apparently also through leaking junctional complexes. A similar situation was observed in developing rat kidney tubules by Horster and Larsson (1976), who found no transtubular passage of protein at normal intraluminal hydrostatic pressures, but rapid penetration of microperoxidase through the junctional complexes at elevated luminal pressure.

Conclusions

(1) Protein present in the lumen of the proximal tubule is normally taken up by endocytosis and transported to the lysosomes for digestion.

(2) Proteins bind reversibly to the peritubular plasma membrane and in certain experimental situations this binding may mimic transtubular transport of protein.

(3) Proteins may be forced through the epithelium by large hydrostatic pressure gradients which cause ruptures of the epithelium or open junctional complexes.

(4) No convincing evidence has been presented for the existence of transcellular transport of intact protein across the wall of the renal proximal tubule.

References

Bernier, G. M. and Conrad, M. E. (1969). Catabolism of human β_2-microglobulin by the rat kidney. *Am. J. Physiol.* **217**, 1359–1362.

Bourdeau, J. E. and Carone, F. A. (1974). Protein handling by the renal tubule. *Nephron* **13**, 22–34.

Bulger, R. E. and Trump, B. F. (1969). A mechanism for rapid transport of colloidal particles by flounder renal epithelium. *J. Morph.* **127**, 205–224.

Chamberlain, M. J. and Stimmler, L. (1967). The renal handling of insulin. *J. clin. Invest.* **46**, 911–919.

Christensen, E. I. and Maunsbach, A. B. (1974). Intralysosomal digestion of lysozyme in renal proximal tubule cells. *Kidney Int.* **6**, 396–407.

Davidson, S. J. (1973). Protein absorption by renal cells. II. Very rapid lysosomal digestion of exogenous ribonuclease *in vitro*. *J. Cell Biol.* **59**, 213–222.

de Duve, C. (1971). Tissue fractionation. Past and present. *J. Cell Biol.* **50**, 20D–55D.

Graham, R. C. Jr and Karnovsky, M. J. (1966). The early stages of absorption of injected horseradish peroxidase in the proximal tubules of mouse kidney. Ultrastructural cytochemistry by a new technique. *J. Histochem. Cytochem.* **14**, 291–302.

Horster, M. and Larsson, L. (1976). Mechanisms of fluid absorption during proximal tubule development. *Kidney Int.* **10**, 348–363.

Johnson, V. and Maack, T. (1977). Renal extraction, filtration, absorption, and catabolism of growth hormone. *Am. J. Physiol.* **233**, F185–F196.

Just, M., Röckel, A., Stanjek, A. and Bode, F. (1975). Is there any transtubular reabsorption of filtered proteins in rat kidney? *Naunyn-Schmiedeberg's Arch. Pharmac.* **289**, 229–236.

Kau, S. T. and Maack, T. (1977). Transport and catabolism of parathyroid hormone in isolated rat kidney. *Am. J. Physiol.* **233**, F445–F454.

Maack, T. (1975). Renal handling of low molecular weight proteins. *Am. J. Med.* **58**, 57–64.

Maack, T. and Kinter, W. B. (1969). Transport of protein by flounder kidney tubules during long-term incubation. *Am. J. Physiol.* **216**, 1034–1043.

Maack, T., Mackensie, D. D. S. and Kinter, W. B. (1971). Intracellular pathways of renal reabsorption of lysozyme. *Am. J. Physiol.* **221**, 1609–1616.

Maude, D. L., Scott, W. N., Shehadeh, I. and Solomon, A. K. (1965). Further studies on the behaviour of inulin and serum albumin in rat kidney tubule. *Pflügers Arch. ges. Physiol.* **285**, 313–316.

Maunsbach, A. B. (1966). Absorption of ^{125}I-labeled homologeous albumin by rat kidney proximal tubule cells. A study of microperfused single proximal tubules by electron microscopic autoradiography and histochemistry. *J. Ultrastruct. Res.* **15**, 197–241.

Maunsbach, A. B. (1969). Functions of lysosomes in kidney cells. In *Lysosomes in Biology and Pathology*, Vol. 1 (J. T. Dingle and D. H. Fell, eds), North-Holland, Amsterdam, pp. 115–154.

Maunsbach, A. B. (1974). Isolation of kidney lysosomes. *Methods Enzymol.* **31**, 330–339.

Maunsbach, A. B. (1976). Cellular mechanisms of tubular protein transport. In *Kidney and Urinary Tract Physiology II* (K. Thurau, ed.), International Review of Science, Physiology, Series 2, Vol. 11, University Park Press, Baltimore, pp. 145–167.

Miller, F. and Palade, G. E. (1964). Lytic activities in renal protein absorption droplets. An electron microscopical cytochemical study. *J. Cell Biol.* **23**, 519–552.

Ottosen, P. D. (1976). Effect of intraluminal pressure on the ultrastructure and protein transport in the proximal tubule. *Kidney Int.* **9**, 252–263.

Ottosen, P. D. (1978). Reversible peritubular binding of a cationic protein (lysozyme) to flounder kidney tubules. *Cell Tissue Res.* **194**, 207–218.

Ottosen, P. D. and Maunsbach, A. B. (1973). Transport of peroxidase in flounder kidney tubules studied by electron microscope histochemistry. *Kidney Int.* **3**, 315–326.

Ottosen, P. D., Bode, F., Madsen, K. M. and Maunsbach, A. B. (1979). Renal handling of lysozyme in the rat. *Kidney Int.* **15**, 246–254.

Rodewald, R. (1973). Intestinal transport of antibodies in the newborn rat. *J. Cell Biol.* **58**, 189–211.

Straus, W. (1964). Cytochemical observations on the relationship between lysosomes and phagosomes in kidney and liver by combined staining for acid phosphatase and intravenously injected horseradish peroxidase. *J. Cell Biol.* **20**, 497–507.

Strober, W. and Waldmann, T. A. (1974). The role of the kidney in the metabolism of plasma proteins. *Nephron* **13**, 35–66.

Wochner, R. D., Strober, W. and Waldmann, T. A. (1967). The role of the kidney in the catabolism of Bence Jones proteins and immunoglobulin fragments. *J. exp. Med.* **126**, 207–221.

Part IV

Interstitium

28
Functional Aspects of the Renal Interstitium

A. Erik G. Persson

Introduction

The structure and function of the space between the tubular and vascular structures, the interstitial space, are poorly known. Recent experiments indicate, however, that significant modulation of renal function can result from changes in the interstitium. In an attempt to explain how modulation of renal function might occur through changes in the interstitium, one can divide the nephron schematically into two portions. The first is a volume-regulating segment consisting of the glomerulus, proximal tubule, loop of Henle and distal tubule to the macula densa, at which point a tubulo-glomerular feedback control of glomerular filtration is possible. The second segment is a fine-adjusting segment for electrolyte and water excretion and consists of the distal tubule and collecting ducts. In this presentation only the volume-regulating unit will be dealt with.

Measurements of Interstitial Pressures

Several recent observations have suggested that the pressure and volume conditions in the interstitial space might modulate renal tubular function in response to disturbances in fluid balance. To study the pressure conditions in the interstitial space, small catheters (20–80 μm in diameter) can be introduced into the subcapsular space. This space communicates with at least the wide interstitium (Pedersen *et al.*, Chapter 32 in this volume) and the lymphatic system (Wunderlich, 1971). Through these catheters hydrostatic pressure can be measured and samples withdrawn for protein analysis. A hydrostatic pressure of about 3 mm Hg and a protein concentration of about 2 g per cent, equal to that in lymph, were found under control conditions. During saline volume expansion the hydrostatic pressure rose to high values of 5–10 mm Hg, while the protein concentration fell to about 0·5 g per cent (Wolgast *et al.*, 1973).

By dripping albumin solutions with different protein concentrations onto the renal capsule above a pressure-recording catheter in the subcapsular space, the protein concentration that did not change the subcapsular hydro-static pressure could be determined. With this *in vivo* oncometric method the subcapsular oncotic pressure can be calculated (Wolgast *et al.*, 1973). It was found that the oncotic pressure was always higher than that calculated from the protein concentration alone. This indicates that factors other than protein concentration can influence oncotic pressure. One such factor could be the hyaluronic acid in the interstitial ground substance (Laurent and Ogston, 1953). The ready communication between the vascular and interstitial com-partment was indicated by rapid transient changes in hydrostatic pressure in the interstitial space on aortal injections of albumin or saline solutions (Persson and Selén, 1979). From these measurements the combined hydro-static and oncotic pressure gradient directed to the interstitium across the proximal tubular wall was calculated to be 20–25 mm Hg under control conditions. During saline volume expansion this control value was approxi-mately halved.

Driving Forces for Proximal Tubular Fluid Transport

A large fraction of the fluid filtered in the glomerulus will be reabsorbed during the passage through the proximal tubule by a multifactorial process. There is considerable divergence in opinion concerning the driving forces for this fluid transport. Some investigators believe that fluid transfer across the wall occurs mainly by means of active sodium transport (Green *et al.*, 1974; Burg and Orloff, 1973), while others suggest that acid ion secretion involved in bicarbonate reabsorption plays a large part (Rector *et al.*, 1966; Ullrich *et al.*, 1971). It has also been proposed that chloride diffusion resulting from an increased intraluminal chloride concentration on reabsorption of bi-carbonate, is an important driving force (Baratt *et al.*, 1974). The hydro-static and oncotic pressure difference across the proximal tubular wall may also be significant in this respect (Bresler, 1970; Persson *et al.*, 1972).

Despite these divided opinions about the mechanisms involved in fluid transport, most authors agree that a rise in colloid oncotic pressure of the peritubular capillary blood leads to an increased rate of reabsorption, while a reduction in the capillary colloid concentration will reduce fluid transport

(Lewy and Windhager, 1968). It is reasonable to assume that the capillary protein concentration influences fluid absorption via a change in the interstitial pressure and volume conditions, which in turn alters the structural components, which may affect the physiological properties of the fluid transport routes. Ågerup and Persson (1979) recently found, in fact, that the hydraulic conductivity of the proximal tubular wall was reduced to half its control value when the capillary was artificially perfused with a fluid with a low colloid concentration. As mentioned above, the fluid balance situation will influence the pressure conditions in the interstitium. Thus, during saline volume expansion the reduction in pressure gradient and hydraulic conductivity might in turn give rise to a reduction in that component of fluid transport that appears to be driven directly by the combined pressure gradient.

The Tubulo-glomerular Feedback Mechanism

Evidence for feedback mechanism
The anatomical feature of the nephron that makes the existence of the tubulo-glomerular feedback mechanism at least possible was described by Peter (1907) at the beginning of the century. He found that nephrons are arranged in such a way that the ascending limb of the loop of Henle passes close to its own glomerulus. Peter found this to be a regular feature of all nephrons. Zimmerman (1933) observed that the group of cells in the part of the distal tubule adjacent to the glomerulus has a characteristic appearance, and called this region the macula densa. As early as in the 1930s Goormaghtigh (1932) suggested that the composition of the distal tubular urine might in some way affect the tonus of the glomerular arteriole, with a resulting change in glomerular blood flow and filtration rate. Early micropuncture experiments gave conflicting results (Schnermann *et al.*, 1970; Morgan, 1971). However, in subsequent experiments in rats, proximal tubules were blocked with highly viscous silicone oil while the distal segment was perfused with an end-proximal Ringer solution (Schnermann *et al.*, 1973). Proximal to the oil block the tubular stop-flow pressure was recorded, as a relative measure of glomerular capillary pressure. It was found that when the flow was increased above the normal end-proximal rate of 15 nl/min the glomerular capillary pressure declined in a non-linear way. This behaviour is shown in Fig. 1. When the flow was reduced from the normal rate to zero no change in glomerular capillary pressure was detected. However, when a 300 mM mannitol solution was used to perfuse the distal nephron, no change in glomerular capillary pressure was observed even at high flow rates. From these studies it appears that some ionic constituent in the Ringer solution may release a flow-dependent signal.

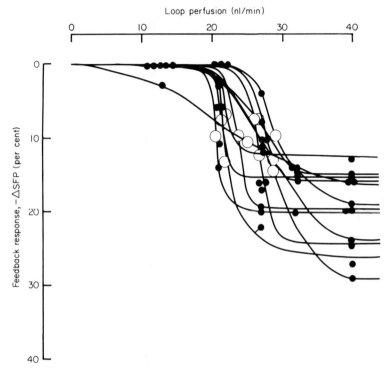

FIG. 1. *Percentage change in glomerular capillary pressure in individual nephrons estimated from the proximal tubular stop-flow pressure at different rates of Ringer perfusion of the loop of Henle. The unfilled circles show the flow rate at which 50 per cent of the maximal stop-flow response was obtained.*

Flow signal

Some investigators have reported that calcium ions seem to be necessary for the release of the feedback response (Burke *et al.*, 1974). However, later studies have revealed that the response can be elicited in the absence of calcium ions (Schnermann and Hermle, 1975). In fact, it has not been clear whether the flow-dependent signal is released by an anion or a cation. To investigate this question Wright and Persson (1974) clamped the distal tubular electrical potential with microelectrodes while at the same time the proximal tubular stop-flow pressure was measured and the distal nephron was perfused at a normal rate with a Ringer solution. By sending a current through one of the microelectrodes the tubular lumen at the macula densa could be made a few millivolts more negative or positive. A feedback response was elicited when the tubular lumen was made more negative. In this situation the driving force for outward movement of anions is increased. This finding supports the view that the transport of negatively charged ions such as chloride into the macula densa cells constitutes the flow-dependent signal. This concept is also supported by results of ionic substitution experiments (Müller-Suur *et al.*, 1973; Schnermann *et al.*, 1976).

Activation and Resetting of Feedback Mechanism

As mentioned above, it was found that there was no increase in glomerular capillary pressure when the distal delivery was reduced from normal to zero. This observation indicates that under control conditions the tubulo-glomerular feedback control is not activated to reduce the glomerular filtration rate. The question then arises, under what physiological circumstances is the feedback control mechanism activated to reduce the glomerular filtration rate? In earlier experiments it appeared that only rats on a low sodium diet (Dev *et al.*, 1974) or undergoing diuresis with acetazolamide (Persson and Wright, 1974) exhibited signs of a reduction in the glomerular filtration rate released by the feedback. In the dog the characteristics of the feedback may be different (Burke *et al.*, 1974). In theory a feedback response should be elicited either by a reduced tubular reabsorption, which would increase fluid delivery, or by an increase in sensitivity, with a lower threshold and a higher maximal response, so that a normal or subnormal load to the distal nephron will be large enough to release a response. Signs of resetting of the feedback were found in experimental animals undergoing saline volume expansion (Persson *et al.*, 1974), the maximal feedback response being reduced on volume expansion. This result indicates that a larger load to the distal nephron may be allowed by the macula densa without the release of a feedback response.

Resetting mechanism
To investigate the nature of the resetting mechanism, rat experiments were performed in which the peritubular capillary network supplying the macula densa area was artificially perfused in nephrons with the glomerulus on the surface (Persson *et al.*, 1976). In these artificially perfused nephrons, feedback characteristics, the maximal stop-flow pressure response and the end-proximal flow rate at which 50 per cent of the maximal response was obtained, were determined before, during and after capillary perfusion. It was found, as shown in Fig. 2, that when the peritubular capillary colloid concentration was decreased the feedback response was greatly reduced or abolished, as indicated by a reduced maximal feedback response and an increased flow threshold. An increase in the capillary colloid concentration, on the other hand, increased the feedback response, as shown by an increased

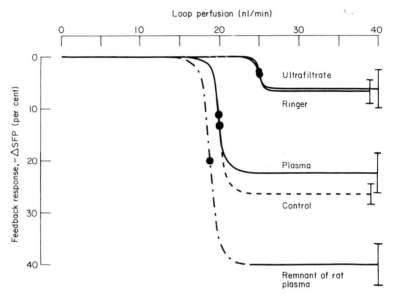

FIG. 2. *Change in proximal tubular stop-flow pressure ($\triangle SFP$, expressed in per cent of normal stop-flow pressure ± S.E.M.) at different rates of Ringer perfusion of the loop of Henle while the capillary network supplying the macula densa area of the investigated nephron was artificially perfused with different solutions. The perfusion solutions used were Ringer solution, ultrafiltrate of rat plasma, rat plasma and remnant of rat plasma after ultrafiltration (protein concentration about 10 g per cent). The curves were derived from the maximal drop in stop-flow pressure and the tubular flow rate at which 50 per cent of the maximal stop-flow pressure response was obtained. The hatched line at remnant perfusion indicates that the flow rate with 50 per cent reduction of maximal feedback response was not determined with sufficient safety. (From Persson et al. (1979).)*

maximal feedback response. It was suggested that the change in feedback response was mediated to the macula densa cells via pressure or volume changes in the interstitial space. A rise in peritubular capillary oncotic pressure will increase the reabsorption of fluid from the interstitial space, with a decline in interstitial hydrostatic pressure and volume, while the interstitial oncotic pressure might rise. At a low colloid perfusion, on the other hand, capillary fluid uptake will be reduced and the interstitial hydrostatic pressure and volume will increase while the oncotic pressure will be lowered. From this study it appeared possible that in conditions with a low interstitial pressure and volume and a high interstitial oncotic pressure, as in dehydration or in arterial hypotension, the feedback sensitivity should be increased. On the other hand, in situations with increased interstitial pressure and volume and with a low interstitial oncotic pressure, as in volume expansion, the feedback sensitivity should be decreased.

Dehydrated animals

Recent experiments by Persson *et al.* (1977) on dehydrated rats (24 h without food and water) have shown that under these conditions the feedback activity is increased, judged both from an increased maximal feedback response and a reduced flow threshold for feedback activation, also resulting in a feedback-elicited reduction in the glomerular filtration rate (Fig. 3). Saline volume expansion in these animals depressed the feedback sensitivity, as indicated

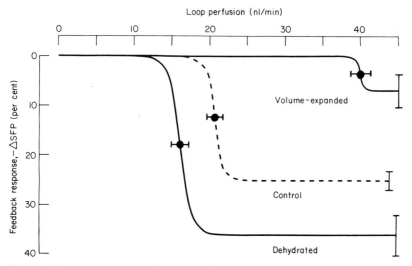

FIG. 3. *Change in proximal tubular stop-flow pressure ($\triangle SFP$, expressed in per cent of normal stop-flow pressure $\pm$ s.e.m.) at different rates of Ringer perfusion of the loop of Henle in rats under three different sets of conditions: dehydrated animals (deprived of food and water for 24 h); volume-expanded animals (saline, 5 per cent of BW to dehydrated animals); and control animals. The curves were derived from the maximal stop-flow pressure response and the tubular flow rate at which 50 per cent of the maximal response was obtained.*

both by a reduction or disappearance of the feedback response and by an increased flow threshold for feedback activation. These events allow the load to the distal nephron to increase without a reduction in the glomerular filtration rate.

Transplanted kidneys of uninephrectomy

In experiments on transplanted kidneys in rats with one transplanted kidney and one remnant kidney the tubulo-glomerular feedback activities were determined directly or 15 h after transplantation (Norlén *et al.*, 1978; Müller-Suur *et al.*, 1977). An intact normal feedback response was found directly after transplantation, indicating that the renal nerves are not essential for the release of a feedback response. However, the transplanted kidneys were initially diuretic and lost volume. Fifteen hours after transplantation the animals became dehydrated. In this situation the tubulo-glomerular feedback sensitivity was increased as shown in Fig. 4, the increase being indicated by a reduced flow threshold for feedback activation, which caused a reduction in the glomerular filtration rate. However, when the remnant kidney was

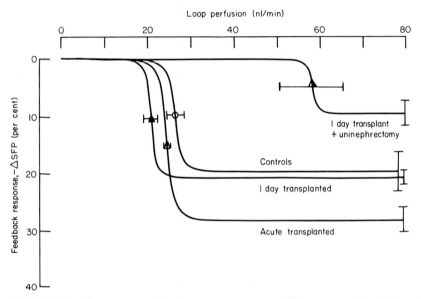

FIG. 4. *The change in stop-flow pressure* $\pm$ S.E.M. *at different rates of perfusion of the loop of Henle in rats. The curves were derived from the maximal stop-flow pressure response and the flow rate* $\pm$ S.E.M. *at which 50 per cent of the maximal response was obtained. Feedback characteristics were determined in transplanted kidneys directly after transplantation* ($\triangle$) *and 1 day later* ($\blacktriangle$), *and in the latter group after removal of the remnant native kidney* ($\blacktriangle$), *and compared with control animals* ($\bigcirc$).

removed, the feedback was reset to a very low sensitivity after 20 min, with a low maximal feedback response and a high flow threshold for feedback activation. This resetting allowed the glomerular filtration rate to rise (Müller-Suur *et al.*, 1977). To investigate the nature of this resetting process following nephrectomy, the subcapsular interstitial hydrostatic pressure was recorded in the transplanted kidney after removal of the rats' own remnant kidney. In all experiments the subcapsular hydrostatic pressure invariably rose by at least 50 per cent within 15 min, indicating changes in interstitial pressure–

volume conditions in parallel with a change in feedback sensitivity (Hahne et al., 1979).

It has been suggested that local renal hormones such as prostaglandins might influence the tubulo-glomerular feedback control (Larsson and Änggård, 1974). In experiments in which rats were injected with indo-methazine (2 mg/kg body weight) it was found that the resetting of the feed-back sensitivity in the transplanted kidney after removal of the remnant native kidney was abolished (Hahne et al., 1979). In another series of experi-ments the addition of PGI_2 to the tubular perfusate or the infusion of arachidonic acid into the renal artery completely blocked the feedback response, while the addition of PGE_2 or PGF_{2_a} did increase the feedback sensitivity. Thus, it seems that arachidonic acid and prostaglandins are able to reset the tubulo-glomerular feedback, but the physiological importance cannot yet be evaluated owing to the lack of knowledge about the prosta-glandin concentration in the fluid of different tubular segments.

Reduced arterial perfusion pressure

A decrease in arterial pressure is yet another situation in which an increased feedback response might be expected. Experiments were designed to study this situation (Persson and Selén, 1979). An aortic clamp below the region of the right renal artery was used to reduce the left renal arterial pressure to 75 mm Hg. The result is shown in Fig. 5. In the first 15 min after clamping, no change in feedback sensitivity was detected as compared with the controls. After 15–60 min of clamping an increased sensitivity, with an increased percentage of maximal feedback response and decreased flow threshold, was noted. In the period 0–15 min after declamping, the feedback sensitivity was still increased, while in the period 15–60 min after declamping it was reduced to preclamping values. These results indicate that on reduction of the arterial blood pressure the interstitial hydrostatic pressure and volume will be reduced and the feedback sensitivity increased after some delay of 15–30 min.

Conclusions

Measurements of interstitial pressure and proximal tubular hydraulic con-ductivity suggest that the reduction in fluid reabsorption during saline volume expansion can be explained by a reduction of that component of fluid transport that is directly driven by the combined transtubular pressure gradient.

The existence of an interstitial pressure or volume receptor mechanism in the juxtaglomerular apparatus is indicated from feedback experiments. When the load on the distal nephron is sensed at the macula densa site the response

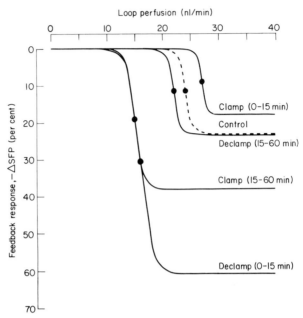

FIG. 5. *The change in tubular stop-flow pressure (in per cent of normal stop-flow pressure) at different rates of perfusion of the loop of Henle when the arterial pressure of the left kidney was reduced to 75 mm Hg by clamping the aorta. The curves were derived from the maximal stop-flow pressure response and the flow rate at which 50 per cent of the maximal response was obtained. These characteristics were determined in controls, 0–15 min and 15–60 min after clamping, and 0–15 min and 15–60 min after declamping.*

from the juxtaglomerular apparatus is dependent on the stimulation from the interstitium. In a situation with volume depletion or arterial hypotension, the feedback sensitivity is augmented and consequently the feedback will be activated and will reduce the glomerular filtration rate, even though the distal load might be normal or subnormal. Thus, the feedback control is activated as a consequence of the extracellular fluid needs and blood pressure level, and not merely as a result of an increase in distal fluid delivery.

Thus, it appears as if the interstitial pressure–volume conditions might modulate both the proximal tubular reabsorption rate and the setting of the sensitivity of the tubulo-glomerular feedback. Such mechanisms represent an automatic means of modulating renal function without the use of hormonal or nervous pathways.

References

Baratt, L. J., Rector, F. C., Kokko, J. P. and Seldin, D. W. (1974). Factors governing the transpeithelial potential difference across the proximal tubule of the rat kidney. *J. clin. Invest.* **53**, 454–464.

Bresler, E. H. (1970). Aspects of tubular reabsorption revisited. *Chest* **58**, 261–270.

Burg, M. and Orloff, J. (1973). Perfusion of isolated renal tubules. In *Handbook of Physiology*, Sect. 8, *Renal Physiology* (J. Orloff and R. W. Berliner, eds), American Physiological Society, Washington, DC, pp. 145–159.

Burke, T. J., Navar, G., Clapp, J. R. and Robinson, R. R. (1974). Response of single nephron glomerular filtration rate to distal nephron microperfusion. *Kidney Int.* **6**, 230–240.

Dev, B., Drescher, C. and Schnermann, J. (1974). Resetting of tubulo-glomerular feedback sensitivity by dietary salt intake. *Pflügers Arch. ges. Physiol.* **346**, 263–277.

Green, R., Windhager, E. E. and Giebisch, G. (1974). On protein oncotic effects on proximal tubular movement in the rat. *Am. J. Physiol.* **226**, 265–276.

Goormaghtigh, N. (1932). Les segments neuro-myo-artériels, juxtaglomérulaires de réin. *Archs Biol., Liège* **43**, 575–591.

Hahne, B., Selén, G. and Persson, A. E. G. (1979). In *Proceedings of the IIIrd European Colloquium on Renal Physiology, Saltsjöbaden*, p. 24.

Larsson, C. and Ånggård, E. (1974). Increased juxtamedullary blood flow on stimulation of intrarenal prostaglandin biosynthesis. *Eur. J. Pharmac.* **25**, 326–334.

Laurent, T. C. and Ogston, A. G. (1953). The interaction between polysaccharides and other macromolecules. 4. The osmotic pressure of mixtures of serum albumin and hyaluronic acid. *Biochem. J.* **89**, 249–253.

Lewy, J. E. and Windhager, E. E. (1968). Peritubular control of proximal tubular fluid reabsorption in the rat kidney. *Am. J. Physiol.* **214**, 943–954.

Morgan, T. (1971). A microperfusion study of influence of macula densa on glomerular filtration rate. *Am. J. Physiol.* **220**, 186–190.

Müller-Suur, R., Gutsche, H. U. and Hegel, U. (1973). Triggering factors of the tubulo-glomerular feedback. *Pflügers Arch. ges. Physiol.* **343**, R45.

Müller-Suur, R., Norlén, B. J. and Persson, A. E. G. (1977). Reseting of tubulo-glomerular feedback in transplanted rat kidneys. In *Proceedings of the International Congress of Physiologists, Paris 1977*, p. 533.

Norlén, B. J., Müller-Suur, R. and Persson, A. E. G. (1978). Tubulo-glomerular feedback response and excitatory characteristics of the transplanted rat kidney. *Scand. J. Urol. Nephrol.* **12**, 27–33.

Persson, A. E. G. and Selén, G. (1979). In *Proceedings of the IIIrd European Colloquium on Renal Physiology, Saltsjöbaden*, p. 60.

Persson, A. E. G. and Wright, F. S. (1974) Reduction of glomerular filtration rate by intrarenal feed-back during acetazolamid administration. In *Federation Proceedings. Federation of Societies for Experimental Biology, Atlantic City*, p. 806.

Persson, A. E. G., Ågerup, B. and Schnermann, J. (1972). The effect of luminal application of colloids on rat proximal tubular net fluid flux. *Kidney Int.* **2**, 203–213.

Persson, A. E. G., Müller-Suur and R. Selén, G. (1976). Peritubular capillary oncotic pressure as a modifier of tubulo-glomerular feedback. *Kidney Int.* **10**, 595.

Persson, A. E. G., Müller-Suur, R. and Selén, G. (1979). Capillary oncotic pressure as a modifier for tubuloglomerular feedback. *Am. J. Physiol.* **236**, F97–F102.

Persson, A. E. G., Selén, G. and Müller-Suur, R. (1977). Activation of the tubu-loglomerular feedback in dehydrated animals. In *Proceedings of the International Congress of Physiologists, Paris 1977*, p. 589.

Persson, A. E. G., Schnermann, J. and Wright, F. S. (1974). The effect of saline expansion on the glomerular-tubular feedback. In *Proceedings of the International Congress of Physiologists, India*, p. 357.

Peter, K. (1907). Die Nierenkanälchen des Menschen und einiger Säugetiere. *Anat. Anz.* **30**, 114–124.

Rector, F. C., Mártinez-Maldonado, M., Brunner, F. P. and Seldin, W. D. (1966). Evidence for passive reabsorption of NaCl in proximal tubule of rat kidney. *J. clin. Invest.* **45**, 1060–

Schnermann, J., Wright, F. S., Davis, J. M., Stackelberg and Grill, G. (1970). Regula-tion of superficial nephron filtration rate by tubulo-glomerular feedback. *Pflügers Arch. ges. Physiol.* **318**, 147–175.

Schnermann, J., Persson, A. E. G. and Ågerup, B. (1973). Tubuloglomerular feedback: nonlinear relation between glomerular hydrostatic pressure and loop of Henle perfusion. *J. clin. Invest.* **52**, 862–869.

Schnermann, J. and Hermle, M. (1975). Maintenance of feedback regulation of filtration dynamics in the absence of divalent anions in the lumen of the distal tubule. *Pflügers Arch. ges. Physiol.* **358**, 311–323.

Schnermann, J., Ploth, D. W. and Hermle, M. (1976). Activation of tubulo-glomerular feedback by chloride transport. *Pflügers Arch. ges. Physiol.* **362**, 229–240.

Ullrich, K. J., Radke, H. W. and Rumrich, G. (1971). The role of bicarbonate and other buffers on isotonic absorption in the proximal convolution of the rat kidney. *Pflügers Arch. ges. Physiol.* **330**, 149–160.

Wolgast, M., Persson, A. E. G., Schnermann, J., Ulfendahl, H. and Wunderlich, P. (1973). The colloid osmotic pressure of the subcapsular interstitial fluid of rat kidneys during hydropenia and volume expansion. *Pflügers Arch. ges. Physiol.* **340**, 123–135.

Wunderlich, P., Persson, A. E. G., Schnermann, J., Ulfendahl, H. R., and Wolgast, M. (1971). Hydrostatic pressure in the subcapsular interstitial space of rat and dog kidney. *Pflügers Arch. ges. Physiol.* **328**, 307–319.

Zimmermann, K. W. (1933). Uber den Bau des Glomerulus der Säugerniere. *Z. mikrosk.-anat. Forsch.* **32**, 176–278.

Ågerup, B. and Persson, A. E. G. (1979). In *Proceedings of the IIIrd European Colloquium on Renal Physiology, Saltsjöbaden*, p. 2.

29
Interstitial Albumin Pool in the Renal Cortex: Its Turnover and the Permeability of Peritubular Capillaries

G. G. Pinter, P. D. Wilson, D. R. Bell, J. L. Atkins and J. E. Stork

Introduction

"To be perfectly frank, I will not venture to express anything more definite than probabilities about the function of this fluid . . ." So wrote Olof Rudbeck in 1653 in his *Nova excercitatio anatomica, exhibens ductus hepaticos aquosos et vasa glandularum serosa* about the fluid in the hepatic lymphatics, the discovery of which he had just described (see Nielsen, 1942).

From the distance of more than three centuries one is struck by the astuteness of this remark, and in this presentation we intend to follow his example.

The subject of this presentation is renal lymph. Although much has been written about it, the role of lymph in renal function is still less than well known. On the one hand, the outstanding reviews and monographs by Mayerson (1963), Rusznyák, Földi and Szabo (1967) and Yoffey and Courtice (1971) survey many experimental and clinical observations and theories on the importance of renal lymph drainage in health and disease. On the other hand, answers to some questions of fundamental importance are still a matter of controversy. For example, where does the renal lymph originate, and how does the drainage system of the medullary interstitium work? In this paper we do not attempt to answer these fundamental questions. Instead, we will focus on one specific role of renal lymph: namely that it is a potential source of information about the cortical interstitium. Is there any reason to expect that the interstitium has important information to offer? This question is justified from the functional point of view because of the well established anatomical findings that tubules and peritubular capillaries are at several points closely apposed—sometimes to the point of sharing a common basement membrane. If all or most of the tubular reabsorbate should flow into the peritubular capillaries at such sites without sweeping across the interstitial spaces, the interstitial fluid would be a stagnant pool unrelated to the main stream, and information from the interstitium would be unrelated to tubular reabsorption. Important data on this question have been presented recently by Kriz and Napiwotzky (1978) of the University of Heidelberg and by Rittinger, Pfaller and Deetjen (1978) of the University of Innsbruck. These authors used a morphometric technique to estimate the apposed tubular and capillary surface areas. The results of Kriz and Napiwotzky showed that approximately one-fourth of the total tubular surface is covered with capillary walls—including all the sites in which the basement membranes were apposed, or adjacent with a very narrow slit between them. Rittinger *et al.* (1978) estimated that approximately 6 per cent of the basement membrane surface of the tubules appeared to be fused with that of the capillaries. These observations suggest that much of the tubular reabsorbate flows through the interstitium and, in turn, that lymph contains information about tubular reabsorption. We also have observations which constitute tentative functional evidence that this is the case: When tracer glucose is given as a pulse intravenous (i.v.) injection, a characteristic concentration versus time pattern of the tracer is seen in renal lymph. After injection of phlorizin the pattern showed a change indicating an absence of reabsorbed glucose in the interstitial fluid. A less specific finding pointing to the same conclusion is a consistent increase of lymph flow during acetylcholine infusion into the renal artery (D. A. Reese and G. G. Pinter, in preparation).

It appears, therefore, that the renal lymph does carry functionally important signals from the interstitium, and the remainder of this presentation will focus on our method of reading these signals. The assumption has often been made that concentrations of various substances, in particular of macromolecules, are equal in interstitial fluid and lymph. Recently, however, some observations pointed to the conclusion that interstitial fluid and lymph may, under certain circumstances, have different compositions. This point has been reviewed recently by Földi (1977). Pertaining to the kidney, of particular interest is the experimental finding of Källskog and Wolgast (1973) which showed that subcapsular fluid and lymph had similar protein concentrations in the concentrating kidney, but the concentrations appeared different after saline infusion. It is not unexpected that water and other small molecules should approach equilibrium across the wall of small lymphatics with the environment which prevails around these vessels. Thus lymph concentrations of small molecules should reflect the environment through which permeable portions of the lymphatic vessels pass; and even the concentration of macromolecules is subject to change because of the movement of water across the wall of collecting lymphatics.

To overcome this difficulty we have developed a technique which utilizes specific activity of a macromolecule, rather than its concentration, as the means of information carried by lymph from the interstitium. This information pertains to the renal cortex, since there is strong evidence that lymphatics are absent from the renal medulla (Kriz and Dieterich, 1970). We focused on plasma albumin, which being the most abundant protein component in the plasma with a relatively small molecular weight, plays the most important role in the colloid osmotic effect across the peritubular capillary wall. Our method involves determination of the specific activity of albumin in plasma and renal lymph under both transient and steady state conditions. Using these measurements we estimated the following characteristics of the interstitial albumin pool and microcirculation in the renal cortex: (1) size of the pool; (2) turnover rate of the pool; (3) unidirectional clearance of albumin across the peritubular capillary wall; (4) reflection coefficient of the peritubular capillary wall to albumin; (5) heterogeneity of the interstitial albumin pool. Some parts of this work have already been published (Bell, Pinter and Wilson, 1978) and others are still in progress. We will attempt to review each point briefly.

The Size of the Interstitial Pool of Albumin

We measured the distribution volume of interstitial albumin as the difference between the total (steady state) and intravascular distribution volumes of tagged albumin. Two tracers of human plasma albumin were used: one labelled with ^{125}I and the other with ^{131}I. In separate experiments we ascertained for each shipment of pairs of tracer preparations that the two tracers were equivalent (Bell et al., 1977), and that the inorganic iodine radioactivity did not exceed 1 per cent of the total. One of the tracers, usually ^{125}I-tagged albumin, was injected i.v. in a rat and about 3 h was allowed for equilibration with the total renal albumin pool. ^{131}I-tagged albumin was then injected and allowed to mix with the albumin pool for about 3–4 min. During this time it equilibrated with intravascular plasma, and, to some degree, it also penetrated into the interstitial part of the albumin pool. The latter fraction would have made the estimation of the vascular volume inaccurate and required a correction. We assumed that the specific activity of lymph follows that of the interstitial pool and calculated the distribution volume of the interstitial albumin (V_i) by the following formula:

$$V_i = \frac{V - V(t)}{1 - L(t)/P(t)},$$

(1)

where V and $V(t)$ are the distribution volumes of the steady state (3 h equilibration time) and non-steady state (3–4 min mixing time) tracers, respectively. $L(t)$ is the specific activity of lymph albumin, and $P(t)$ is the specific activity of arterial plasma albumin at the time of tying off the renal pedicles. Derivation of this formula is shown in appendix II of the paper by Bell *et al.* (1978).

In developing equation (1) no assumption is made about equality of lymph and the interstitial albumin concentrations; instead equality of specific activities is assumed.

We calculated that the volume of distribution of albumin in the interstitial space of the renal cortex of 2–3 months old Sprague-Dawley rats amounts to about 1·7 ml/100 g tissue. The physical volume in which this albumin is distributed is not known. If we assume that the concentration of albumin in lymph provides a rough estimate of the average interstitial concentration, the physical interstitial volume containing this amount of albumin would correspond to some 5–10 ml/100 g tissue.

Transit Time of Albumin from Plasma to Lymph

To facilitate the measurement of albumin specific activity in both lymph and plasma, two albumin tracers again were used. A dose of ^{125}I-labelled albumin was injected intravenously immediately after induction of anesthesia. This tracer was allowed to equilibrate with both plasma and renal lymph albumin. A hilar lymphatic vessel was cannulated. The measurement of transit times was then carried out by injecting ^{131}I-tagged albumin and determining the ratio of ^{131}I/^{125}I activities in arterial plasma and renal lymph. Figure 1 shows the results of one of these experiments. The specific activity of lymph albumin increased gradually, and by about 90 min, when this experiment was terminated, the specific activities were nearly equal.

The tracer molecules arriving in lymph have crossed the capillary wall and the interstitial space in succession. The time taken by each albumin tracer molecule to make the journey from arterial plasma to lymph is variable and can be described statistically by a probability density function (p.d.f.) of transit times, which may be obtained by deconvolution of the plasma and lymph specific activity versus time curves, and which has its mean value equal to the mean transit time. We have derived this mean value by using several

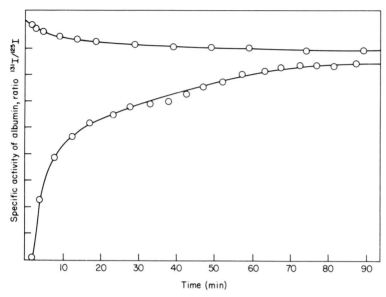

FIG. 1. *Ordinate shows specific activities of albumin in arterial plasma (upper curve) and renal hilar lymph (lower curve) as measured by tracer activity ratios. For details, see text.*

different approaches. Two of these we mention here; a third one will be discussed below in the section on the heterogeneity of the interstitial space.

One of the approaches was directly from the results of the numerical deconvolution. This is the least restrictive and requires only that the tracer system interposed between plasma and lymph be linear and stationary; no compartmental structure is assumed. The mean transit time calculated by using this approach was 28 min. However, the experiments were terminated after about 94 min, and this figure was obtained as the mean of a truncated p.d.f. of transit times. Due to truncation, the area under the p.d.f. was near 0·9 instead of 1·0. It is therefore apparent that the mean transit time calculated by this method underestimated the true transit time.

The second approach was to assume that the system under study consisted of a single rapidly mixed compartment. We do not propose any *a priori* justification for the assumption of instantaneous mixing in the interstitial space. Rather, by looking at the reconstruction of the response of the lymph specific activity versus time function to a step function change in the plasma albumin specific activity, we concluded that the assumption of a single well mixed compartment seems to provide a roughly acceptable fit to the experimental data. The mean transit time calculated by using this model was 33 min. This estimate differs from the previous one in that it is not from a truncated p.d.f. and cannot be said to be an underestimate due to truncation.

We shall discuss another approach for calculating the mean transit time of albumin from plasma to lymph in connection with the heterogeneity of the interstitial albumin pool.

Calculation of the Unidirectional Clearance of Albumin from the Peritubular Capillaries into the Interstitium

To carry out this calculation we invoke the central volume theorem, which states for a system in dynamic equilibrium that the product of the flow rate through the system multiplied by the mean residence time of the molecules flowing through the system is equal to the volume of the system. With reference to the interstitial albumin pool this theorem is stated as

$$\tau\phi = \mu, \tag{2}$$

where τ is the mean residence time (in minutes), ϕ is the unidirectional flow (in milligrams per minute), and μ is the mass of albumin in the interstitial pool (in milligrams). After dividing both sides of equation (2) by the arterial plasma albumin concentration, c_p, one obtains

$$\tau\phi/c_p = \mu/c_p. \tag{2a}$$

Here, ϕ/c_p is the unidirectional clearance of albumin and μ/c_p is the interstitial distribution volume of albumin. Although this clearance is similar to the PS product of Renkin (1964), PS represents a net clearance and ϕ/c_p is unidirectional. To emphasize this difference we refer to ϕ/c_p as ψ. Therefore,

$$\psi \equiv \phi/c_p = (\mu/c_p)\,(1/\tau). \tag{2b}$$

In an earlier section, we described the interstitial distribution volume measurement V_i, and we have justified elsewhere (Bell *et al.*, 1978) the use of this measurement to represent μ/c_p. In the section on transit time we described the computation of $\bar{t}$, the mean transit time of albumin from plasma to lymph. Providing that $\bar{t}$ is equivalent with τ in equation (2b), the experimentally defined measurement

$$V_i/\bar{t} \tag{3}$$

is equivalent to ψ, and the unidirectional clearance of albumin across the peritubular capillary wall can be calculated from equation (3). Regarding the assumption of equality of $\bar{t}$ and τ, we note that τ, the mean residence time of albumin, and $\bar{t}$, the mean transit time of albumin from plasma to lymph, are equal only if two specific conditions are met: (i) all molecules in the entire interstitial albumin pool have a nonzero probability of exiting through the lymph, and (ii) the mean transit time observed at the lymph exit is the same as at any other possible exit for albumin molecules (such as a potential re-entry into the capillaries). As we have discussed in a recent publication (Bell *et al.*, 1978), these conditions appear to be met in our experiments on normal rats. However, in general, we observe that under different experimental conditions the equality of ψ and ψ' should be specially ascertained.

The unidirectional clearance of albumin calculated by using equation (3) was $(10\cdot2 \pm 1\cdot4) \times 10^{-4}$ ml/s in 100 of tissue, and $(8\cdot4 \pm 1\cdot2) \times 10^{-4}$ ml/s in 100 g tissue, respectively, when the values for $\bar{t}$ were utilized as determined with the method of numerical deconvolution and single compartmental assumption.

The Solvent Drag Reflection Coefficient of the Capillary Wall to Albumin

The data allow the calculation of a lower limiting value of the solvent drag reflection coefficient for the reabsorbing surface of the peritubular capillary wall for albumin. The lower limiting value follows from the following inequality: the rate of entry of albumin into the interstitium from the peritubular capillaries is greater than the rate at which albumin is dragged back by the convective flow of tubular reabsorbate into the capillaries. This statement is justified by the fact that some of the albumin which enters the interstitial space is removed by way of lymphatic drainage. This statement is formulated as

$$|\phi| > |J_v|(1 - \sigma)\bar{c}, \tag{4}$$

where ϕ is the unidirectional flow of albumin into the interstitium, J_v is the rate of tubular fluid volume reabsorption, σ is the solvent drag reflection coefficient of the capillary wall to albumin, and $\bar{c}$ is the average concentration of albumin in the capillary wall. According to Katchalsky and Curran (1965), $\bar{c}$ may be approximated as the arithmetic mean of concentrations on both sides of the membrane, i.e. $\bar{c} \doteq (c_i + c_p')/2$, where c_i and c_p' refer to the unknown concentrations of albumin on the interstitial and plasma sides respectively of the peritubular capillaries. Rearrangement of equation (4), and using this approximation for $\bar{c}$, yields

$$1 - \sigma < \frac{|\phi|}{|J_v|\bar{c}} \doteq \frac{2|\phi|}{|J_v|(c_i + c_p')} < \frac{2|\phi|}{|J_v|c_p}, \tag{5}$$

where the last inequality is obtained by employing the inequalities $c'_p > c_p$ and $c_i > 0$, which imply that $c_i + c'_p > c_p$. Finally, using the fact that $\phi = \psi' c_p$ and rearranging, one obtains the approximate lower bound

$$\sigma > 1 - 2\frac{|\psi'|}{|J_v|}. \tag{6}$$

By estimating the rate of tubular reabsorption as 60 ml/min = 1 ml/s in 100 g of renal cortex and substituting the estimate of $\psi' = 10 \times 10^{-4}$ ml/s in 100 g of renal cortex, the lower limiting value for the estimate of σ is

$$\sigma > 0{\cdot}998.$$

Provided that the osmotic reflection coefficient is equal to the solvent drag reflection coefficient, it is apparent that the effective colloid osmotic force is not diminished to any significant degree resulting from a concentration difference of albumin. It should be emphasized that this calculation is valid specifically for the reabsorbing surface of the capillaries as, in this model, the sites of albumin entry from the capillary into the interstitium are considered to be separate from the reabsorbing portions of the capillary surface.

Heterogeneity of the Interstitial Space in the Renal Cortex

In the section on transit time we discussed two approaches to the study of the kinetics of albumin specific activity in lymph. The need for a model other than that of a single well mixed compartment arose from our perception that the latter was not entirely satisfactory as regards the physiological and anatomical circumstances known to exist in the interstitium of the renal cortex or in its fit to the experimental data.

However, we found particularly intriguing the observation that the kinetics of the interstitial albumin pool show some agreement with those of a single instantaneously mixed compartment since, structurally, the interstitial space is spread over the cortical tissue in such a way that it can be considered as consisting of microscopically small subunits with little or no communication between distant subunits.

This consideration promoted further exploration of a model in which the interstitial albumin pool is assumed to be a composite of a very large number of small subunits, each of which have single compartment kinetics, and with the rate constants statistically distributed over the subunits. It has become apparent that in order to proceed with the model, it was necessary to specify the p.d.f. of this distribution.

Selection of such a p.d.f. proved to be a difficult task as neither the known anatomical features, nor the known properties of combined convection and diffusion of molecules provided unequivocal guidance. For this reason we have chosen a particular p.d.f. arbitrarily; first we specified the criteria compatible with such a p.d.f. and then selected the simplest one among those that fulfill such criteria.

The following criteria were set:

(a) Only positive values exist for the rate constants. Therefore, the p.d.f. should be positive only for positive rate constants.

(b) Since each subunit is characterized as a single well mixed compartment, the model should revert to that of a single well mixed compartment when all rate constants are equal.

(c) The p.d.f. should be able to take on a rich variety of shapes depending on parameter values.

(d) The average response of the collection of subunits (averaged over the distribution of rate constants) should fit well the empirical response obtained from numerical deconvolution.

Among the possible options we have picked the gamma distribution because of its simplicity.

The gamma p.d.f. has two parameters denoted here as α and λ, such that the mean value of the p.d.f. is α/λ and the variance is α/λ^2. If each subunit behaves independently as a well mixed compartment, with step response $H(t) = 1 - e^{-xt}$, and if the rate constants $\{x\}$ are distributed over subunits according to the gamma distribution, then it follows that the average step response of the ensemble of subunits is

$$\text{Av}[H(t)] = 1 - \left(\frac{\lambda}{\lambda + t}\right)^{\alpha}. \tag{7}$$

The fit of the model of equation (7) to the experimental data of two rats is shown in Fig. 2. The two rats whose analysis is shown here were selected to be those for whom the model of equation (7) provided the worst fit. Judging by the mean square error, the fit of the model of equation (7) to the experimental data was always much better than that of a single well mixed compartment. The mean transit time averaged over nine experiments obtained by this approach was 35·6 min. Fits of the equation (7) model providing individual values of α and λ were calculated from each individual experiment. A typical gamma distribution was created by using the mean values of α and λ averaged over the nine rats. For this gamma distribution we calculated the 17th and 83rd percentiles. These correspond to 86·6 min and 22·7 min, respectively, after inverting rate constant to yield mean transit time. These figures indicate that, although single compartment kinetics can provide a representation of the data, by using a statistically distributed model a much better fit to the data was obtained, and a greater than fourfold variation

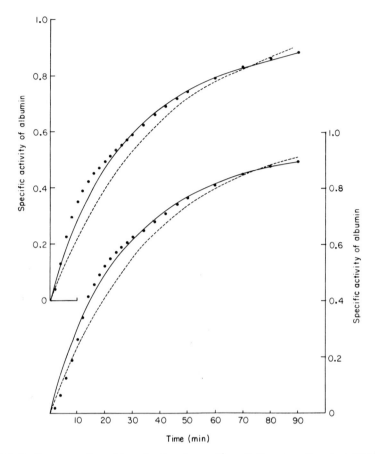

FIG. 2. *Response of renal lymph albumin specific activity versus time to a step input in plasma albumin specific activity. Dots represent experimental points showing empirical step response obtained by numerical deconvolution. Dashed and solid lines represent the fits to the data of two models:* -----, *Fit of* $1 - e^{-xt}$ *(the entire interstitial space is assumed to be a single well mixed compartment)* ——, *fit of* $1 - (\lambda/(\lambda + t))^a$ *(microscopic subunits of the interstitial pool are assumed to be well mixed but their rate constants are not uniform; the rate constants are assumed to be distributed as a gamma probability density function). For details, see text.*

was detected among the turnover rates of the individual subunits. This point deserves emphasis, particularly because of the attractiveness of representing the interstitial kinetics of various substances by a lumped model of a single well mixed compartment. Moreover, because a very large number of somewhat independent interstitial subunits appears to be a more valid representation of the physical reality, the distributed model might be considered as an alternative to the single well mixed compartment.

Conclusions

We have measured the specific activities of albumin in renal lymph and arterial plasma both in steady state and transient conditions. By using the results of these measurements and various models, we have calculated both the size and the turnover rate of the interstitial albumin pool in the renal cortex and determined the unidirectional clearance and a limiting value for the reflection coefficient for albumin and the peritubular capillary wall. By applying a probabilistic model to the data, using the gamma distribution, we obtained a better fit than by the deterministic single compartment assumption. This probabilistic model allowed us to draw some conclusions about the heterogeneity of the interstitial space in the renal cortex.

It is our hope that the genius of Olof Rudbeck will not be offended by our discussion of lymph and probability in a context different from his.

References

Bell, D. R., Pinter, G. G. and Wilson, P. D. (1978). Albumin permeability of the peritubular capillaries in rat renal cortex. *J. Physiol., Lond.* **279**, 621–640.

Bell, D. R., Wilson, P. D., Rasmussen, S. N. and Pinter, G. G. (1977). Comparison of plasma albumin preparations labelled with radioactive iodine. *Int. J. nucl. Med. Biol.* **4**, 43–46.

Földi, M. (1977). The lymphatic system, A review. *Z. Lymphol.* 2 1, 44–56.

Källskog, Ö. and Wolgast, M. (1973). Driving forces over the peritubular capillary membrane in the rat kidney during antidiuresis and saline expansion. *Acta physiol. scand.* **89**, 116–125.

Katchalsky, A. and Curran, P. F. (1965). *Nonequilibrium Thermodynamics in Biophysics*, Harvard University Press, Cambridge, Mass.

Kriz, W. and Dieterich, H. J. (1970). Das Lymphgefäszsystem der Niere bei einigen Säugetieren. Licht und elektronenmicroskopische Untersuchungen. *Z. Anat. EntwGesch.* **131**, 111–147.

Kriz, W. and Napiwotzky, P. (1978). Direct capillary–tubular relations: a judgement of their possible relevance. In *Proceedings of an International Symposium on the Vascular and Tubular Organization of the Kidney*, Harvard Medical School, Boston, p. 51.

Mayerson, H. S. (1963). The physiologic importance of lymph. In *Handbook of Physiology*, Sect. 2, Vol. II (W. F. Hamilton, ed.), American Physiological Society, Washington, DC, pp. 1035–1074.

Nielsen, A. E. (1942). A translation of Olof Rudbeck's *Novo excercitatio anatomica* announcing the discovery of the lymphatics (1653). *Bull. Hist. Med.* **11**, 304–339.

Renkin, E. M. (1964). Transport of large molecules across capillary walls. *Physiologist* **7**, 13–28.

Rittinger, M., Pfaller, W. and Deetjen, P. (1978). Quantitative-structural organization of the different nephron segments. In *Proceedings of an International Symposium on the Vascular and Tubular Organization of the Kidney,* Harvard Medical School, Boston, pp. 5–9.

Rusznyák, J., Földi, M. and Szabó, G. (1967). *Lymphatics and Lymph Circulation. Physiology and Pathology,* Pergamon Press, New York.

Yoffey, J. M. and Courtice, F. C. (1970). *Lymphatics, Lymph and the Lymphomyeloid Complex,* Academic Press, New York.

30
Interstitial Albumin Pool in the Renal Cortex: The Permeability of the Peritubular Capillaries in Experimental Diabetes Mellitus

J. E. Stork, P. D. Wilson and G. G. Pinter

Introduction

In the previous paper (Pinter *et al.*, Chapter 29 in this volume) we described a new approach to studying the interstitial albumin pool and drew some conclusions regarding the permeability of the peritubular capillaries to albumin in renal cortex of rats. In this report we give a preliminary account of using these techniques in experiments that were carried out on diabetic and control animals.

An important clinical complication of diabetes mellitus is microvascular disease, which develops primarily in the juvenile form of the disease. Diabetic microangiopathy has an immense literature. Both morphological (Østerby-Hansen, 1965; Siperstein *et al.*, 1968) and functional (Parving and Rossing, 1973; Trap-Jensen and Lassen, 1970) alterations of the capillary bed in various organs have been well established. In the present experiments our goal was to study the development of functional abnormalities in experimental diabetes mellitus in relation to both duration and severity of the disease. We consider this report as preliminary on experiments still in progress. Nevertheless, some trends are already discernible.

Materials and Methods

Male Sprague-Dawley rats, 25 days of age, were injected intravenously with

45 mg/kg body weight of streptozotocin. Animals from the same litter were kept as controls, and some of these received the solvent buffer injection. As no effect of the buffer solution alone was seen, its injection was not consistently administered.

Four weeks after the injections glucose tolerance was tested on all animals. Those animals that showed abnormal glucose tolerance were classified into two groups: The first group, clinical diabetics, was characterized by retarded body weight gain, high water consumption, and high urine flow rate. After about 6 months these rats developed cataracts. The second group included animals which showed no other sign of diabetes except abnormal glucose tolerance. They were termed subclinical diabetics.

The experimentation on capillary permeability was carried out at 6, 9 and 12 months after the injection of streptozotocin. We refer to this time factor as age. Nine groups of animals were studied: controls, subclinically diabetic animals, and clinically diabetic animals in each age group. Our results thus fall into a two-way classification with three levels in each classification. They were evaluated statistically by the method of analysis of variance with unequal numbers of replications in each cell (Table I).

TABLE I

Number of animals in experiments on capillary permeability after injection of streptozotocin[a]

Months after injection	Control	Subclinical diabetes	Clinical diabetes
6	11 (6)	10 (4)	4 (4)
9	6 (12)	11 (12)	3 (5)
12	7 (9)	5 (8)	2 (2)

[a] In each cell the number of animals in the mean transit time experiments is shown without parentheses; the number in the volume of distribution experiments is shown in parentheses.

Results and Discussion

Table II shows the findings on lymph flow from a single cannulated renal lymphatic vessel. Two-way analysis of variance indicated that age had no effect, whereas severity of the disease denoted as "condition" had a highly significant effect. The higher lymph flow in diabetic rats was a consistent finding and amounted to 5–10 times the flow seen in control rats.

Table III shows the lymph-to-plasma albumin concentration ratios in these rats. Here age had a highly significant effect, but the severity of the diabetic condition did not show association with the lymph-to-plasma albumin con-

TABLE II

Lymph flow from one renal lymphatic vessel in microlitres per minute after injection of streptozotocin (means ± S.E.M., analysis of variance)

Months after injection	Control	Subclinical diabetes	Clinical diabetes
6	1·8 ± 0·3	2·1 ± 0·3	8·8 ± 4·1
9	1·4 ± 0·3	2·0 ± 0·4	7·0 ± 2·4
12	1·5 ± 0·5	2·1 ± 0·7	19·7 ± 9·1

Age: $0.27 < p$. Condition: $p < 0.0001$.

TABLE III

Lymph/plasma albumin concentration ratio (means ± S.E.M., analysis of variance)

Months after injection	Control	Subclinical diabetes	Clinical diabetes
6	0·35 ± 0·03	0·37 ± 0·04	0·37 ± 0·11
9	0·48 ± 0·07	0·53 ± 0·06	0·44 ± 0·10
12	0·99 ± 0·17	0·72 ± 0·16	0·65 ± 0·19

Age: $p < 0.001$.   Condition: $0.38 < p$.

centration ratios. It appears that the aging process itself leads to a higher rate of extravasation of albumin, and that in the old control animals increasing the concentration of albumin in lymph was sufficient to drain the extravasated albumin without increase in the lymph flow. In the old diabetics, however, as seen in Table II, increasing flow of lymph was also present in addition to increased lymph/plasma albumin ratio.

Table IV shows the data on the extravascular distribution volume of albumin. The analysis of these data is complicated by the fact that, both with

TABLE IV

Interstitial distribution volume (V) in millilitres per 100 g cortex (means ± S.E.M., analysis of variance)

Months after injection	Control	Subclinical diabetes	Clinical diabetes
6	0·6 ± 0·1	1·2 ± 0·9	2·0 ± 0·8
9	1·3 ± 0·5	2·3 ± 1·0	5·8 ± 4·9
12	2·3 ± 1·5	2·4 ± 1·1	17·6 ± 16·9

Age: $0.16 < p$.   Condition: $0.02 < p < 0.03$.

increasing age and severity of the diabetic condition, there was an increasing concentration of albumin in the urine. Therefore, in the aging and diseased kidneys, there was a substantial amount of intratubular tracer included in the measurement of extravascular albumin volume of distribution. By using a covariance analysis, we made corrections for the intratubular albumin; the variable used for this purpose was the ratio of albumin concentration in the urine to that in plasma. The correction was severe, as indicated by the following comparison: In the normal controls at 6 months, the extravascular pool is shown on Table IV as 0·6 ml/100 g cortex. But in the previous paper, the 10–12 week old control rats (in which the tracer albumin in the urine hardly exceeded trace amounts and where no correction was needed for the intratubular fraction) had a distribution volume of 1·7 ml/100 g cortex. Moreover, it is important to note that urinary albumin increased with age as well as with the severity of the diabetic condition, and the uncorrected values of extravascular distribution volumes tended to increase the same way. The figures corrected by covariance analysis shown in Table IV, however, do not indicate a significant effect of age; yet they do point up an effect of the diabetic condition. Thus, the experimental method and analysis appear to be sensitive enough to discern differences in the effects of aging and diabetic disease in respect to the several variables studied.

TABLE V

Mean transmit time from plasma to lymph ($\bar{t}$) in minutes (means $\pm$ s.e.m., analysis of variance)

Months after injection	Control	Subclinical diabetes	Clinical diabetes
6	21·9 ± 1·2	20·7 ± 0·9	16·7 ± 1·9
9	20·1 ± 1·8	15·3 ± 1·9	17·2 ± 2·0
12	17·4 ± 2·2	16·6 ± 1·1	10·6 ± 2·7

Age: $p = 0.005$.   Condition: $0.05 < p < 0.06$.

Table V depicts the mean transit times of albumin from plasma to lymph as calculated by the method of numerical deconvolution. Although these figures represent the mean values of truncated probability density functions, they are roughly comparable among themselves. First we note that the 21·9 min found in the 6 month old controls is shorter than the 28 min obtained by the same method in the 2–3 month old control rats reported in the preceding paper (Pinter *et al.*, Chapter 29 in this volume). We attribute this to the difference in age, as the decrease of $\bar{t}$ values in the controls seems to be progressive. Next, with regard to condition, the reduction of mean transit time approaches the 5 per cent level of statistical significance, and with regard to age a decrease in $\bar{t}$ seems to be definite.

Table VI represents the unidirectional clearance values of albumin from the plasma into the interstitium. Since, with increasing age and disease, albumin is present in the tubular lumen in ever-increasing quantity, it is possible that some of the albumin entered the interstitium by means of glomerular filtration and tubular reabsorption. Thus far we have been unable to find the means quantitatively to partition the increased clearance of albumin into components according to capillary and tubular sources. We observed that the inorganic isotope content of the cortical tissue was somewhat elevated; in normal controls it was below 5 per cent, whereas in diabetic animals it was occasionally as high as 7 per cent. This relative rise in inorganic tracer may indicate that both reabsorption and metabolism of albumin molecules by the tubular cells have increased, although we cannot give a quantitative estimate.

TABLE VI

Unidirectional clearance of albumin (ψ') in millilitres per second $\times$ 10^{-4} per 100 g cortex (means $\pm$ S.D., analysis of variance using log ψ')

Months after injection	Control	Subclinical diabetes	Clinical diabetes
6	$4\cdot7 \pm 0\cdot8$	$9\cdot2 \pm 7\cdot1$	$20\cdot2 \pm 8\cdot4$
9	$10\cdot6 \pm 4\cdot3$	$25\cdot3 \pm 11\cdot5$	$55\cdot7 \pm 48$
12	$22\cdot6 \pm 14\cdot8$	$24\cdot2 \pm 11\cdot5$	278 ± 275

Age: $0\cdot03 < p < 0\cdot04$.   Condition: $0\cdot02 < p < 0\cdot03$.

As noted on Table VI, the statistical analysis was carried out on the ψ' values after logarithmic transformation. The original values and their standard deviations are shown in the table. It is seen that the variances are not homogeneous to the extent that a basic assumption underlying the analysis of variance was not met. After log transformation the heteroscedasticity no longer precluded the analysis. Both age and severity of the diabetic condition turned out to be significant factors which affect the unidirectional clearance of albumin across the renal interstitium.

We have also made preliminary calculations by using the distributed model which implies that the small components of the interstitial albumin pool are not uniform but the rate constants are statistically distributed over the subunits according to the gamma distribution. By fitting this model, we obtained the mean and the standard deviation of the rate constants for the assembly of subunits within each rat. We find two points worthy of note:

(1) The correlation coefficient between the mean transit times calculated by this method and by numerical deconvolution was 0·93.

(2) The standard deviation of the rate constants within kidney tended to be smaller in the normal controls than in the diabetic animals, as borne out by a non-parametric statistical test. This point is consistent with the hypothesis that the damage caused by the disease process is not uniform throughout the organ.

Conclusions

This paper reports some preliminary results of our experiments in progress on rats made diabetic by streptozotocin injection. We carried out measurements on the interstitial albumin pool of the renal cortex and on renal lymph. Duration and severity of the disease were the experimental variables studied. As littermate control rats showed, the aging process itself produced significant changes in the lymph-to-plasma albumin concentration ratio and the turnover of the interstitial albumin pool. The alterations were more extensive in the diabetic animals. The flow rate of renal lymph was significantly increased in diabetes, and the extravascular pool of albumin showed a tendency to increase in size. The unidirectional clearance of albumin through the interstitial pool was increased with increasing age, and the increase was greatly exaggerated by the disease. There was great variability among animals in the same group.

In studying the kinetics of the extravascular albumin pool in the renal cortex, we have used a new model which permits estimation of the heterogeneity of the turnover among the subunits of the pool. Application of this model in conjunction with the experimental data lead us to the conclusion that, while in a normal control rat variability does exist, in diabetic animals the variability is definitely greater.

Acknowledgement

The excellent technical assistance of Ms G. L. Cook is gratefully acknowledged. This research was supported by USPHS Grant AM 17093.

References

Parving, H. M. and Rossing, N. (1973). Simultaneous determination of the transcapillary escape rate of albumin and IgG in normal and long-term diabetic subjects. *Scand. J. clin. Lab. Invest.* **32**, 239–244.

Siperstein, M. D., Unger, R. H. and Madison, L. L. (1968). Studies of muscle capillary basement membranes in normal subjects, diabetic and prediabetic patients. *J. clin. Invest.* **47**, 1973–1999.

Trap-Jensen, J. and Lassen, N. A. (1979). Capillary permeability for smaller hydrophilic tracers in exercizing skeletal muscle in normal man and in patients with long-term diabetes mellitus. In *Capillary Permeability* (C. Crone and N. A. Lassen, eds), Proceedings of the Alfred Benson Symposium II, Munksgaard, Copenhagen, pp. 135–152.

Østerby-Hansen, R. (1965). A quantitative estimate of the peripheral glomerular basement membrane in recent juvenile diabetes. *Diabetologia* **1**, 97–100.

31
Renal Interstitium Ultrastructure and Capillary Permeability

Karl Heinz Langer

Introduction

The renal interstitium can be subdivided in different parts (Table I). The peritubular interstitium with its two components, the capillaries and the extracapillary interstitial space can be regarded as the specific interstitium of the kidney. Only this part of the interstitium will be discussed here, but it is of interest to compare the interstitial components of cortex with those of medulla because of their different structure and function.

TABLE I

Classification of the renal interstitium

I. Interstitium with the arterial and venous vascular system
   (a) Blood vessels
   (b) Extravascular interstitium
II. Peritubular interstitium
   (a) Capillaries
   (b) Extracapillary interstitium
III. Periglomerular interstitium

The following presentation is based on our experiments on rat kidney (for further details and methods see Langer, 1975a, b, c). The findings correspond essentially to those of Bulger and Nagle (1973), who also described the components of the interstitium in all zones of the rabbit kidney.

Ultrastructure of Interstitium in Cortex and Medulla

Cortical peritubular interstitium

In histological sections, the cortical peritubular interstitium was very small, especially after *in vivo* fixation (by dripping the fixative on the surface of the kidney; Fig. 2). At low magnification the open capillaries appeared to represent the peritubular interstitium, corresponding to the *in vivo* situation, in which the tubules are lying between the abundant peritubular vascularization (Fig. 1). However, at higher magnification cells were recognized outside the capillaries in a wedge shaped region (Fig. 3). This type of location, observable even by histological observation, demonstrates an important principle in the cortex, namely the immediate neighbourhood of tubules and capillaries. Therefore, the interstitial cells, especially the cytoplasm with the nucleus, are situated outside the tubulo-capillary neighbourhood, and are often associated with endothelial cells which showed their greatest cross-section around the nucleus.

The cortical interstitial cells were characterized by small processes which were poor in cytoplasmic organelles and which extended outside the wedge shaped regions. Most of the cytoplasmic constituents, sometimes large Golgi complexes, lysosome-like bodies and often centrioles, were located in the

---

FIG. 1. In vivo *microphotograph of the rat kidney surface showing tubules and peritubular capillaries.* (*From Langer* (*1975a*).)

FIG. 2. *After* in vivo *fixation, the histological section of the cortex corresponds to the* in vivo *situation in Fig. 1; in both, the open capillaries appeared to represent the peritubular interstitium.* (*From Langer* (*1975a*).) × 100.

FIG. 3. *Light micrograph of the cortex, showing a narrow extracapillary interstitium between expanded tubulo-capillary areas and broader areas with cells in a wedge shaped order* (*encircled*). × 380.

FIG. 4. *Contrary to the cortex, interstitial cells* (*arrows*) *and broad interstitial spaces are intercalated between tubules and capillaries in the medulla.* × 950.

FIG. 5. *Electron micrograph showing the ultrastructural appearance of the broad area of the cortical interstitium, which corresponds with the enclosed areas of Fig. 3. IC, interstitial cell; G, Golgi complex; CL, capillary lumen; IS, interstitial space with microfibrils and ground substance.* (*From Langer* (*1975a*).) × 10 000.

FIG. 6. *Electron micrograph of the medulla, showing the broader peritubular interstitium between capillary and tubules; a few processes of interstitial cells* (*asterisks*) *are lying in the dense ground substance. CL, capillary lumen; IS, interstitial space.* × 57 000.

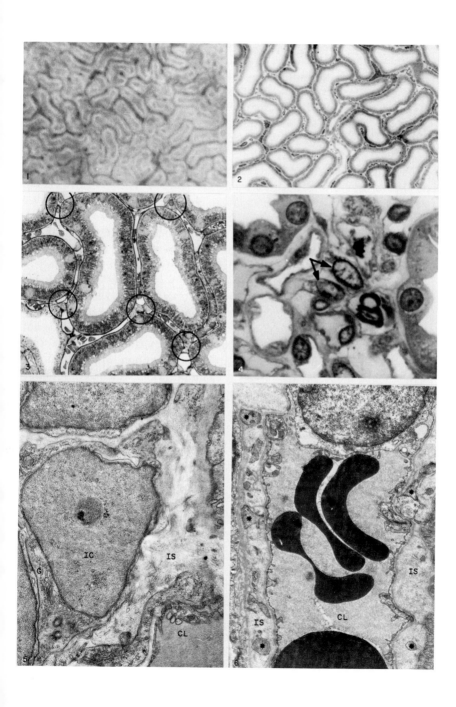

region of the nucleus (Fig. 5). Concerning the functional properties of the cells, Romen and Thoenes (1970) demonstrated in tracer experiments with ferritin that the cells were capable of ferritin storage. In keeping with the well known fibrocytic quality, the authors concluded that the cortical interstitial cells are of a uniform type with bi- (or multi-) functional properties, thus showing fibrocytic as well as histiocytic activities depending upon the prevailing conditions. The alternative interpretations "uniformity of the cell type with different functional stages" and "different cells with separate functions" were discussed by Romen and Thoenes (1970) and Bulger and Nagle (1973).

The remaining two interstitial components, the so-called ground substance and the fibrils, are located around the cells (Fig. 5). The ground substance was observed as a flocculent or moderately dense material. The fibrils were mostly without a periodic substructure and were only 200 Å in diameter (Fig. 7) and are therefore different from typical collagenous fibrils, which were abundant in the large expanded areas of the extravascular and periglomerular interstitium (see Table I). We think that the microfibrils represent mainly the ultrastructural appearance of the so-called "reticulin fibres" in histological silver staining and prefer the term "reticular microfibrils", which revives the early histological term "reticulin" (see Maximow, 1927; Möllendorff, 1930), and is in good agreement to considerations of Osvaldo and Latta (1966b).

In contrast to the zones of interstitial cells, the expanded tubulo-capillary areas contained only a narrow extracapillary interstitium, which was limited by the tubular and capillary basement membranes and which only contained small processes of the interstitial cells or some microfibrils of the reticular type (Figs 3, 11).

FIG. 7. *Electron micrograph showing "reticular microfibrils", i.e. the ultrastructural appearance of reticulin fibres in light microscopy, which are common in the peritubular interstitium.* × 27 200.

FIG. 8. *Peritubular interstitium of the inner medulla with basement membrane-like material, partly in continuity with the basement membrane of a capillary. CL, capillary lumen.* × 20 200.

FIG. 9. *5–10 min after injection of horse-radish peroxidase, the infoldings of the proximal tubules are without reaction product after in vivo fixation, contrary to immersion fixation; inset demonstrates the similar observation in a semithin section. (From Langer (1975c).)* × 11 200; inset × 1000.

FIG. 10. *Inner medulla. Reaction product of peroxidase is located in the capillary, at lower concentration in the peritubular interstitium, and in the infoldings and intercellular space of a collecting duct. CL, capillary lumen; CD, collecting duct.* × 12 800.

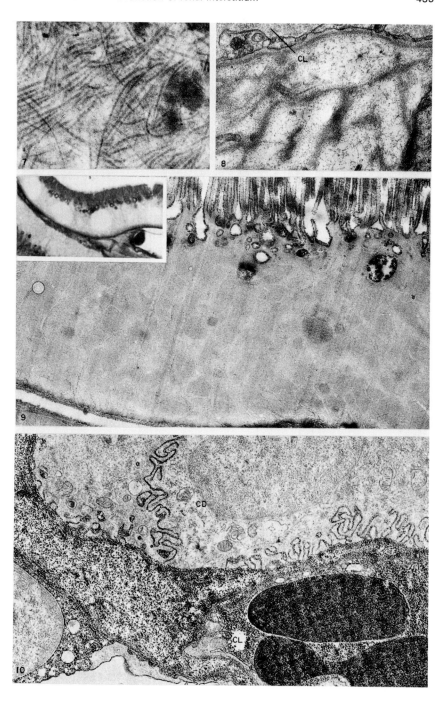

Medullary peritubular interstitium

The arrangement of the cortical peritubular interstitium in broad areas with cells and small tubulo-capillary zones without cells cannot be detected in the medullary interstitium. Instead, the interstitial cells were intercalated between tubules or between tubules and capillaries (Fig. 4) and usually oriented perpendicular to the axis of the tubule. The fine structure of these cells was different from that of the cortical interstitial cells as described by Bohman (Bohman, Chapter 33 in this volume). The other components of the medullary interstitium are well known, since the first ultrastructural descriptions by Lapp and Nolte (1962) and Osvaldo and Latta (1966*a, b*). It seems important to emphasize that the microfibrils were reduced more and more in frequency from the outer to the inner medulla and that the microfibrils were absent in the inner medulla (Fig. 6). A further characteristic feature of the interstitium in the medulla was a basement membrane-like material, which traversed the interstitium, sometimes unrelated to the tubules and sometimes in continuity with basement membranes of tubules or capillaries (Fig. 8).

Comparison of cortical and medullary interstitium

The following important differences can be recognized between medullary and cortical peritubular interstitium: (1) the extracapillary areas are in general broader in the medullary than in the cortical interstitium; (2) characteristic differences exist between cortex and medulla with respect to the composition and distribution of all interstitial components, i.e. interstitial cells, microfibrils, and ground substance.

Considering the fact that great fluid quantities must be moved in a tubulo-capillary direction in the cortex, the ultrastructure of the cortical interstitium seems especially suitable for the so-called *"Endstreckentransport"* (Thoenes, 1961), which is the passive fluid movement from tubular infoldings (lateral intercellular spaces) to capillaries (Ruska *et al.*, 1957; Curran and McIntosh, 1962). This pathway is not interrupted by cells. The abundance of ground substances and basement membrane-like material may be important with regard to the fluid movements in the medullary interstitium, but direct experimental evidence supporting this assumption is lacking. However, in view of the specific differences in the peritubular interstitium of cortex and medulla, the distribution in the peritubular interstitium of blood proteins or experimentally injected tracer proteins deserves particular attention.

Distribution of Tracers and Capillary Permeability

The localization of ferritin and horse-radish peroxidase was determined 5–10 min after intra-aortal infusion of the tracers (for details see Langer, 1975*b*, *c*). Similar studies have previously been reported by Straus (1971, 1972) and Bentzel *et al.* (1971) using horse-radish peroxidase, Oliver and Essner (1972) using tyrosinase, and Venkatachalam and Karnovsky (1972) using catalase and ferritin. When comparing these different studies, interest should be focused on the fixation procedures, since our comparative observations after immersion and *in vivo* fixation (Langer, 1975*c*) showed that they influenced the result in some details.

Figure 10 illustrates the medulla following immersion fixation, 5–10 min after peroxidase infusion. The highest concentration of the reaction product of peroxidase was located in the capillaries. Peroxidase at a lower concentration was distributed outside the capillaries in the interstitium in a uniform manner, and permeated the infoldings and lateral intercellular spaces of the tubules. Similar observations were made after ferritin infusion, although the extracapillary concentration of ferritin was evidently lower than in the capillary lumen (Fig. 15). In the cortex, peroxidase was located in the small portions of the peritubular interstitium, and also in the infoldings of the proximal and distal tubules. Comparable results were obtained after ferritin infusion.

The above observations were made after immersion fixation. After *in vivo* fixation, the infoldings of the proximal tubules did not contain peroxidase and the reaction product was lower in the distal labyrinth (Fig. 9). Obviously, the permament bulk flow of water *in vivo* from the labyrinth (lateral intercellular space) to the capillaries prevented the tracer proteins from entering the infoldings. Only *in vivo* fixation revealed this tracer localization because of the quick equilibration of fluids immediately after termination of the circulation. Our observations are consistent with those of Thoenes (1968), who described a high ferritin content in the infoldings of the proximal tubules after *in vivo* fixation, when the renal vein was clamped during ferritin infusion. Thoenes concluded that this localization was a sequence of an elevated hydrostatic capillary pressure. On the other hand, when the fluid reabsorption was inhibited after ischaemic injury, protein tracers permeated the peritubular interstitium more rapidly than under normal conditions. Thus, after ischaemia and *in vivo* fixation, ferritin or peroxidase (Figs 18 and 19) was demonstrated in proximal labyrinth spaces (lateral intercellular spaces) which were often widened (Langer, 1971).

In the cortex, ferritin molecules showed a higher concentration in the broad areas around the interstitial cells (Fig. 16) than in the small interstitial areas between tubules and capillaries (Fig. 15). It is assumed that the molecules are preferentially permeating from the smaller to the broader areas, because the endothelium along the latter often lacks endothelial pores. The uptake of ferritin molecules by endocytosis in interstitial cells demonstrates the histiocytic activity of these cells (inset in Fig. 16) as early as 5–10 min after intraaortal infusion. It may be speculated that the molecules escape via the lymphatic capillaries, which contain a modified filtrate derived from peritubular blood capillaries (Gärtner et al., 1968; Vogel et al., 1969; McIntosh and Morris, 1971).

Localization of capillary barriers

The observed differences in the concentrations of tracer proteins raise the question of the localization of the structural barriers for the capillary passage. The endothelium of the cortical and most of the medullary capillaries is of a fenestrated type with diaphragms (Figs 11–13; for a characterization of blood capillaries, see Hammersen, 1977). Since ferritin molecules could be demonstrated immediately before, between and behind the diaphragms (Fig. 15), but not along intercellular clefts, it is concluded that these pores were the only structures that allowed ferritin molecules to pass the endothelial wall. On the other hand, the reaction product of peroxidase filled the intercellular spaces, although the staining density was lower than intra- and extracapillary staining density. Nevertheless, we conclude that the peroxidase, like ferritin, mainly penetrated through endothelial pores since (1) the intercellular clefts were very scanty in comparison with the pores and (2) it is likely that the pores are permeable to the peroxidase molecules with a diameter of about 50 Å because they are permeable to ferritin molecules, which are about 110 Å in diameter.

The concentration gradient between capillary lumen and interstitial space

---

FIGS 11–13. *Ultrastructural appearance of the peritubular capillaries with relatively symmetrical 500 Å pores and with diaphragms; arrows in Fig. 11 shows the beginning of the narrow extracapillary cortical interstitium, which is limited by the tubular and capillary basement membranes. CL, capillary lumen. (Figs 12 and 13 from Langer (1975a).) Fig. 11, × 7000; Fig. 12, × 80 000; Fig. 13, × 25 500.*

FIGS 14 and 15. *A concentration gradient exists between capillary lumen (CL) and interstitial space (IS) for both peroxidase (Fig. 14) and ferritin (Fig. 15); Fig. 15 from an unstained section. Fig. 14, × 9700; Fig. 15, × 67 800.*

FIG. 16. *A broader area of cortical peritubular interstitium outside the tubulo-capillary neighbourhood, showing the relatively high content of ferritin. The inset shows ferritin molecules in vacuoles of an interstitial cell, which demonstrates an uptake of ferritin by endocytosis 5–10 min after intra-aortal infusion. CL, capillary lumen; E, endothelial cell. × 47 200; inset 61 600.*

FIG. 17 *Ferritin molecules penetrate to a greater extent pores of glomerular capillaries, which are lacking diaphragms in contrast to peritubular capillaries; the lamina densa (LD) of the glomerular basement membrane prevents a further entrance of molecules. × 65 000.*

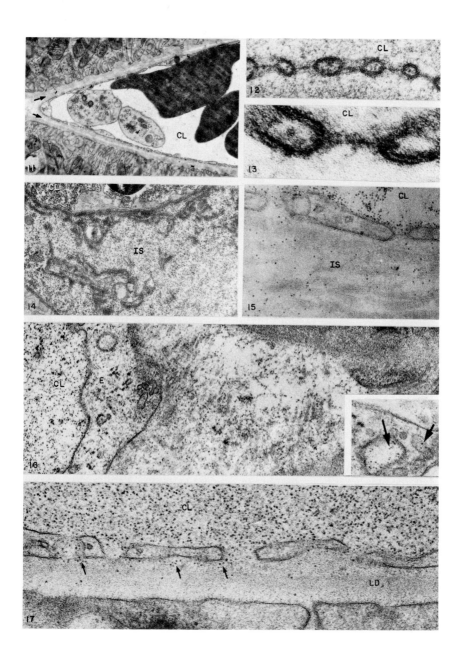

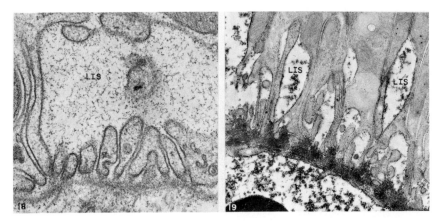

FIGS 18 and 19. *After ischaemia, ferritin molecules (Fig. 18) and peroxidase (Fig. 19) were demonstrated in often widened proximal labyrinth spaces (lateral intercellular spaces, LIS) after in vivo fixation contrary to normal conditions (Fig. 9). (Fig. 19 from Langer (1971).) Fig. 18, × 34 000, Fig. 19 × 13 300.*

for peroxidase as well as ferritin (Figs 14, 15) suggests that the pores of fenestrated capillaries act as a diffusion barrier. This assumption is based on the pore structure, in particular the relatively symmetrical 500 Å openings (Fig. 12) and the presence of diaphragms (Fig. 13), which may be highly organized structures (Maul, 1971). The pore theory of diffusion across endothelial cells assumes two sets of pores in the endothelium (Pappenheimer et al., 1951; Renkin, 1954; Landis and Pappenheimer, 1963). In the endothelium studied here it is likely that the postulated two sets of pores are localized in the same structure, i.e. the endothelial pores (Langer, 1975b).

With regard to the ultrastructural localization of the pores the literature is quite controversial. Thus, Karnovsky (1967) identified the intercellular spaces as the sites of small pores in muscle capillaries and the cytopemptic vesicles as the sites of large pores, while in capillaries of the small intestine, Clementi and Palade (1969) described the fenestrated pores as small pores and the pores without diaphragms as large pores. Venkatachalam and Karnovsky (1972) compared the permeation of catalase and ferritin in kidneys, pancreas, and small intestine, and described passage of tracers largely through endothelial pores and to a lesser extent via cylindrical channels. (In our opinion, the latter structures are scanty in the kidney after in vivo fixation.) At present, the morphological findings have not resolved the problems brought up by the pore theory, and further investigations are necessary to reconcile the morphological and physiological data. The importance of the diaphragms in endothelial pores is evident from the fact that ferritin molecules penetrated capillaries to a greater extent through pores lacking diaphragms, such as in glomerular capillaries (Fig. 17), where the basement membrane prevented a further entrance of ferritin molecules. In contrast, the diaphragms represented a diffusion barrier in peritubular capillaries where the underlying basement membrane did not seem to impede diffusion.

References

Bentzel, C. J., Tourville, D. R., Parsa, B. and Tomasi, T. B. (1971). Bidirectional transport of horse-radish peroxidase in proximal tubule of *Necturus* kidney. *J. Cell Biol.* **48**, 197–202.

Bulger, R. E. and Nagle, R. B. (1973). Ultrastructure of the interstitium in the rabbit kidney. *Am. J. Anat.* **136**, 183–204.

Clementi, F. and Palade, G. E. (1968). Intestinal capillaries. I. Permeability to peroxidase and ferritin. *J. Cell Biol.* **41**, 35–58.

Curran, P. F. and McIntosh, J. R. (1962). A model system for biological water transport. *Nature, Lond.* **193**, 347–348.

Gärtner, K., Vogel, G. and Ulbrich, M. (1968). Untersuchungen zur Penetration von Makromolekülen (Polyvinylpyrrolidon) durch glomeruläre und postglomeruläre Capillaren in den Harn und die Nierenlymphe und zur Größe der extravasalen Umwälzung von ^{131}I-Albumin im Interstitium der Niere. *Pflügers Arch. ges. Physiol.* **298**, 305–321.

Hammersen, F. (1977). Bau und Funktion der Kapillaren. In *Handbuch der allgemeine Pathologie*, III/7, *Mikrozirkulation* (H. Meessen, ed.), Springer, Berlin, Heidelberg, New York, pp. 135–229.

Karnovsky, M. J. (1967). The ultrastructural basis of capillary permeability studied with peroxidase as a tracer. *J. Cell Biol.* **35**, 213–236.

Landis, E. M. and Pappenheimer, J. R. (1963). Exchange of substances through the capillary walls. In *Handbook of Physiology*, Sect. 2, *Circulation II*, American Physiology Society, Washington, DC, pp. 961–1034.

Langer, K. H. (1971). Zum Inhalt erweiterter Labyrinthspalten im proximalen Nierentubulus. *Virchows Arch. B, Zellpath.* **8**, 357–360.

Langer, K. H. (1975a). Niereninterstitium—Feinstrukturen und Kapillarpermeabilität. I. Feinstrukturen der zellulären und extrazellulären Komponenten des peritubulären Niereninterstitiums. *Cytobiologie* **10**, 161–184.

Langer, K. H. (1975b). Niereninterstitium—Feinstrukturen und Kapillarpermeabilität. II. Elektronenmikroskopische Permeabilitätsstudien an peritubulären Kapillaren der Niere (zugleich ein Beitrag zur kapillären Porentheorie). *Cytobiologie* **10**, 185–198.

Langer, K. H. (1975c). Niereninterstitium—Feinstrukturen und Kapillarpermeabilität. III. Untersuchungen über die Verteilung von Tracerproteinen im peritubulären Interstitium und tubulären Labyrinth. *Cytobiologie* **10**, 199–216.

Lapp, H. and Nolte, A. (1962). Vergleichende elektronenmikroskopische Untersuchungen am Mark der Rattenniere bei Harnkonzentrierung und Harnverdünnung. *Frank. Z. Path.* **71**, 617–633.

McIntosh, G. H. and Morris, B. (1971). The lymphatics of the kidney and the formation of renal lymph. *J. Physiol., Lond.* **214**, 365–376.

Maul, G. G. (1971). Structure and formation of pores in fenestrated capillaries. *J. Ultrastruct. Res.* **36**, 768–782.

Maximow, A. (1927). Bindegewebe und blutbildende Gewebe. In *Handbuch der mikroskopishe Anatomie das Menschen*, II/1, *Die Gewebe*, Springer, Berlin, pp. 232–583.

Möllendorff, W. von (1930). Der Exkretionsapparat. In *Handbuch der mikroskopische Anatomie das Menschen*, VII/1, *Harn- und Geschlechtsapparat*, Springer, Berlin, pp. 1–328.

Oliver, C. and Essner, E. (1972). Protein transport in mouse kidney utilizing tyrosinase as an ultrastructural tracer. *J. exp. Med.* **136**, 291–304.

Osvaldo, L. and Latta, H. (1966a). The thin limbs of the loops of Henle. *J. Ultrastruct. Res.* **15**, 144–168.

Osvaldo, L. and Latta, H. (1966b). Interstitial cells of renal medulla. *J. Ultrastruct. Res.* **15**, 589–613.

Pappenheimer, J. R., Renkin, E. M. and Borrero, L. M. (1951). Filtration, diffusion and molecular sieving through peripheral capillary membranes. A contribution to the pore theory of capillary permeability. *Am. J. Physiol.* **167**, 13–46.

Renkin, E. M. (1954). Filtration, diffusion and molecular sieving through porous cellular membranes. *J. gen. Physiol.* **38**, 225.

Romen., W. and Thoenes, W. (1970). Histiocytäre und fibrocytäre Eigenschaften der interstitiellen Zellen der Nierenrinde. *Virchows Arch. B, Zellpath.* **5**, 365–375.

Ruska, H., Moore, D. H. and Weinstock, J. (1957). The base of the proximal convoluted tubule cells of rat kidney. *J. biophys. biochem. Cytol.* **3**, 249–254.

Straus, W. (1971). Comparative analysis of the concentrations of injected horseradish peroxidase in cytoplasmic granules of the kidney cortex, in the blood, urine, and liver. *J. Cell Biol.* **48**, 620–632.

Straus, W. (1972). Cytochemical observations on the transport of horseradish peroxidase in different segments of the nephron. *Histochem. J.* **4**, 517–529.

Thoenes, W. (1961). Die Mikromorphologie des Nephron in ihrer Beziehung zur Funktion. II. Funktionseinheit: Henle Schleife-Sammelrohr. *Klin. Wschr.* **39**, 827–839.

Thoenes, W. (1968). Neue Befunde zur Beschaffenheit des basalen Labyrinths im Nierentubulus. *Z. Zellforsch. mikrosk. Anat.* **86**, 351–363.

Venkatachalam, M. A. and Karnovsky, M. J. (1972). Extracellular protein in the kidney. An ultrastructural study of its relation to renal peritubular capillary permeability using protein tracers. *Lab. Invest.* **27**, 435–444.

Vogel, G., Ulbrich, M. und Gärtner, K. (1969). Über den Austausch des Plasma-Albumin (^{131}I-Albumin) der Niere mit dem Blut und den Abfluß von Mikromolekülen (Polyvinylpyrrolidon) mit der Nierenlymphe bei normaler und durch Furosemid gehemmter tubulärer Reabsorption. *Pflügers Arch. ges. Physiol.* **305**, 47–64.

32
Ultrastructure and Quantitative Characterization of the Cortical Interstitium in the Rat Kidney

Jens Chr. Pedersen, A. Erik G. Persson and Arvid B. Maunsbach

Introduction

The renal cortical interstitium has an important role for the function of the renal tubules since it mediates changes in peritubular capillary oncotic and hydrostatic pressures which modulate the proximal tubular reabsorption rate (Spitzer and Windhager, 1970; Schnermann et al., 1974). However, only a few investigations have dealt specifically with the ultrastructure of the cortical interstitium and the relations between capillaries and tubules (Langer, 1975a; Bulger and Nagle, 1973). Furthermore, little is known about the quantitative ultrastructural characteristics of the interstitium, although attention has recently been focused on this question (Pedersen and Maunsbach, 1973; Pfaller and Rittinger, 1977; Pedersen, 1978; Kriz and Napiwotzky, 1978; Pedersen et al., 1978). Quantitative studies by light microscopy have also emphasized the importance of the interstitium in human renal pathology (Bohle et al., 1977a, b; Mackensen-Haen et al., 1979).

In this investigation we have analysed the relations between tubules and capillaries and determined morphometrically some interstitial compartments of physiological interest. In addition we have studied the lymphatic capillaries and the cortical distribution of ferritin following subcapsular infusion of the tracer.

Methods

Kidneys of male Wistar rats were fixed for electron microscopy by perfusion with 1 per cent glutaraldehyde in Tyrode's solution containing three-quarters of the regular amount of sodium chloride (Maunsbach, 1966) and 2·25 per cent dextran T 40 (Pharmacia, Uppsala, Sweden) (Bohman and Maunsbach, 1970). The kidneys were postfixed in OsO_4, dehydrated and embedded in Epon or Vestopal. Ultrathin sections were analysed in a JEOL 100 B electron microscope.

In five rats the cortical zone extending between 100 and 300 μm below the renal surface was investigated by morphometry. The relative volumes of the cortical components listed in Table I were estimated by point counting.

The relative areas of the walls of proximal tubules and peritubular capillaries facing the narrow and the wide interstitium, respectively (for definitions see below), were estimated by intersection counting using a curvilinear Merz grid (Merz, 1968). By the same method, the relative areas of fenestrated and non-fenestrated parts (see below) of the capillary wall were estimated within the capillary wall facing both the narrow and the wide interstitium.

Subcapsular catheterization was carried out in six kidneys as previously described (Wunderlich et al., 1971). A hole was made in the renal capsule and a subcapsular channel formed using a glass rod with a small spherical tip. A fine polyvinylchloride (PVC) catheter with an outer tip diameter of 40–90 μm was introduced into the channel and the hole in the capsule closed with polymerizing silicon rubber (Ringsted and Semler, Copenhagen). Ferritin (100 mg/ml in 0·9 per cent sodium chloride) was infused into the subcapsular space at a rate of 25–50 nl/min for 1–2 h, and the kidneys were then fixed for electron microscopy as described above.

Results and Discussion

Ultrastructural definition of interstitial compartments
The renal cortical interstitium, which is located between the tubules and the blood capillaries, can, on the basis of ultrastructure and the relations between tubules and capillaries, be divided in two different compartments which are characterized by different volumes and shapes: a *narrow interstitium* between very closely apposed and largely parallel tubular and capillary walls and an irregular *wide interstitium* limited by non-apposed tubular and capillary walls (Figs 1 and 2).

Wide cortical interstitium
The wide interstitium (Fig. 3) is irregular in shape and contains many

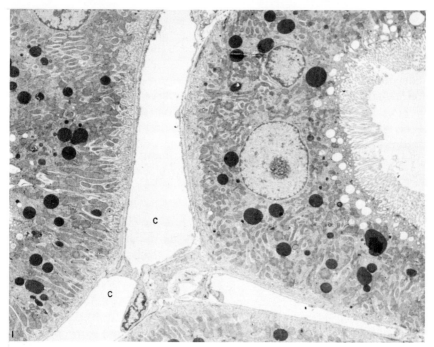

FIG. 1. *Survey electron micrograph of rat kidney cortex illustrating the relationships between proximal tubules, peritubular capillaries (C) and interstitium and emphasizing the close apposition of capillaries and proximal tubular walls.* × *3100.*

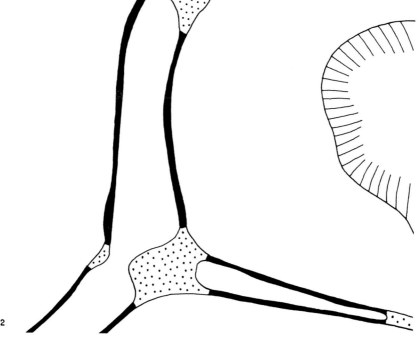

FIG. 2. *Schematic drawing of the area shown in Fig. 1 and outlining the two interstitial compartments: the narrow interstitium (filled) and the wide interstitium (dotted).*

interstitial cells. The cells often have long cytoplasmic processes which pass through the interstitium and adjacent interstitial cells may show sites of close apposition. Some processes are closely apposed to those parts of the capillary walls which face the wide interstitium. In fact, our observations indicate that the interstitial cells form a three-dimensional network within the interstitium. The extracellular matrix of the wide interstitium consists of a dispersed flocculent precipitate and thin fibrils, 150–250 Å, occurring singly or in small bundles.

Narrow cortical interstitium
The main structural components within the narrow interstitium (Fig. 4) are the tubular and capillary basement membranes which show areas of very close apposition. However, they are usually separated by a narrow space which may appear empty or contain a few fibrils of the same dimensions as the fibrils seen in the wide interstitium. Similar observations have been made by Langer (1975a) in the rat renal cortex and by Bulger and Nagle (1973) in the rabbit. A similar narrow interstitium is present around parts of the distal tubules.

Capillary walls
As observed in the electron microscope the capillary wall can be divided in thin fenestrated areas and non-fenestrated areas (Figs 3 and 4). The fenestrated areas consist of thin sheats of endothelial cytoplasm, which are penetrated by pores closed by a thin diaphragm (Rhodin, 1963; Maul, 1971). Occasionally two diaphragms are present in one pore. The non-fenestrated areas are interposed between the fenestrated areas and show ribosomes, mitochondria and the nuclear region. The cytoplasm adjacent to junctions between endothelial cells does not exhibit pores.

Lymphatic capillaries
Lymphatic capillaries were observed close to the interlobular vessels and were characterized, as in other tissues (Casley-Smith and Florey, 1961) by the absence of pores and a basement membrane (Rhodin, 1965) (Fig. 5). As previously described (Kriz and Dieterich, 1970; Rojo-Ortega, 1973; Ohkuma,

---

FIG. 3. *The wide cortical interstitium with parts of several interstitial cells. There is often close apposition between the interstitial cell processes (arrows), and between endothelial and interstitial cells. A floccular matrix material is present throughout the interstitium (✳). × 12 500.*

FIG. 4. *The narrow interstitium between endothelial and tubular walls, containing the endothelial basement membrane (arrow) closely apposed to the tubular basement membranes. × 52 000.*

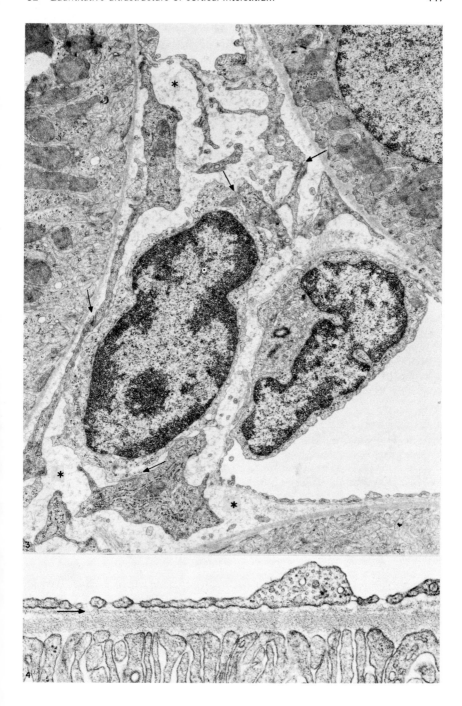

1973; Gorgas, 1978), the lymphatic capillary wall varied in thickness and contained in places single mitochondria, rough endoplasmic reticulum, free ribosomes and Golgi regions (Fig. 6). Many vesicles were seen in the cytoplasm, and the luminal cell membrane showed many endocytic invaginations (Figs 6 and 7). The endothelial junctions varied from simple end-to-end contacts to interdigitating forms (Rojo-Ortega *et al.*, 1973; Ohkuma, 1973; Kriz and Dieterich, 1970).

Volumes of cortical interstitial compartments and capillaries
The relative volumes of the different structural components of the renal cortex are shown in Table I. The proximal and distal tubules together composed 86·2 per cent of the renal cortex and the remaining 13·8 per cent consisted of glomeruli, capillaries (6·5 per cent) and the interstitium, including the two

TABLE I
Relative volumes of compartments of rat superficial renal cortex[a]

Proximal tubules	72·0 ± 2·7	
Distal tubules	14·2 ± 2·4	
Glomeruli	0·6 ± 0·4	
Capillaries	6·5 ± 0·3	
Capillary lumens		5·5 ± 0·2
Endothelial cells		1·0 ± 0·1
Interstitium	6·7 ± 0·2	
Wide interstitial space		3·4 ± 0·2
Narrow interstitial space		0·7 ± 0·09
Interstitial cells		2·6 ± 0·1

[a] Values are expressed as per cent of cortical volume and represent means of five animals ± S.E.M.

FIG. 5. *Lymphatic capillary (L) without basement membrane adjacent to blood capillary (C) with a basement membrane. The capillary wall is of variable thickness and shows no fenestrae. Intercellular contacts (arrows) are present in the lymphatic capillary wall. × 9500.*

FIG. 6. *Golgi apparatus in cell of lymphatic capillary wall. Ferritin particles are seen in the lymphatic capillary lumen (L). × 30 300.*

FIG. 7. *Endocytic uptake of ferritin by the lymphatic capillary wall. Ferritin is present in lymphatic capillary lumen (L) and in endocytic invaginations (arrows) as well as in cytoplasmic vacuoles. × 28 000.*

FIG. 8. *Ferritin in the lumen of a lymphatic capillary (L). An endothelial Junction is present in the capillary wall. The interstitium (✳) contains some ferritin and an interstitial cell process. Fenestrae are seen in the wall of the blood capillary (C). × 40 000.*

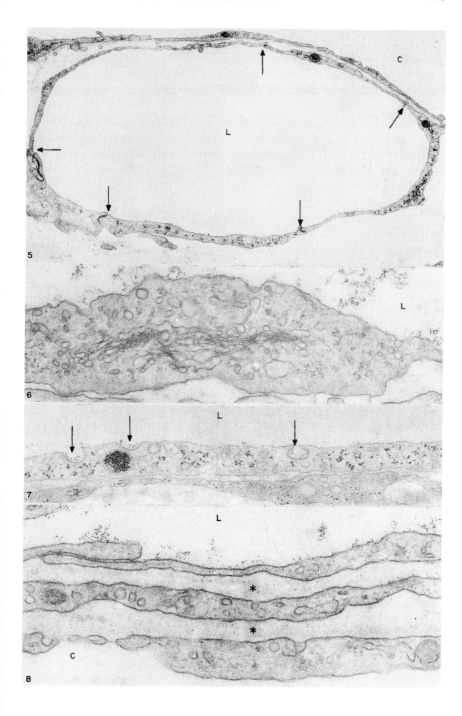

interstitial spaces (6·7 per cent). Pfaller and Rittinger (1977) and Kriz and Napiwotzky (1978) reported a similar quantitative composition of the outer cortex, but did not distinguish between wide and narrow interstitium. Relative volumes of the rat renal cortex, measured by light microscopy, have also been reported. Christensen and Madsen (1978) found a relative volume of capillaries and interstitium of 15·8 per cent, which is close to the presently reported value, and Kügelgen and Braunger (1962) a relative volume of the interstitium and greater vessels of 17 per cent in the dog kidney. In contrast, Faarup et al. (1971) found that the interstitial space alone had a volume of 14 per cent. This discrepancy may be due to the fact that Faarup et al. used kidneys which were excised before freezing and freeze drying.

Quantitative relationships between interstitial spaces, capillary walls and proximal tubules

The capillary wall faced both the narrow and the wide interstitial space (Figs 1 and 2). The proportions of the capillary wall facing the two interstitial spaces were quite different (Table II). Thus, 59·6 per cent of the capillary surface

TABLE II

Relations and ultrastructure of the peritubular capillary wall[a]

Capillary wall facing narrow interstitium around proximal tubules	59·6 ± 1·8	
Fenestrated areas		67·9 ± 0·5
Non-fenestrated areas		32·1 ± 0·5
Capillary wall facing wide interstitium	33·4 ± 2·1	
Fenestrated areas		37·1 ± 3·1
Non-fenestrated areas		62·9 ± 3·1
Capillary wall facing narrow interstitium around distal tubules	7·0 ± 0·6	

[a] Values are expressed as per cent of capillary circumference and represent means of five animals ± S.E.M.

faced the narrow interstitium around proximal tubules, while a significantly ($2p < 0.001$) smaller part, 33·4 per cent, faced the wide interstitium. These two parts of the capillary wall also showed differences in ultrastructure. The capillary wall facing the narrow interstitium was thin and fenestrated in 67·9 per cent of its area, while only 37·1 per cent of the capillary wall facing the wide interstitium was fenestrated ($2p < 0.001$).

This difference in ultrastructure of the capillary wall is partially due to the localization of the nuclear region, which usually faces the wide interstitium. Further analysis of the relations of the fenestrated areas of the capillary wall showed that a total of 76·6 per cent of these areas faced the narrow interstitium around proximal tubules, while the remaining 23·4 per cent faced the wide interstitial space ($2p < 0.001$). Thus, 59·6 per cent of the capillary wall, containing 76·6 per cent of the total fenestrated area, faced the narrow interstitium around proximal tubules, while 33·4 per cent of the capillary wall containing 23·4 per cent of the total fenestrated areas faced the wide interstitium.

The proximal tubule also showed characteristic relationships to the two divisions of the interstitial space. Thus, the smallest part of the circumference of the tubule wall, 42·5 ± 2·8 per cent (S.E.M.) ($n = 5$), faced the narrow interstitium while a significantly greater part, 57·5 ± 2·8 per cent (S.E.M.) ($n = 5$), was related to the wide interstitium ($2p < 0.02$). Kriz and Napiwotzky (1978) found that only 26 per cent of total outer tubular surface was directly related to capillaries.

It appears very likely that the quantitative ultrastructural relationships described above have a functional significance. Our observations suggest that there are potentially two distinctly different pathways for water and solutes from the peritubular surface to the capillary lumen, a long and complex pathway and a short and direct pathway. The long pathway extends from the largest part of the peritubular surface of the proximal tubule and passes through a large interstitial compartment and a capillary wall where pores are sparse. The short pathway passes from a minor part of the peritubular surface through a very narrow interstitial compartment which faces a large part of the capillary surface with a large fraction of the endothelial pores.

Functional communication between interstitium and subcapsular space
Ferritin was observed in the wide interstitium following subcapsular infusion, thus demonstrating a communication between the subcapsular space and the interstitium (Figs 9 and 10). Ferritin was distributed throughout this compartment, but few ferritin molecules were located in the tubular basement membranes. Ferritin was also endocytosed by interstitial cells (Fig. 9) (Romen and Thoenes, 1970) and observed in the narrow interstitium (Fig. 11). The latter observation suggests a communication between the narrow and wide interstitium, although the concentration of ferritin molecules was lower in the narrow than in the wide interstitium and in the former mainly localized in the narrow space between the tubular and capillary basement membranes. The access of the interstitial space from the blood capillaries have previously been demonstrated for protein tracers following intraaortal infusion of ferritin and peroxidase in rats (Langer, 1975b; Thoenes, 1968), and after intravenous infusion of ferritin and catalase in mice (Venkatachalam and Karnovsky, 1972).

Following subcapsular infusion of tracer, ferritin also appeared in the lumen of lymphatic capillaries (Figs 6, 7, 8) and the lymphatic capillary wall showed endocytic uptake of the protein (Fig. 7). A similar endocytic uptake of ferritin by lymphatic endothelial cells has been reported by Casley-Smith (1964) in mice diaphragms after intraperitoneal injections, and by Leak (1971) in ears of guinea-pigs after interstitial injections. Ohkuma (1970) observed carbon particles in lymphatic endothelial cells after intracortical injection in rat kidneys. In the dog kidney, however, Nordquist *et al.* (1973) did not observe lymphatic endocytic uptake of carbon particles after retrograde injections in capsular lymphatic vessels.

The present tracer demonstration of communications between the sub-capsular space, the interstitium and the lymphatic capillaries supports the suggestion by Wolgast *et al.* (1973) that nearly identical protein concentration in fluid samples simultaneously collected from hilar lymphatics and the sub-capsular space reflects the protein concentration in the interstitium. However, this protein concentration probably represents an average value and the protein concentration in the wide and the narrow interstitium might well be different. The present ultrastructural observations also suggest the possibility that the content of the narrow interstitium is more readily equilibrated with the capillaries than is the wide interstitium. A discrepant equilibration between the capillaries and the wide interstitium may explain the observations by Ågerup (1975) that subcapsular perfusion with solutions containing a high concentration of colloids did not significantly alter proximal tubular fluid reabsorption, while similar solutions applied into the peritubular capillaries induced large variations in the tubular reabsorption. It is possible that tubular reabsorption rate to a large extent is determined from the narrow interstitial space that is rapidly equilibrated from the capillary side. Future studies should elucidate the functional importance of the different compartments within the interstitial space.

Conclusions

(1) The renal cortical interstitium can be divided in two structurally different compartments: a narrow interstitium interposed between apposed proximal tubules and the capillary walls and composing 0·6 per cent of the cortical volume and a wide interstitium occupying 3·4 per cent of the cortical volume.

FIGS 9 and 10. *Ferritin in the wide interstitium* (✲) *after subcapsular infusion. The tracer is also taken up by interstitial cells and is present in cytoplasmic vacuoles* (*arrows*). *Fig. 9,* × 28 700; *Fig. 10,* × 30 300.

FIG. 11. *Ferritin in the narrow interstitium after subcapsular injection.* × 46 200.

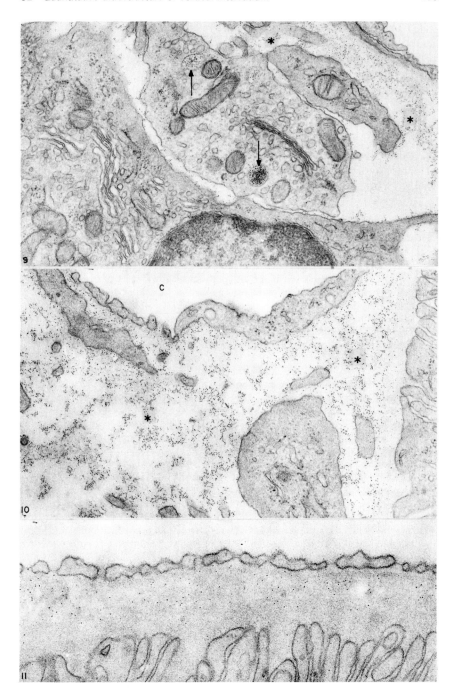

(2) The capillary wall facing the narrow interstitium is significantly more fenestrated than the capillary wall facing the wide interstitium. The periphery of the proximal tubule faces the wide interstitium to a larger extent than the narrow interstitium.

(3) Protein tracer injected in the subcapsular space flows into the wide as well as the narrow interstitium, and can also be found in lymphatic capillaries.

(4) The present ultrastructural observations strongly suggest that the diffusion pathways from the tubular periphery to the capillary lumen follow at least two distinctly different routes which differ with respect to length as well as characteristics of the interposed interstitial components and capillary walls.

References

Bohle, A., Grund, K. E., Mackensen, S. and Tolon, M. (1977a). Correlations between renal interstitium and level of serum creatinine. Morphometric investigations of biopsies in perimembranous glomerulonephritis. *Virchows Arch. A Path. Anat. Histol.* **373**, 15–22.

Bohle, A., Glomb, D., Grund, K. E. and Mackensen, S. (1977b). Correlations between relative interstitial volume of the renal cortex and serum creatinine concentration in minimal changes with nephrotic syndrome and in focal sclerosing glomerulonephritis. *Virchows Arch. A Path. Anat. Histol.* **376**, 221–232.

Bohman, S.-O. and Maunsbach, A. B. (1970). Effects on tissue fine structure of variations in colloid osmotic pressure of glutaraldehyde fixatives. *J. Ultrastruct. Res.* **30**, 195–208.

Bulger, R. E. and Nagle, R. B. (1973). Ultrastructure of the interstitium in the rabbit kidney. *Am. J. Anat.* **136**, 183–204.

Casley-Smith, J. R. (1964). Endothelial permeability—the passage of particles into and out of diaphragmatic lymphatics. *Q. Jl exp. Physiol.* **49**, 365–383.

Casley-Smith, J. R. and Florey, H. W. (1961). The structure of normal small lymphatics. *Q. Jl exp. Physiol.* **46**, 101–117.

Christensen, E. I. and Madsen, K. M. (1978). Renal age changes. Observations on the rat kidney cortex with special reference to structure and function of the lysosomal system in the proximal tubule. *Lab. Invest.* **39**, 289–297.

Faarup, P., Selan, H. and Ryø, G. (1971). Correlation between tubules and capillaries and size of interstitial space in the functioning rat kidney. *Acta path. microbiol. scand.* **79**, 607–616.

Gorgas, K. (1978). Structure and innervation of the juxtaglomerular apparatus of the rat. *Adv. Anat. Embryol. Cell Biol.* **54**, 7–84.

Kriz, W. and Dieterich, H. J. (1970). Das Lymphgefässsystem der Niere bei einigen Säugetieren. Licht- und elektronenmikroskopische Untersuchungen. *Z. Anat. EntwGesch.* **131**, 111–147.

Kriz, W. and Napiwotzky, P. (1978). Direct capillary–tubular relations: a judgement of their possible relevance. In *Proceedings of an International Symposium on Vascular and Tubular Organization of the Kidney*, Harvard Medical School, Boston, p. 51.

Kügelgen, A. V. and Braunger, B. (1962). Quantitative Untersuchungen über Kapillaren und Tubuli der Hundeniere. *Z. Zellforsch. mikrosk. Anat.* **57**, 766–808.

Langer, K. H. (1975*a*). Niereninterstitium—Feinstrukturen und Kapillarpermeabilität. I. Feinstrukturen der zellulären und extrazellulären Komponenten des peritubulären Niereninterstitiums. *Cytobiologie* **10**, 161–184.

Langer, K. H. (1975*b*). Niereninterstitium—Feinstrukturen und Kapillarpermeabilität. III. Untersuchungen über die Verteilung von Tracerproteinen im peritubulären Interstitium und tubulären Labyrinth. *Cytobiologie* **10**, 199–216.

Leak, L. V. (1971). Studies on the permeability of lymphatic capillaries. *J. Cell Biol.* **50**, 300–323.

Mackensen-Haen, S., Grund, K. E., Schirmeister, J. and Bohle, A. (1979). Impairment of the glomerular filtration rate by glomerular and interstitial factors in membranoproliferative glomerulonephritis with normal serum creatinine concentration. *Virchows Arch. A Path. Anat. Histol.* **382**, 11–19.

Maul, G. G. (1971). Structure and formation of pores in fenestrated capillaries. *J. Ultrastruct. Res.* **36**, 768–782.

Maunsbach, A. B. (1966). The influence of different fixatives and fixation methods on the ultrastructure of rat kidney proximal tubule cells. I. Comparison of different perfusion fixation methods and of glutaraldehyde, formaldehyde and osmium tetroxide fixatives. *J. Ultrastruct. Res.* **15**, 242–282.

Merz, W. A. (1968). Streckenmessung an gerichteten Strukturen im Mikroskop und ihre Anwendung zur Bestimmung von Oberflächen-Volumen-Relationen im Knochengewebe. *Mikroskopie* **22**, 132–142.

Nordquist, R. E., Bell, R. D., Sinclair, R. J. and Keyl, M. J. (1973). The distribution and ultrastructural morphology of lymphatic vessels in the canine renal cortex. *Lymphology* **6**, 13–19.

Ohkuma, M. (1970). Fine structure and function of cutaneous and renal lymphatic capillary. *Bull. Tokyo med. dent. Univ.* **17**, 103–111.

Ohkuma, M. (1973). Electron microscopic observation of the renal lymphatic capillary after injection of ink solution. *Lymphology* **6**, 175–181.

Pedersen, J. C. (1978). Quantitative ultrastructural analysis of rat renal cortex. *J. Ultrastruct. Res.* **63**, 91.

Pedersen, J. C. and Maunsbach, A. B. (1973). Ultrastructural characteristics of peritubular capillaries and interstitium in rat renal cortex. *J. Ultrastruct. Res.* **42**, 401.

Pedersen, J. C., Persson, E. and Maunsbach, A. B. (1978). Ultrastructure and quantitative characterization of compartments in renal cortical interstitium. In *Proceedings of an International Symposium on Correlation of Renal Ultrastructure and Function*, University of Aarhus, Aarhus, p. 56.

Persson, A. E., Müller-Suur, R. and Selén, G. (1979). Capillary oncotic pressure as a modifier for tubuloglomerular feedback. *Am. J. Physiol.* **5**, F97–F102.

Pfaller, W. and Rittinger, M. (1977). Quantitative Morphologie der Niere. *Mikroskopie* **33**, 74–79.

Rhodin, J. A. G. (1963). Structure of the Kidney. In *Diseases of the Kidney* (Strauss and Welt, eds), Little, Brown and Co., Boston, pp. 1–29.

Rhodin, J. A. G. (1965). Fine structure of the peritubular capillaries of the human kidney. In *Progress in Pyelonephritis* (E. H. Kass, ed.), F. A. Davis Co., Philadelphia, pp. 391–397.

Rojo-Ortega, J. M., Yeghiayan, E. and Genest, J. (1973). Lymphatic capillaries in the renal cortex of the rat. *Lab. Invest.* **29**, 336–341.

Romen, W. and Thoenes, W. (1970). Histiocytäre und fibrocytäre Eigenschaften der interstitiellen Zellen der Nierenrinde. *Virchows Arch. B Zellpath.* **5**, 365–375.

Schnermann, J., Persson, A. E. G. and Ågerup, B. (1974). Proximal tubular fluid reabsorption—a multifactorial process. In *Proceedings of the Vth International Congress of Nephrology, Mexico, 1972*, Vol. 2, Karger, Basel, pp. 32–41.

Spitzer, A. and Windhager, E. E. (1970). Effect of peritubular oncotic pressure changes on proximal tubular fluid reabsorption. *Am. J. Physiol.* **218**, 1188–1193.

Thoenes, W. (1968). Neue Befunde zur Beschaffenheit des basalen Labyrinthes im Nierentubules. *Z. Zellforsch. mikrosk. Anat.* **86**, 351–363.

Venkatachalam, M. A. and Karnovsky, M. J. (1972). Extravascular protein in the kidney. An ultrastructural study of its relation to renal peritubular capillary premeability using protein tracers. *Lab. Invest.* **27**, 435–444.

Wolgast, M., Persson, E., Schnermann, J., Ulfendahl, H. and Wunderlich, P. (1973). Colloid osmotic pressure of the subcapsular interstitial fluid of rat kidneys during hydropenia and volume expansion. *Pflügers Arch. ges. Physiol.* **340**, 123–131.

Wunderlich, P., Persson, E. Schnermann, J., Ulfendahl, H. and Wolgast, M. (1971). Hydrostatic pressure in subcapsular interstitial space of rat and dog kidneys. *Pflügers Arch. ges. Physiol.* **328**, 307–319.

Ågerup, B. (1975). Influence of peritubular hydrostatic and oncotic pressures on fluid reabsorption in proximal tubules of the rat kidney. *Acta physiol. scand.* **93**, 184–194.

33
The Ultrastructure and Function of the Interstitial Cells of the Renal Medulla with Special Regard to Prostaglandin Synthesis

Sven-Olof Bohman

Introduction

The interstitial cells of the renal medulla are located in the wide medullary interstitium between the collecting ducts, loops of Henle and capillaries, and their cytoplasm contains abundant lipid inclusions (Fig. 1). They have attracted much attention during recent years, mainly because they have been suggested to be endocrine cells secreting some types of lipid hormone.

A secretory function for the interstitial cells was first suggested on the basis of ultrastructural studies (Novikoff, 1960; Gloor and Neiditsch-Halff, 1965; Osvaldo and Latta, 1966; Bulger and Trump, 1966) and the possibility that the cytoplasmic lipid droplets represent a secretory product was discussed (Osvaldo and Latta, 1966). This hypothesis gained much support when it was found that large quantities of prostaglandins could be extracted from renal medullary but not from cortical tissue (Lee *et al.*, 1963, 1967). The presence of an obviously lipid-rich cell type in that part of the kidney which had a high prostaglandin content seemed more than a coincidence, and it was speculated that there was a connection between the interstitial cells and the renal prostaglandin production (Muehrcke *et al.*, 1965). The lipid droplets were suggested to represent a storage of prostaglandins (Nissen, 1967). Reports on variations in the number of lipid droplets induced by experimental hypertension (Mandal *et al.*, 1967) and by changes in salt or water balance of the animals (Nissen, 1968*a*, *b*) were taken to support the suggested connection between the interstitial cells and prostaglandins, since the latter had been found to have effects on blood pressure as well as on sodium and

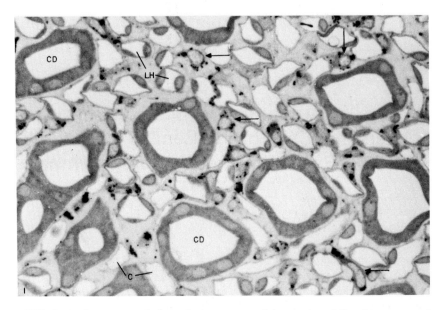

FIG. 1. *Light micrograph from the inner zone of the renal medulla of an untreated rat. In the interstitium between capillaries (C), thin limbs (LH) and collecting ducts (CD) there are numerous interstitial cells (arrows). They contain heavily stained bodies which are the lipid droplets. 1 µm Vestopal section, p-phenylenediamine staining. × 500.*

water excretion. The interstitial cells were proposed to be endocrine cells which produced and secreted the prostaglandins of the renal medulla (Muehrcke *et al.*, 1965; Mandal *et al.*, 1967; Nissen, 1968b; Nissen and Andersen, 1968). This theory has since gained a widespread acceptance although no direct evidence for its correctness has been presented.

Our work in this field has been carried out in order to provide more information about the ultrastructure and function of the interstitial cells and in particular to elucidate the question about their possible prostaglandin synthesizing and secretory functions.

Ultrastructure of the Interstitial Cells in Untreated Animals

Fixation
Because of the special osmotic conditions prevailing in this tissue, the ultrastructure of the renal medulla including the interstitial cells is best studied when the kidneys have been perfusion-fixed with a hypertonic fixative. The exact osmolality of the fixative has to be adjusted according to the species of the animal and its diuretic state, as well as the exact level of the medulla

to be studied (Bohman, 1974; Bohman and Jensen, 1978). Normally only one level of the medulla is optimally preserved with a given fixative solution.

Cell types
The lipid-containing interstitial cells or type 1 interstitial cells (Bohman, 1974) are abundant in the inner stripe of the outer zone as well as in the inner zone of the rat renal medulla. Very similar cells have also been described in other animal species (Bohman and Jensen, 1978) and in man (Bulger *et al.*, 1967). Interstitial cell type 2, a lymphocyte-like cell and type 3, a pericyte, are present in the outermost layer of the inner zone and in the outer zone of the rat and rabbit renal medulla (Bohman, 1974; Bulger and Nagle, 1973). In the major part of the inner zone of the rat, rabbit and gerbil medulla, however, all interstitial cells are of type 1, and only this type will be discussed below, while types 2 and 3 will not be further considered.

Cell shape and topography
The type 1 interstitial cells have an irregular shape with long cytoplasmic processes which are often closely apposed to the basal laminae of the surrounding loops of Henle and capillaries (Fig. 2). In contrast, a close relationship between interstitial cells and collecting tubules is virtually never seen. Some interstitial cells have a flattened shape and surround part of the circumference of one thin limb or capillary, while the majority of interstitial cells have a stellate shape with projections making contact with several of the surrounding structures. Close to the tip of the papilla, many of the interstitial cells have a round shape with few and short cytoplasmic projections. In longitudinal sections the interstitial cells are seen to extend between the parallel rows of loops and capillaries at rather regular distances, like the rungs of a ladder. The processes of the interstitial cells very rarely penetrate the basal laminae of the loops or capillaries. Cytoplasmic processes from two interstitial cells may show areas of close contact with tight junction-like surface specializations (Bulger and Trump, 1966). Occasionally, a single cilium is seen to extend from the surface of the cell body (Bulger and Trump, 1966). Inside the plasma membrane of the cytoplasmic processes there are bundles of 50 Å filaments running parallel to the cell surface, mainly in the horizontal plane.

Nucleus
The nucleus may have different shapes, according to the general shape of the cell. In the rabbit it is often lobulated. Some investigators have found a widely expanded perinuclear cisterna to be characteristic of the interstitial cells (Osvaldo and Latta, 1966) but this is probably a fixation artefact (Bohman, 1974).

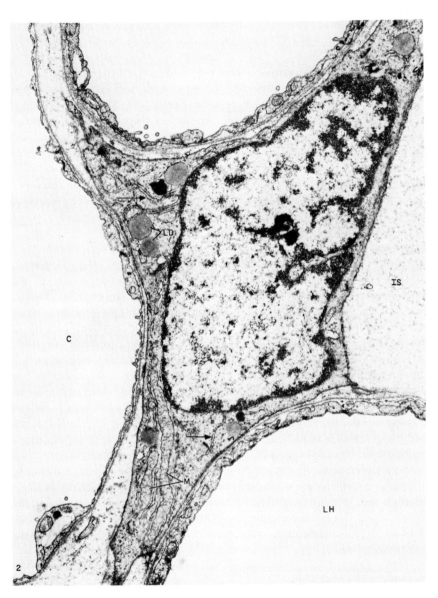

FIG. 2. *Interstitial cell from the middle level of the inner zone of the renal medulla of untreated rat. Note the close relationship to capillaries (C) and loops of Henle (LH). In the cytoplasm there are lipid droplets (LD), elongated mitochondria (M) and some rough endoplasmic reticulum (arrows). IS, interstitial space. × 12 000.*

Lipid droplets

The two most characteristic cytoplasmic features of the interstitial cells are the abundant lipid droplets and the well developed endoplasmic reticulum. As discussed below, it is possible that these two components are functionally related, but they may also reflect different functions of the interstitial cells.

The lipid droplets are usually round and smooth in contour in perfusion-fixed tissue (Figs 2 and 3). Their mean diameter is in the order of 0·4–0·5 μm in the rat (Bohman and Jensen, 1976), while in rabbits and gerbils they are somewhat smaller (Bohman and Jensen, 1978). The content of the lipid droplets usually appears homogeneous and has a moderate electron density, but the latter may vary with fixation method, section thickness, staining procedure and possibly also with the physiological state of the animal. The lipid droplets do not have a surrounding triple-layered membrane (Fig. 3) (Osvaldo and Latta, 1966). Instead they are limited by a somewhat irregular 20–50 Å thick, electron-dense outer zone (Bohman and Maunsbach, 1972). The absence of a surrounding membrane comparable in ultrastructure to that of the plasma membrane or that surrounding the secretory granules of many endocrine and exocrine glands speaks strongly against the theory that the lipid droplets can be released from the interstitial cells by way of exocytosis (Mandal *et al.*, 1975). Furthermore, extracellularly located lipid droplets are virtually never seen in well fixed medullary tissue.

Inside the electron-dense outer zone of the lipid droplets clusters of 50–200 Å large, highly electron-dense and partly confluent granules may be seen (Fig. 3) (Bohman and Jensen, 1978). In addition, a lamellar material is sometimes seen at the droplet periphery. It consists of alternating electron-dense and electron-lucent layers with a periodicity of about 40 Å. In the rat and rabbit the lamellar material is relatively sparse and present only along the periphery of some lipid droplets. In many cells no lamellar material can be seen, and only rarely are large accumulations of lamellar material seen in these species. In the gerbil medulla, however, large masses of the lamellar material are present in a significant proportion of the cells. It usually surrounds very large, so-called "giant lipid droplets" with a diameter up to 5 μm and appears to fill a large part of the interstitial cell cytoplasm (Bohman and Jensen, 1978). The ultrastructure of the lamellar material closely resembles that of so called "myelin figures" which can be made from phospholipid–water mixtures, and this suggests that the lipid droplets may have some relation to phospholipid synthesis or metabolism in the renal medulla.

The lipid droplets may be present in different parts of the cytoplasm, both close to the nucleus and in the cytoplasmic processes. No specific orientation of the lipid droplets in relation to the cell surface can be seen. In contrast

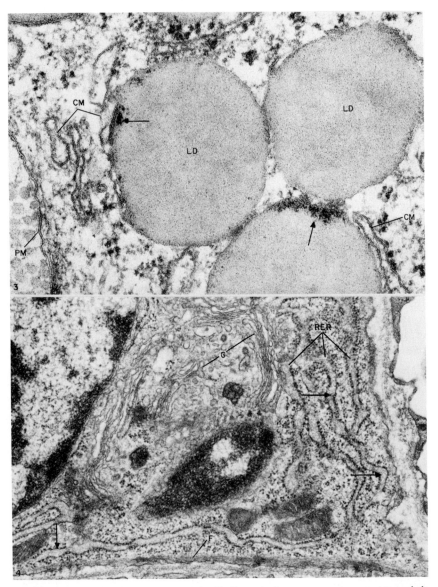

FIG. 3. *Lipid droplets in interstitial cell. Note the homogenous appearance and the lack of a surrounding membrane comparable to the plasma membrane (PM) or the cytomembranes (CM). In certain areas there are accumulations of highly electron-dense granular material at the droplet periphery (arrows). Smooth cytomembranes (CM) are in some places close to the droplet surface.* × 75 000.

FIG. 4. *Part of an interstitial cell from the outermost level of the inner zone of the rat renal medulla. There is a well developed rough endoplasmic reticulum (RER), the cisternae of which are filled with a material of moderate electron density (arrows). A large Golgi complex (G) as well as a peripheral bundle of microfilaments (F) are also seen.* × 32 000.

to the lipid droplets of some other cell types, like hepatocytes or heart muscle cells, the interstitial cell lipid droplets are *not* preferentially associated with mitochondria. This observation, together with the special fatty acid composition of the lipid droplets (Nissen and Bojesen, 1969), as well as the relatively low fatty acid oxidation in the medulla, makes it appear unlikely that the lipid droplets simply represent metabolic energy stores.

Endoplasmic reticulum

The presence of numerous cisternae of rough endoplasmic reticulum is a constant finding in the cytoplasm of the interstitial cells. In the rat the rough endoplasmic reticulum is especially well developed in cells located in the outer levels of the inner zone and in the outer zone of the medulla (Fig. 4). Frequently the cisternae are expanded and filled with a flocculent material of moderate electron density (Novikoff, 1960). This material thus bears some resemblance to the extracellular material surrounding the interstitial cells, and it has been repeatedly suggested that the interstitial cells sythesize and secrete interstitial substances. However, direct proof of such a synthesis has never been presented.

On rare occasions bundles of long, parallel, cylindrical bodies with a diameter of 0·1–0·2 μm are found in the cytoplasm of interstitial cells. They were first described by Bulger *et al.* (1966) who found them to be continuous with membranes of the rough endoplasmic reticulum and to be particularly abundant in dehydrated animals. The latter finding has not been confirmed, however, and the functional significance of these unusual structures remains unknown.

Smooth cytomembranes are also often seen in the interstitial cells. They do not form the common, branched tubular type of smooth endoplasmic reticulum but are usually seen as large sheaths or sometimes as small vesicular profiles. Direct continuity between smooth membranes and the rough-surfaced endoplasmic reticulum can be seen, the smooth-surfaced areas often being close to the surface of lipid droplets (Fig. 3) (Bohman and Jensen, 1978). Occasionally, several concentric layers of smooth-surfaced 60–70 Å thick membranes form a "whorl" around one or a few lipid droplets (Bulger and Trump, 1966). The innermost layer of membranes is in some places closely apposed to the lipid droplet surface (Bohman, 1974). Typically, the lamellar and/or granular electron-dense material of the lipid droplets is found at places where the smooth cytomembranes in the form of sheaths, vesicles or "whorls" are close to the droplet surface. This may reflect a functional relationship and it can be speculated that these cytomembranes contain enzymes involved in the turnover of the stored lipids (Bohman and Jensen, 1978).

Mitochondria, Golgi apparatus and lysosomes

In the cytoplasm there is a moderate number of usually elongated

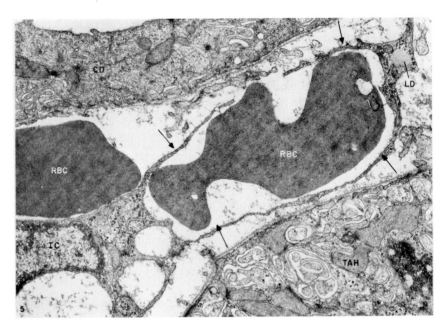

FIG. 5. *Interstitial cell (IC) in the inner stripe of the outer medulla of an untreated rat. Two red blood cells (RBC) are lying in the interstitium and thin cytoplasmic projections from the interstitial cell (arrows) almost completely enclose one of them. LD, lipid droplet; TAH, thick ascending limb of Henle; CD, collecting duct. × 15 000.*

mitochondria (Fig. 2), some lysosomes and a relatively well developed Golgi apparatus (Fig. 4). The latter is usually located in the vicinity of the nucleus. There is also a small number of free ribosomes. Cytoplasmic vacuoles as well as plasma membrane invaginations are few and small, indicating that endocytosis is not very active under normal conditions. However, when the interstitial cells are exposed to foreign substances like horse-radish peroxidase the latter is actively taken up and large vacuoles appear in the interstitial cell cytoplasm (S.-O. Bohman, unpublished). In one preparation there were images suggesting the engulfment of extravasated red blood cells by interstitial cells (Fig. 5).

Experimental Variations in the Structure of the Interstitial Cells

Hypertension
Mandal *et al.* (1967) were the first to report on changes in the number of interstitial cell lipid droplets in experimentally hypertensive animals. These

findings stimulated much new research concening the relationship between interstitial cells and hypertension.

Diuresis

Nissen (1968*a*, *b*), in light microscopic studies, found that salt repletion in salt-depleted rats, and also acute hydration in dehydrated rats, caused an increase in lipid droplets. In the latter type of experiment, rats were deprived of water for 24 h and then given 4 ml of water 1 h before being killed. We performed an ultrastructural stereological study (Bohman and Jensen, 1976) to compare the amount of lipid droplet material in (a) dehydrated rats, deprived of drinking water for 24 h; (b) acutely hydrated rats, treated according to Nissen (1968*b*); and (c) water-loaded rats allowed free access to water and in addition given a total of 12 ml of water before being killed. The electron microscopic stereological method, where the volume density or volume fraction of lipid droplets is determined, has the advantage over previously used methods that the data are quantitative and take into account changes in both size and number of the lipid droplets. No differences were found between animals of groups (a) and (b), with respect to either urine osmolality or amount of lipid in the interstitial cells. However, the water-loaded animals, excreting a urine of relatively low concentration, had more than twice the amount of lipid droplet material than the dehydrated rats (Table I). This difference was due to an increase in both size and number

TABLE I

Interstitial cell lipid droplets of rats in different diuretic states

	Urine osmolality (mosmol/kg water $\pm$ S.E.M.)	Volume density of lipid droplets (per cent $\pm$ S.E.M.)
Dehydrated animals	2180 ± 117	$1 \cdot 9 \pm 0 \cdot 37$
Water-loaded animals	630 ± 124	$4 \cdot 2 \pm 0 \cdot 44$

of the lipid droplets in the water-loaded rats. These results seem to indicate a functional relationship between the interstitial cells and the urinary concentrating mechanism, although the exact mechanism behind the alterations in the lipid droplets is still unknown.

When exactly the same experiment was carried out with rabbits and gerbils (Bohman and Jensen, 1978) the changes in the lipid droplets were smaller in magnitude and opposite in direction to those seen in the rats. These species differences show that great caution is necessary when interpreting changes in the number of lipid droplets in terms of functional roles for the interstitial cells.

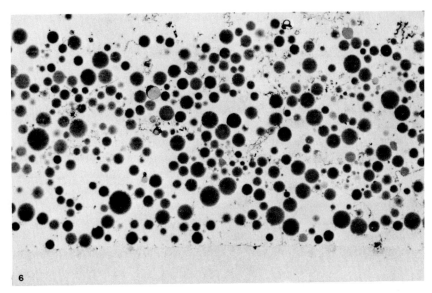

6

FIG. 6. *Lipid droplet fraction isolated from rat renal medulla by ultracentrifugation. The isolated droplets closely resemble the interstitial cell lipid droplets* in situ *and the amount of contaminating material is small.* × 7000.

The Composition of the Lipid Droplets

The lipid droplets of the interstitial cells can be isolated from renal medulla homogenates by a floatation technique in the ultracentrifuge (Bohman and Maunsbach, 1969, 1972; Nissen and Bojesen, 1969) (Fig. 6).

The lipid droplets consist mainly of triglycerides with a variety of esterified fatty acids. In addition there are smaller amounts of free fatty acids, cholesterol esters and phospolipids, but the results from different laboratories vary somewhat with respect to the exact contribution of these components (Änggård *et al.*, 1972; Bojesen, 1974; Comai *et al.*, 1975). In the first analyses of isolated lipid droplets some prostaglandins also seemed to be present (Bohman and Maunsbach, 1969; Nissen and Bojesen, 1969), but this was probably due to contamination from the prostaglandin-rich supernatant since prostaglandins were quantitatively removed by washing of the lipid droplets (Änggård *et al.*, 1972). In the rat lipid droplets, arachidonic acid, the main prostaglandin precursor, was found to make up 15 per cent of the total fatty acids, suggesting that the lipid droplets could serve as a store of prostaglandin precursor (Nissen and Bojesen, 1969). However, considerably lower proportions of arachidonic acid (2–6 per cent) are present in the lipid droplets of other species investigated (Änggård *et al.*, 1972; Bojesen, 1974).

For comparison it can be mentioned that the polar lipids from rabbit medulla microsomes and mitochondria contain 13–15 per cent arachidonic acid (Änggård et al., 1972). Thus, although the absolute amount of arachidonic acid in the lipid droplets is high, they show no enrichment of this fatty acid.

Comai et al. (1975) have investigated the changes in the composition of the lipid droplets isolated from rabbit medulla when the total amount of lipid material was increased by either indomethacin treatment or hydronephrosis. In both cases the proportion of triglycerides was increased (90–95 per cent) compared to controls (72 per cent). Of the total fatty acids, the proportion of adrenic acid (c. 22:4) was decreased. In the hydronephrotic kidneys there was also a relative increase in linoleic acid (c. 18:2), but in the indomethacin-treated animals there were no other significant changes in the fatty acid composition. Neither indomethacin treatment nor hydronephrosis induced any changes in the relative amount of arachidonic acid (c. 20:4).

Thus, the analyses of isolated lipid droplets have so far failed to demonstrate a direct relationship between the lipid droplets and renal prostaglandin formation. Furthermore, it is generally agreed that the arachidonic acid used for prostaglandin synthesis in vivo is mainly derived from phospholipids through cleavage by phospholipase A, and this appears to be the case also in the kidney (Nishikawa et al., 1977).

The Cellular Site of Prostaglandin Synthesis in the Renal Medulla

As discussed above, the interstitial cells were early suggested to be the site of synthesis of the renomedullary prostaglandins. In different, later studies, circumstantial evidence for this theory has been presented and it has become very widely held, although contradictory results have also appeared.

Hypertension

Mandal et al. (1967) reported on changes in the number of interstitial cell lipid droplets in experimentally hypertensive rats and proposed a connection between the lipid droplets and the renal prostaglandins since the latter were known to have a vasodepressor action. However, the role of the renal prostaglandins in blood pressure regulation is still controversial (Dunn and Hood, 1977) and there is no solid support for the proposed relation. Furthermore, later studies have indicated that the changes of the lipid droplets observed in hypertension are not directly related to the increased blood pressure, but to secondary phenomena such as derangements in the renal medullary blood flow and/or the medullary osmotic gradient (Muehrcke *et al.*, 1969; Tobian *et al.*, 1969).

Muirhead *et al.* (1975) have shown that subcutaneous implants of a cultured cell line morphologically identified as the interstitial cell have the ability to lower the blood pressure in various types of experimental hypertension. It was first believed that secretion of prostaglandins was of major importance for this antihypertensive action, but later experiments showed that this is probably not the case (Muirhead *et al.*, 1975). Instead, the endocrine secretion of a so-called antihypertensive neutral renomedullary lipid (ANRL) has been implicated. The precise nature of this substance and its mode of action is still unknown.

Diuresis

Nissen (1968*b*) suggested that an increase in the number of lipid droplets which he observed during hydration of dehydrated rats was related to the previously demonstrated effects of prostaglandins on ADH-stimulated fluid transport. However, since the role of prostaglandins in renal physiology is still unclear (Dunn and Hood, 1977), it is not possible, on the basis of these experiments, to determine if a relation exists between the lipid droplets and prostaglandin synthesis.

Tissue culture

Muirhead *et al.* (1972) demonstrated that prostaglandins could be synthezised in tissue cultures of cells identified as renomedullary interstitial cells. This should not be interpreted to indicate that the capacity to produce prostaglandins is a specific feature of the interstitial cells, since possible prostaglandin synthesis in other medullary cell types was not investigated.

Bartter's syndrome

Verberckmoes *et al.* (1976) have recently reported on a hyperplasia of the interstitial cells of the renal medulla in a patient with Bartter's syndrome. In this rare electrolyte disorder increased amounts of prostaglandins are excreted in the urine and treatment with indomethacin has been found to be effective. Thus, an increase in renal prostaglandin systhesis seems to be an important pathogenetic factor and Verberckmoes *et al.* suggested that hyperplasia of the interstitial cells was the cause of this overproduction. The hyperplasia of interstitial cells has not been convincingly documented, however. A light micrograph of the renal medulla of the patient investigated was published but the tissue preservation is poor and it is very difficult to identify the different cell types in this micrograph. No cell counts were made nor was any normal kidney tissue presented for comparison.

Indomethacin treatment

Studies on the effect of indomethacin treatment on the interstitial cells are contradictory. Injection of indomethacin into rabbits results in a considerable increase in the number of lipid droplets (Comai *et al.*, 1975), while in rats lipid droplets are reduced in number (Limas *et al.*, 1976). In both cases the results have been interpreted to support the hypothesis that the lipid droplets are directly related to prostaglandin synthesis, but it cannot be excluded that the changes observed were due to secondary effects from the inhibition of the prostaglandin synthesis, such as alterations in the salt or water balance of the animals, which are known to influence the number of lipid droplets (Nissen, 1968*a*; Bohman and Jensen, 1976). As described above, alterations in the water balance induce changes in opposite directions in rats and rabbits (Bohman and Jensen, 1978). Muirhead *et al.* (1975) reported an indomethacin-induced increase in size and number of lipid droplets in *in vitro* cultures of rat cells identified as interstitial cells. The opposite effect is seen in the rat cells *in vivo* (Limas *et al.*, 1976). This may be taken to support the above suggestion that the effect of indomethacin on the lipid droplets, at least *in vivo*, is an indirect one.

Histochemical studies

Histochemical methods based on the oxidation of 3,3'-diaminobenzidine (Janszen and Nugteren, 1973) or on specific immunofluorescence directed against the fatty acid cyclooxygenase (Smith and Wilkin, 1977) have detected prostaglandin synthetase virtually only in the collecting duct cells in the renal medulla. The method based on the benzidine reaction (Janszen and Nugteren, 1973) has been subjected to serious criticism, however, and may in fact not demonstrate prostaglandin synthetase activity (Bohman, 1977; Litwin, 1977). The immunofluorescence method (Smith and Wilkin, 1977) appears more promising, but the results obtained are in complete contradiction to the theory that the interstitial cells are responsible for the production of prostaglandins in the renal medulla.

Direct biochemical measurements

In order to solve some of the above controversy, a study was undertaken to test the possibility that prostaglandin synthesis in the renal medulla is confined to one cell type only (Bohman, 1977). Slices with a thickness of 200–300 μm were cut from the rabbit renal papilla perpendicular to the course of the medullary tubules and immersed in a hypertonic saline medium. Under a stereomicroscope the cross-sectioned collecting ducts were easily identified on the cut surface (Fig. 7) and the collecting duct cells were removed by suction through a micropipette (tip diameter 40–50 μm) mounted on a micro-

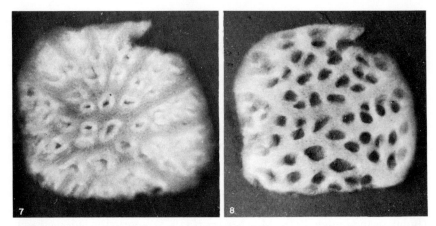

FIG. 7. *Tissue slice cut from the rabbit renal papilla, immersed in a hypertonic saline medium ("dissection medium") and photographed through the stereomicroscope. The cross-sectioned collecting ducts are seen as light rings on the cut surface.* × 25.

FIG. 8. *Dissected slice. The same slice as in Fig. 7, but after the removal of the collecting duct cells by the technique described in the text. By electron microscopy it could be shown that the collecting duct basal laminae were always retained in the dissected slices, explaining the smooth contours of the resulting "holes".* × 25.

manipulator. The removed cellular material (collecting duct fraction) was trapped in a small test tube. By light microscope stereology it could be shown that 92 per cent of the collecting duct cells were removed from the slices. The remainders of the slices, referred to as dissected slices, were essentially devoid of collecting duct cells and thus contained three main cell types: the epithelial cells of the thin limb of Henle's loop, the endothelial cells and the interstitial cells (Fig. 8).

A sensitive quantitative radioactive substrate assay for prostaglandin synthetase was developed (Bohman and Larsson, 1975; Bohman, 1977) and the following four preparations were subjected to such analysis using ^{14}C-labelled arachidonic acid as substrate: collecting duct fraction, dissected slices, samples of the medium used for immersion of the slices during dissection, and whole slices treated like the dissected ones except that the collecting duct cells were not removed.

The distribution of prostaglandin synthetase between the different fractions is shown in Fig. 9. The isolated collecting duct fraction contained 39 ± 4.5 (s.e.m.) per cent of the recovered activity, the dissected slices (cells of Henle's loop, endothelial cells, interstitial cells) contained 53 ± 4.8 (s.e.m.) per cent and the dissection medium contained 7 ± 2.8 (s.e.m.) per cent. When a correction is made for the remnants (8 per cent) of collecting duct cells that were retained in the dissected slices, the proportion of the prostaglandin

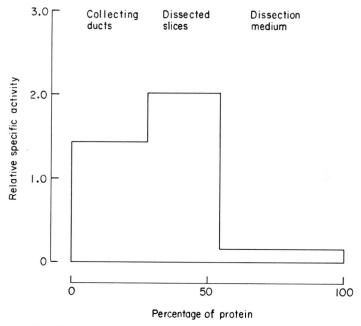

FIG. 9. *Distribution of prostaglandin synthetase and protein in tissue slices from the rabbit renal papilla. The proportion of the total enzyme activity present in a given fraction corresponds to the area of the diagram under this fraction. The recovery of prostaglandin synthetase was 88 ± 10 per cent (S.E.M.) and of protein 110 ± 13 per cent (S.E.M.). Relative specific activity is defined as percentage of total activity/percentage of total protein.*

synthetase activity present in the collecting ducts is increased to 42 per cent and the proportion present in the other cell types is correspondingly reduced to 50 per cent. In addition, the activity recovered in the dissected medium was probably derived from damaged cells of different types.

The above results are not in complete agreement with the results obtained by Smith and Wilkin (1977), who found a positive immunofluorescence staining for fatty acid cyclooxygenase (the first step of the prostaglandin synthetase) only in the collecting ducts when rabbit renal medulla was studied. The reason for this discrepancy is not apparent, but it is suggested that negative immunofluorescence staining in certain tissue components is not indicative of the absence of the enzyme. However, it seems not simply to be a matter of sensitivity, since by direct biochemical assay about half of the enzyme activity was found outside the collecting ducts and in this location the specific activity of the enzyme was higher than in the collecting ducts (Fig. 9).

The collecting duct cells contain close to half of the renal medullary prostaglandin synthetase. Since in these experiments the activities related to cells of the thin limbs, endothelial cells and interstitial cells were not distinguished, the interstitial cells may well contain prostaglandin synthetase, but this clearly is a property shared by other medullary cells. At present, therefore, there seems to be no basis for considering the interstitial cells as specialized prostaglandin-producing cells. However, as discussed above, it is possible that hormone-like substances other than prostaglandins may be secreted by the interstitial cells.

Conclusions

The interstitial cells of the renal medulla have topographical and ultra-structural features which distinguish them from other types of interstitial and connective tissue cells and it appears likely that they represent a unique cell type.

The ultrastructural observations suggest that the interstitial cells are capable of a high protein synthesis as well as lipid synthesis, and the turnover of their abundant neutral lipids appear to be closely related to the urinary concentrating mechanism. A possible release of lipids from the interstitial cells does not appear to take place by way of exocytosis of whole lipid droplets.

The interstitial cells have a capacity for endocytosis, but the endocytic mechanism is not very active.

The hypothesis that the interstitial cells represent a specialized prosta-glandin-secreting cell type appears unlikely to be true, and the lipid droplets may not be directly related to prostaglandin synthesis. Other functions for the interstitial cells must be considered and the possibility that they are endocrine cells producing other hormone-like substances deserves further attention.

Acknowledgements

The original research reported here was supported by the Danish Medical Research Council.

References

Änggård, E., Bohman, S.-O., Griffin, J. E., III, Larsson, C. and Maunsbach, A. B. (1972). Subcellular localization of the prostaglandin system in the rabbit renal papilla. *Acta physiol. scand.* **84**, 231–246.

Bohman, S.-O. (1974). The ultrastructure of the rat renal medulla as observed after improved fixation methods. *J. Ultrastruct. Res.* **47**, 329–360.

Bohman, S.-O. (1977). Demonstration of prostaglandin synthesis in collecting duct cells and other cell types of the rabbit renal medulla. *Prostaglandins* **14**, 729–744.

Bohman, S.-O. and Jensen, P. K. A. (1976). Morphometric studies on the lipid droplets of the interstitial cells of the renal medulla in different states of diuresis. *J. Ultrastruct. Res.* **55**, 182–192.

Bohman, S.-O. and Jensen, P. K. A. (1978). The interstitial cells in the renal medulla of rat, rabbit and gerbil in different states of diuresis. *Cell Tissue Res.* **189**, 1–18.

Bohman, S.-O. and Larsson, C. (1975). Prostaglandin synthesis in membrane fractions from the rabbit renal medulla. *Acta physiol. scand.* **94**, 244–258.

Bohman, S.-O. and Maunsbach, A. B. (1969). Isolation of the lipid droplets from the interstitial cells of the renal medulla. *J. Ultrastruct. Res.* **29**, 569.

Bohman, S.-O. and Maunsbach, A. B. (1972). Ultrastructure and biochemical properties of subcellular fractions from rat renal medulla. *J. Ultrastruct. Res.* **38**, 225–245.

Bojesen, I. (1974). Quantitative and qualitative analyses of isolated lipid droplets from interstitial cells in renal papillae from various species. *Lipids* **9**, 835–843.

Bulger, R. E. and Nagle, R. B. (1973). Ultrastructure of the interstitium in the rabbit kidney. *Am. J. Anat.* **136**, 183–204.

Bulger, R. E. and Trump, B. F. (1966). Fine structure of the rat renal papilla. *Am. J. Anat.* **118**, 685–721.

Bulger, R. E., Griffith, L. D. and Trump, B. F. (1966). Endoplasmic reticulum in rat renal interstitial cells: molecular rearrangement after water deprivation. *Science, N.Y.* **151**, 83–86.

Bulger, R. E., Tisher, C. C., Myers, C. H. and Trump, B. F. (1967). Human renal ultrastructure II. The thin limb of Henle's loop and the interstitium in healthy individuals. *Lab. Invest.* **16**, 124–141.

Comai, K., Farber, S. J. and Paulsrud, J. R. (1975). Analyses of renal medullary lipid droplets from normal, hydronephrotic, and indomethacin treated rabbits. *Lipids* **10**, 555–561.

Dunn, M. J. and Hood, V. L. (1977). Prostaglandins and the kidney. *Am. J. Physiol.* **233**, F169–F184.

Gloor, F. and Neiditsch-Halff, L. A. (1965). Die interstitiellen Zellen des Nierenmarkes der Ratte. *Z. Zellforsch. mikrosk. Anat.* **66**, 488–495.

Janszen, F. H. A. and Nugteren, D. H. (1973). A histochemical study of the prostaglandin biosynthesis in the urinary system of rabbit, guinea pig, golden hamster and rat. *Adv. Biosci.* **9**, 287–292.

Lee, J. B., Hickler, R. B., Saravis, C. A. and Thorn, G. W. (1963). Sustained depressor effect of renal medullary extract in the normotensive rat. *Circulation Res.* **13**, 359–366.

Lee, J. B., Crowshaw, K., Takman, B. H. and Attrep, K. A. (1967). The identification of prostaglandins E_2, $F_{2\alpha}$ and A_2 from rabbit kidney medulla. *Biochem. J.* **105**, 1251–1260.

Limas, C., Limas, C. J. and Gesell, M. S. (1976). Effects of indomethacin on renomedullary interstitial cells. *Lab. Invest.* **34**, 522–528.

Litwin, J. A. (1977). Does diaminobenzidine demonstrate prostaglandin synthetase? *Histochemistry* **53**, 301–315.

Mandal, A. K., Muehrcke, R. C., Epstein, M. and Volini, F. I. (1967). Relationship of the renomedullary interstitial cells to experimental hypertension. *J. Lab. clin. Med.* **70**, 872–873.

Mandal, A. K., Frohlich, E. D., Chrysant, K., Nordquist, J., Pfeffer, M. A. and Clifford, M. (1975). A morphological study of the renal papillary granule: analysis in the interstitial cell and in the interstitium. *J. Lab. clin. Med.* **85**, 120–131.

Muehrcke, R. C., Rosen, S. and Volini, F. I. (1965). The interstitial cells of the renal papilla: Light and electron microscopic studies. In *Progress in Pyelonephritis* (E. H. Kass, ed.), F. A. Davis Co., Philadelphia, pp. 422–433.

Muehrcke, R. C., Mandal, A. K., Epstein, M. and Volini, F. I. (1969). Cytoplasmic granularity of the renal medullary interstitial cells in experimental hypertension. *J. Lab. clin. Med.* **73**, 299–308.

Muirhead, E. E., Germain, G. S., Armstrong, F. B., Brooks, B., Leach, B. E., Byers, L. W., Pitcock, J. A. and Brown, P. (1975). Endocrine-type antihypertensive function of renomedullary interstitial cells. *Kidney Int.* **8**, S271–S282.

Muirhead, E. E., Germain, G., Leach, B. E., Pitcock, J. A., Stephenson, P., Brooks, B., Brosius, W. L., Daniels, E. G. and Hinman, J. W. (1972). Production of renomedullary prostaglandins by renomedullary interstitial cells grown in tissue culture. *Circulation Res.* **30** and **31**, Suppl. II, 161–172.

Nishikawa, K., Morrison, A. and Needleman, P. (1977). Exaggerated prostaglandin biosynthesis and its influence on renal resistance in the isolated hydronephrotic rabbit kidney. *J. clin. Invest.* **59**, 1143–1150.

Nissen, H. M. (1967). On lipid droplets in renal interstitial cells. I. A histochemical study. *Z. Zellforsch. mikrosk. Anat.* **83**, 76–81.

Nissen, H. M. (1968*a*). On lipid droplets in renal interstitial cells. II. A histological study on the number of droplets in salt depletion and acute salt repletion. *Z. Zellforsch. mikrosk. Anat.* **85**, 483–491.

Nissen, H. M. (1968*b*). On lipid droplets in renal interstitial cells. III. A histological study on the number of droplets during hydration and dehydration. *Z. Zellforsch. mikrosk. Anat.* **92**, 52–61.

Nissen, H. M. and Andersen, H. (1968). On the localization of a prostaglandin-dehydrogenase activity in the kidney. *Histochemie* **14**, 189–200.

Nissen, H. M. and Bojesen, I. (1969). On lipid droplets in renal interstitial cells. IV. Isolation and identification. *Z. Zellforsch. mikrosk. Anat.* **97**, 274–284.

Novikoff, A. B. (1960). The rat kidney: cytochemical and electron microscopic studies. In *Biology of Pyelonephritis* (E. L. Quinn and E. H. Kass, eds), Little, Brown and Co., Boston, pp. 113–144.

Osvaldo, L. and Latta, H. (1966). Interstitial cells of the renal medulla. *J. Ultrastruct. Res.* **15**, 589–613.

Smith, W. L. and Wilkin, G. P. (1977). Immunochemistry of prostaglandin endoperoxide-forming cyclooxygenases: the detection of the cyclooxygenases in rat, rabbit and guinea pig kidneys by immunofluorescence. *Prostaglandins* **13**, 873–890.

Tobian, L., Ishii, M. and Duke, M. (1969). Relationship of cytoplasmic granules in renal papillary interstitial cells to "post-salt" hypertension. *J. Lab. clin. Med.* **73**, 309–319.

Verberckmoes, R., van Damme, B., Clement, J., Amery, A. and Michielsen, P. (1976). Bartter's syndrome with hyperplasia of renomedullary cells: successful treatment with indomethacin. *Kidney Int.* **9**, 302–307.

Part V

Concluding Remarks

34
Concluding Remarks

Johannes A. G. Rhodin

A wealth of detailed structural information is now available about almost every part of the kidney. In fact, one sometimes wonders if it would not be better to have less information about all these minute components and more about what they are really doing. This, of course, has been the main theme of this symposium, the correlation of renal ultrastructure and function.

The work presented by many of the participants in this symposium has shown that the most fruitful analysis is done where there is collaboration between the cell biologist and the physiologist. I wish more researchers would follow the approach taken by Arvid Maunsbach and join up with a critical and stimulating physiologist such as Emile Boulpaep, who is not only very knowledgeable, but who can also ask simple—and for the morphologist very irritating—questions at the right time and on the right subject. Personally, I have had the good fortune of working with a physiologist as well as with a physicist during the past several years in the field of vascular reactivity. It is remarkable how this influences an anatomist's way of defining the important issues in terms of clarifying which is of real significance in exploring structural and functional relationships. It is therefore my personal conviction that more valuable information related to renal ultrastructure and function will come out of collaborative work. Another outstanding example was given during this symposium by Marilyn Farquhar, who demonstrated so beautifully the importance of the multilateral, multidirectional approach to a problem.

At the end of each day, we have had a pretty good summation of the important points raised that day. I will not attempt to go over these again, except to point out some of the observations which to me represent some of the highlights of this symposium.

Glomerulus

With regard to the *filtration barrier* of the renal glomerulus, the basal lamina (or, as it used to be called, basement membrane) is still the most likely candidate for determining what is being filtered, and what is not, since the endothelium does not seem to be very actively involved in the filtration process. Indirectly, of course, the epithelial podocytes are involved, since they very likely regulate the metabolism of the basal lamina and its turnover.

Tubules

As to the renal tubules, it is obvious that the extent of the involvement of the so-called *paracellular transport system* is not resolved. The invaginations of the cell membrane and the complicated *cellular interdigitations* are there probably to increase the cell surface, and hence the amount of enzymes or degree of surface area available for enzymic activities. This is a unique situation, and is not found to this extent in any other mammalian organ. As far as the *cellular attachments* are concerned, it is still too early to draw far-reaching conclusions as to their functional significance. Yet it is important that they be explored, and that their three-dimensional orientation is mapped out. Eventually, this information will be very valuable, when taken together with other pieces of information, such as, for instance, the detailed exploration of interendothelial attachment specializations in the various segments of the renal vascular channels.

Concerning the *transepithelial transport system*, it is quite apparent that there are no patent channels present. The exploration of the *endoplasmic reticulum* as a potential candidate for transport is exciting, but with present methods of fixation it does not emerge as a transepithelial channel. The role of the *endocytic vacuoles* near the apical cell surface is clearly to participate in the uptake of proteins and other particles of large molecular size. These are, in turn, passed on to the lysosomal system of the cell for digestion and breakdown. This point was very elegantly demonstrated, when it was shown that sodium maleate interrupts the fusion of the endocytic vacuoles with the lysosomes, thereby preventing protein digestion. It has, so far, not been shown that the endocytic vacuoles serve as transepithelial carriers. *Autophagy* does exist to a large extent in the proximal tubule cells, another major role for the many lysosomes of these cells. There is no evidence for transtubular transport of proteins outside the endocytic vacuoles, except for amino acids. The function of the *brush border extensions* (microvilli) is clearly to serve as an enzymic platform during hydrolysis of small peptides.

Renal Interstitium

This difficult area of the kidney is gradually yielding new information, and there are some first attempts to explore mechanisms of tubulo-glomerular feedback. Also, a better understanding has been gained with reference to the extent of the interstitial albumin pool. The role and function of the lipid-laden interstitial cells is still not resolved, but it is assumed, in some quarters, that they may serve as a source of prostaglandins. Topographic relationship between the interstitial space and the peritubular capillaries apparently differs depending on which side of the capillary faces the interstitium, its fenestrated or its non-fenestrated part.

Future Research Orientation

With the hope of stimulating new approaches to research in this field, the following suggestions are offered.

For a certain problem, try to find the right species before embarking upon a long journey of research. The great renal physiologist Homer W. Smith, whom I had the pleasure and privilege of knowing for some time, claimed that God had, in his wisdom, created an animal or a species which would be ideal for a certain experiment. It was only up to the investigator to match the right experiment with the right animal.

More work should be done with single-nephron perfusion preparations. One must isolate the segment to be studied, using micromanipulation, micropuncture and microperfusion techniques, followed by electron microscope analysis of the identical segment. And the entire procedure must be done under strict physiological control. In this connection, the classical work on tubular microdissections by Jean Oliver (1944), the most outstanding renal pathologist the world has ever known, should be repeated in freshly perfused kidneys.

Very little progress has been done in the area of tubular secretion. Here, one should repeat the early light microscope work done by Roy Forster (Forster and Taggart, 1950) with phenol red secretion, using his technique of fresh kidney slices, combining this with fixation and electron microscope studies. A combination of microangiography (Ljungqvist, 1963) with light microscope and electron microscope studies may clarify many as yet poorly understood relationships between the vascular bed and the nephrons, particularly in the medulla and the papilla of the kidney. Intravital microscopy of cortical nephrons, begun by Steinhausen et al. (1977), using a combination of fluorescein-conjugated, electron-dense markers should be extended to include electron microscopy as well. This may provide information on what really goes through the glomerular filtration membrane with the possible exploration of intraglomerular permeability differences, as well as the discovery of shunts and thoroughfares.

Other areas need much more work. One such field is that of renal pathology (Allen, 1951), both experimental and in humans. Morphometry (Weibel *et al.*, 1969) is a must in future structural studies in order to quantify many of the experimental approaches. Radioautography is a very powerful tool when coupled with electron microscopy, and the techniques of culturing and isolating kidney cells (Karnovsky and Kreisberg, Chapter 8 in this volume) are highly important methods for the correlation of structural and functional parameters of the kidney.

References

Allen, A. C. (1951). *The Kidney*, Grune and Stratton, New York.
Forster, R. P. and Taggart, J. V. (1950). Use of isolated renal tubules for the examination of metabolic processes associated with active cellular transport. *J. cellul. comp. Physiol.* **36**, 251.
Ljungqvist, A. (1963). The intrarenal arterial pattern in the normal and diseased human kidney. A micro-angiographic and histologic study. *Acta med. scand.* **174**, Suppl. 401.
Oliver, J. (1944). New directions in renal morphology: a method, its results and its future. *Harvey Lect.* **40**, 102–115.
Steinhausen, M., Wayland, H. and Fox, J. R. (1977). Renal test dyes. V. Quantitative analysis of tubular passage of FITC-dextrans in kidneys of rats. *Pflügers Arch. ges. Physiol.* **369**, 273–279.
Weibel, E. R., Stäubli, W., Gnägi, H. R. and Hess, F. A. (1969). Correlated morphometric and biochemical studies on the liver cell. I. Morphometric model, stereologic methods, and normal morphometric data for rat liver. *J. Cell Biol.* **42**, 68–91.

Index